Psychiatr

Made Simple

The Made Simple series
has been created
especially for self-education
but can equally well
be used as
an aid to group study.
However complex the subject,
the reader is taken
step by step,
clearly and methodically,
through the course. Each volume
has been prepared by experts,
taking account of
modern educational requirements,
to ensure the most
effective way of
acquiring knowledge.

96

D0582718

In the same series

Accounting
Advertising
Auditing
Biology
Book-keeping
British Constitution
Business Calculations
Business and Enterprise Studies
Business Law
Calculus
Chemistry
Child Development
Commerce
Computer Electronics
Computer Programming
Computer Typing
Cost and Management Accounting
Economic and Social Geography
Economics
Education
Electricity
Electronics
Elements of Banking
English
Financial Management
First Aid
French
German
Graphic Communication

Latin
Law
Management
Marketing
Mathematics
Modern European History
Modern World History
MSX
Music
Office Practice
Personnel Management
Philosophy
Photography
Physical Geography
Physics
Politics
Psychiatry
Psychology
Russian
Salesmanship
Secretarial Practice
Social Services
Sociology
Spanish
Statistics
Teeline Shorthand
Typing

Psychiatry

Made Simple

M. T. Haslam, MA, MD, FRCP, FRCPsych

Second edition

**MADE SIMPLE
BOOKS**

Made Simple Books
An imprint of Heinemann Professional Publishing Ltd
Halley Court, Jordan Hill, Oxford OX2 8EJ

OXFORD LONDON MELBOURNE AUCKLAND SINGAPORE
IBADAN NAIROBI GABORONE KINGSTON

First published 1982
Second edition 1990

British Library Cataloguing in Publication Data
Haslam, M. T.
  Psychiatry.–2nd. ed.
  1. Man. Mental disorders
  I. Title II. Series
  616.89

ISBN 0-7506-0725-4

Revised edition by Key Graphics, Aldermaston, Berkshire
Printed in England by Clays Ltd, St Ives plc, Cornwall

To Michael, Fiona and Melanie

Contents

Part 2:   Psychiatric Syndromes

Preface to the second edition

It is now some eight years since this book was first published and some ten years since it was conceived. During this decade psychiatry has continued to advance. Many changes have taken place in the management and administrative side of the specialty, perhaps less in advances in treatment.

1984, however, saw the implementation of the new Mental Health Act which has had profound implications for some aspects of care. There has also, because of changes in the management structure of hospitals and the continuing desire on the part of many to promote the closure of the mental hospital and the translation of patient care into the community, been a considerable change in outlook amongst professions ancillary to psychiatry, in particular the community psychiatric nurse.

The second edition has taken account of these changes in updating those aspects of patient management, particularly for those who have had psychotic illnesses and have some continued long-term disability. The chapter on the Mental Health Act has been completely revised, and those aspects of treatment which have changed within the decade (particularly alterations in types of medication and their usage) have been updated.

Areas of psychiatry which have been particularly newsworthy in recent years have had devoted to them a larger slice of the book's cake. Thus there has been further focus on child abuse and sexual abuse, the psychiatric problems associated with Aids and tranquilliser abuse.

The general format of the book has, however, been retained and the emphasis remains on a description of the orthodox standard National Health Service practice of the specialty of the type the average individual who needs to have contact with the psychiatric services is likely to experience. The medical model which is happily now regaining some of its prestige after a period in the dark ages, continues to be the author's 'raison d'être'.

M. T. HASLAM

Preface to the first edition

Psychiatry has for many years suffered from two images, diametrically opposed, and both detrimental. On the one hand there is the idea of the alienist sitting in an asylum well away from the community, the doors locked and the patients never seeing the light of day again—all certified and all, as the layman would say, 'mad'—this despite the advances in medical treatment and the introduction in Britain of the Mental Health Act, 1959, which set up establishments totally different from the old concepts. Yet prejudice dies hard.

At the other extreme is the bearded analyst with his couch, the butt of humorists the world over the deriving from the more bizarre off-shoots of Freudian analytical concepts. This image is equally detrimental, for it implies that psychiatry is simply synonymous with psychoanalysis, and that the 'talking cure' is, by and large, what psychiatry is all about. This tends to set it apart considerably from the general field of medicine.

Equally, the more unusual views, particularly of some fringe psychologists and psychiatrists, have been widely publicised and have given the general public an idea that psychiatry is indeed similar to the portrayal which humorists put across. Analytical schools have, of course, held considerable sway in the United States for many years. But it is to some extent true that a criticism often levelled at these therapists—namely, that they only treat cases who are not ill—has in fact some foundation!

How then can this ignorance of the facts be remedied? It has seemed to the author for some time that there exists a gap in the literature available to the non-specialist. In this book an attempt is made to put across, in simple terms, present-day concepts and ideas, and to explain methods of treatment with which the average person will not be familiar. There are highly technical books available for the doctor who is specialising in psychiatry, and there are many books written, often in rather flowery terminology, putting across less orthodox views. The reader has little opportunity, without specialised knowledge, to discover which of these is reasonable and which is not.

Furthermore, a recent survey undertaken by a professional psychiatric association showed tremendous ignorance not only among the general public, but indeed among colleagues in other medical subjects, concerning the role of the psychiatrist and the conditions in the modern psychiatric hospital. This ignorance has not been diminished by unfortunate reports of isolated incidents of an undesirable kind associated with some of the older mental hospitals. While it is, of course, important that such episodes should not go undetected, the publicity has not been favourable and has had an adverse effect on recruitment. It has deterred those who might otherwise have taken an interest in more enlightened attitudes from looking further into the problem, while attracting those with less desirable motives to take an excessive interest in the problem.

The purpose of this book is to attempt to educate, in a form acceptable to the lay public who have an interest in the subject, and also to cater for those students who wish for a simple groundwork in psychiatry before progressing to deeper works, by providing a comprehensive but not over-technical summary of present views and knowledge.

The book has been set out in two parts. Part 1 covers in general terms the problems of classification and discusses concepts concerning causation and treatment. The symptoms and signs of psychiatric illness are discussed and consideration is given to research techniques.

Part 2 is devoted to a discussion of individual psychiatric diseases and syndromes. The author has felt that the orthodox concepts of classification that relate back to ideas formulated 100 years ago are not entirely logical or reliable, and that until the causes of many of these diseases are accurately known, it seems reasonable to attempt to group psychiatric disorders on the basis of symptomatology. It is hoped that the reader will find this book a sound basis for more extensive study.

A glossary of terms is provided at the end of the book for easy reference. Brief bibliographies of further reading are listed at the end of each chapter, as well as questions by which readers may test their understanding of the subject.

M. T. HASLAM

Acknowledgments

Thanks to my colleagues who have given advice on the compilation of this manuscript; to Maureen Hudson who typed the initial manuscript; and to Sybil Vause who typed the final version.

Part 1: Concepts in Psychiatry

1
Definitions

What is Psychiatry?

Psychiatry is that branch of medicine which studies disorders affecting thought and emotion, and, arising out of these, behaviour. There is, of course, a wide variety of diseases that can cause disturbance in these functions. The causes of some are known; the causes of others are not entirely known as yet. We may, however, draw a parallel. It would be possible to write a fairly large treatise on the subject, say, of diseases affecting the big toe. Such diseases as gout and gangrene immediately spring to mind. In the former the main symptoms and signs are pain and swelling of the joint. Further investigation, however, will show that there are changes affecting other aspects of the body's function, particularly biochemical, and treatment, apart from the immediate relief of the pain, must be directed towards alleviating the underlying condition. Gangrene, too, may affect the big toe, but the underlying disease may often prove to be a disorder of the circulation. Nevertheless, it would be possible to write extensively simply on diseases affecting the big toe.

If we come on to a more complicated system—and indeed one can take any system in the body that one cares to choose—such as an endocrine gland like the thyroid, it would be possible to write not only a treatise but a book covering the subject. One might first consider diseases which cause an over-production of thyroid hormone; secondly, those that cause an under-production of thyroid hormone, or where some abnormal hormone secretion was produced in place of the one normally utilised by the body. It would be possible to extend this to any other glandular, hormonal or endocrine system that one cared to choose. Any aspect of the body's functioning can go wrong, in the ways stated above or in other ways.

For some absurd reason there seems, in the minds of many people, to be a change in attitude when we get above the neck. Diseases from the neck upwards have some kind of mystical creation. Now, even if nothing at all were known about the functions of that complex organ, the brain, such a concept would surely strike any serious-minded person as nonsense. **Of all the hormone-producing systems in the body, the brain is the most complex.** It consists of a wide variety of ganglia and nerve centres with a very elaborate interacting system of neurohormones and enzymes. There is no reason to think that these systems cannot go wrong by producing, from time to time, too much, too little or the wrong kind of hormone or enzyme. Should this, indeed, prove to be the case, we must ask ourselves what symptoms and signs these abnormalities would be likely to produce. What does the brain do? Basically it controls thinking, emotion and, arising out of these, behaviour. It is likely, therefore, that any abnormality in these systems will show itself by disturbances affecting the thinking, emotion or behaviour of the patient. As a corollary to this, it is reasonable to argue that a patient showing a disturbance of thought, emotion or behaviour may well have some disturbance in brain function due to an abnormality in the production or utilisation of these brain hormones or enzyme mechanisms.

Detection

The detection of these abnormalities is not easy. One is, as it were, working second-hand by examining the tissues and blood specimens peripherally. It is not possible readily to do biopsies of parts of the brain in the same way as one can with, for example, the pancreatic gland in diabetes. Should a patient visit his doctor complaining of slightly bizarre symptoms—say loss of weight, an excessive thirst and a desire to pass water frequently—the doctor will, as a routine, examine a specimen of urine for sugar. Should this be found, a diagnosis of diabetes can be made, and this can be confirmed by blood tests. At a time before blood and urine tests were available, the diagnosis of these slightly bizarre symptoms would have presented a bigger problem and there would have been room for argument between physicians.

Once a test becomes available, then confirmation of a disease becomes easy. We are still at a stage in psychiatry where not many diseases can be confirmed in such a simple manner. Furthermore, until such tests do become available, the classification of psychiatric diseases has to depend entirely on clinical concepts, fitting together symptom patterns, and observing the outcome.

We are perhaps at the stage where a diagnosis can only be made of 'cough' in a patient who presents himself at the surgery coughing. We know that there are different kinds of cough, but if chest X-rays, sputum cultures and the stethoscope had not been invented, we would have difficulty in distinguishing which resulted from pneumonia, which from asthma and which from tuberculosis. Furthermore, we have to decide on whether to use the equivalents of penicillin, streptomycin or Gee's Linctus!

While the elucidation of many of these symptom complexes will depend on the further research which produces such tests and shows the underlying abnormalities, this should not deter us at present from making the attempt. Indeed, modern methods of treatment have shown this to be a very practical and useful matter, and methods of treatment have become available which make psychiatric diagnosis of importance, and the treatment of the subsequent syndromes much easier.

Who is a Psychiatrist?

We have discussed the concepts surrounding a definition of psychiatry. Let us now turn to the definition of a psychiatrist. A survey recently carried out by members of the Society of Clinical Psychiatrists in the United Kingdom showed that public ignorance on this and related definitions was considerable. The distinction between psychiatry, psychology and psycho-analysis was unclear to many people, and the qualifications required produced even vaguer answers. This is, of course, not particularly surprising, but a knowledge of these distinctions will certainly be of value to anyone who is concerned professionally.

A psychiatrist is a doctor who specialises in diseases which affect thought, emotion and behaviour. He will, as other specialists, have gone through medical school and taken his ordinary medical qualifications—MB, BCh or equivalent. He will have done his year's compulsory house jobs, and at this point he will have to decide whether to specialise in some branch of the hospital service or to go into general practice. Should he decide to specialise in surgery, he will take a trainee post under a consultant surgeon. Should he decide to specialise in psychiatry, he will take a trainee post under a consultant psychiatrist, after perhaps a further year or so of general medical training. As a trainee in psychiatry he will work for a Diploma in Psychiatry or Membership of the Royal College of Psychiatrists, which will extend over a period of some four or five years. With this training and experience he will subsequently, having gone through the usual hospital appointments, attempt to obtain a consultant post, and will himself become a specialist in this particular branch of the hospital service. He is thus a qualified doctor with additional specialist qualifications, as is a consultant physician, a consultant surgeon or a consultant gynaecologist.

A psychologist, on the other hand, is not qualified in medicine but is someone who has taken a degree course at a university or polytechnic in psychology as such, i.e. a study of normal mental processes and behaviour, just as a linguist will study a language in depth or a physiologist the working of the normal body. He may then choose to go into the field of research or the field of education—for example, in the school service as an educational psychologist, or into hospital work as a clinical psychologist. In the latter case he will take a higher degree such as MSc, which demands two or three years' practical experience in a hospital setting. If he takes the latter course he will find himself engaged in testing the mental mechanisms of patients by means of psychological tests, for intelligence, or personality disturbances. He may work with behaviour therapy techniques which are based on psychological theory, in conjunction with, in this case, the psychiatrists in charge. He is thus in a similar situation to a biochemist with a degree in biochemistry who works in a hospital pathology department assisting in the elucidation of organic disturbances in the body chemistry. Many hospitals employ a clinical psychologist on the staff of the Psychiatric Unit.

Psychoanalysis is another and a different matter. A psychoanalyst is a person who has obtained a qualification from the Institute of Psycho-Analysis. He completes a personal training analysis, which covers a period of some two years. A psychoanalyst has no direct association with the medical profession, and while there is nothing to stop a medically qualified person from taking a training analysis at the Institute, many analysts have no medical training; nor do they, therefore, have a qualification in psychiatry. They believe in treatment for psychiatric conditions by methods evolved originally by Freud, a neurologist with an interest in psychiatric problems, who practised in Europe at the end of the nineteenth century. These views have, of course, been modified and modernised, and altered by some analysts, over the years. But the technique remains basically a method of working with the patient over a period of some two years, through the patient's life history, uncovering unconscious motivations, and dealing with the problems which the patient has had from early life in developing personal relationships. During this process a 'transference' may develop between the patient and the analyst and this itself is analysed. This method of treatment has its adherents within the medical profession, but by and large is not available on the Health Service, and would be considered by most psychiatrists as an impractical method of treatment for the general population, as it is expensive and time-consuming. Furthermore, the results do not compare particularly favourably when subjected to a critical comparison with other methods of treatment for the same type of condition; although the analyst might argue that it is not simply the condition which is being treated but the patient's whole personality and life style that one hopes will improve.

The situation in the United States is slightly different in that psychoanalysis is more widely practised there and many psychiatrists have had an analytical training. It is probably fair to say, even so, that the treatment at best is of value only to intelligent patients with a reasonably good previous personality who are suffering only from a psychoneurotic condition.

Terminology—Madness and the Mind

Let us now turn to consider one or two other words commonly used in psychiatry and attempt to define them so that their subsequent usage will become clearer to the reader.

Certain problems arise when medicine and the law tend to cross paths, since the law likes to have clear-cut definitions appertaining, for example, to such questions as the responsibility a patient has for his actions, or the question in marital situations of the problem of 'being incurably of unsound mind'. This perhaps has led to a concept familiarly heard in lay circles, and a common source of anxiety to patients suffering from psychoneuroses: the question of madness. The patient will commonly ask of his doctor: 'Am I going mad?' In this situation the patient is usually asked what they mean by madness. Generally this devolves either upon a fear of losing control, or a fear that one will lose one's memory, or especially a fear of the mind becoming deranged, of ideas foreign to the patient's normal functioning becoming dominant and taking over the patient's thoughts so that the mind becomes out of control. This usually boils down to the patient fearing a diagnosis of schizophrenia. (More will be said about this illness in later chapters.) Much the same fear attaches to this as to cancer in the physical sense. A lack of knowledge and understanding of the disease process and of the likely outcome makes the patient fear that the end result will be permanent incarceration in some psychiatric hospital ward. It is usually possible to reassure these individuals.

It is important to realise that no dichotomy exists in reality between body and mind. The conditions we are about to discuss affect the body. They affect the brain, the central nervous system. This complicated and vast collection of nerve cells, arranged into a variety of ganglia and centres, with a fascinating and fantastic arrangement of interconnections, works at an individual cell level on the basis of electrical conduction of impulses along tiny pathways jumping from one nerve cell to another on the basis of chemical transmitter agents. These can go wrong, and when they do, changes in the brain function are inevitable.

The concept of mind is a more nebulous one, part religious and part philosophical. When we talk of diseases of the mind, we are talking more realistically of diseases which create a disturbance in brain or central nervous system functioning. The mind, as distinct from the purely religious concept of the soul, refers to the manifestation of brain function. It is the way the brain works at a conscious and subconscious level. It embraces the total personality, the character, intellect and emotion, the thinking and behaviour of an individual. Yet it functions through chemicals and electrical impulses, and in trying to understand the ways in which it can malfunction we must understand the way in which its activities are mediated.

That the functions of the brain can be influenced by external environmental factors is undoubted. It must also be clear that it can be affected by internal functions or, more particularly, by dysfunctions. The cause, however, in theory at any rate, may be either internal or external or indeed a combination of the two. Certain it is that a human being above the neck is more complicated but not intrinsically different from one below the neck, and the understanding of mental processes should not be looked upon as if there were some mystique about it, but rather with logical awareness of all aspects of the problem.

Classification

In order to start to make sense of any subject it is necessary to have within one's mind an idea of the range of the subject and how it may be broken down into understandable parts. To say that someone is 'mental' is no more or less useful than to say that someone is 'physical'.

If we take a symptom such as a cough and fail to take steps to distinguish one from another, we fail to elucidate such important conditions as tuberculoses, asthma and pneumonia, and will equally fail to develop a rational cure for any. So it is with psychiatry that if we fail to take account of commonly occurring symptom clusters, and identify them in some way which enables us to research their grouping, and thus to develop methods of relieving these symptoms, we shall get nowhere. This surely points to the absurdity of the arguments of the anti-psychiatry lobby.

We need to develop, therefore, some systems classification which at least, imperfect though it may be, allows us to make some kind of logical sorting, and thus to begin to make sense of the whole through making initial sense of the part. Psychiatry is one part of the system of providing medical care. A system of classification which has stood the test of time and allowed us to develop such concepts is one based on the original ideas of Kraepelin in the late nineteenth century. Though modified and improved, it remains a classic example of deductive thought, which will form the basis of our subdivision into conditions where primary disorders of thinking, emotion and memory are to be found.

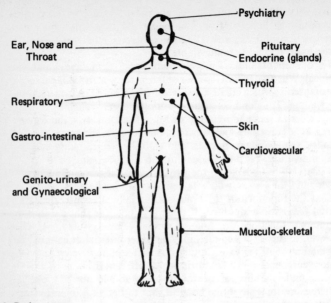

Fig. 1. Body systems.

A simple standard classification following current usage is shown in Fig. 1. Psychiatric conditions form one subgroup of human disease, of which other subgroups might be skin diseases or diseases of the gastro-intestinal tract.

We can subdivide this group of psychiatric problems into certain broad categories, principally the psychoses, the neuroses, disorders of personality, and the so-called organic states, which include dementias. A further large group would be individuals showing mental retardation or subnormality of intellect.

We can subdivide the psychoses into two main types. The first is schizophrenia, and the second the affective psychoses, where the primary disturbance is one of mood.

The neuroses, or psychoneuroses, to give them their full title, embrace states of anxiety, obsessional compulsive behaviour and hysteria. These groups can be further subdivided. Under the personality disorders will come psychopathy, addictions, deviant behaviour, and various social inadequacies which may also come the way of the psychiatrist.

Organic states would include all the possible causes of dementia, delirious reactions and a wide variety of more general bodily diseases that can affect the brain's function directly or indirectly and produce states mimicking the psychoses or dementias. Finally, under subnormality come all the range of conditions inherited, traumatic and acquired either before, during or shortly after birth, which lead to maldevelopment of the brain and, therefore, the intellect.

This is a classification according to syndromes. It would be possible to group illnesses according to their primary symptom, and in psychiatry this might be done by looking at conditions where there was a primary disorder of thought, those where there was a primary disorder of emotional affect,

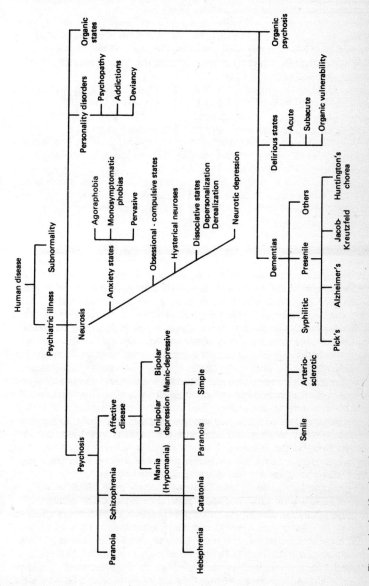

Fig. 2. A classification of psychiatric disorders.

and those where the primary disorder was of intellectual function. One could perhaps expand this to include primary disorders of behaviour and some other smaller categories but working on the main premise that the role of psychiatry is to deal with conditions causing disorders of thinking, emotion and intellect and, arising out of these, behaviour.

It is not yet possible to classify on the basis of aetiology or cause, since in many of the conditions we shall be discussing this remains a relatively unknown quantity. In some bodily systems this is a sensible way to proceed and would include such factors as infection, trauma, endocrine or hormonal imbalance, and degenerative conditions.

The international systems of classification and that adopted by the Registrar General in Britain for statistical purposes tend to follow the first of these three possible types of grouping. We have tried in this book to follow the second as far as it is practical by grouping together conditions where the dominant symptom seems to be a disorder of thinking or of mood, but have included special chapters on specific problems which cannot be subsumed under that general title.

Finally, therefore, in this preliminary chapter let us define some of the key words that we have used in the above paragraphs and shall use later. Others will be found in the glossary at the end of the book.

Definitions

A primary subdivision within psychiatry has been into **psychosis** and **neurosis**. While these terms are somewhat vague, they formed a useful sub-division certainly in pretreatment days. The term psychosis refers to what was a severe form of psychiatric illness in which insight was lost. That is to say, the patients ceased to be aware of the disturbance in their thinking or emotion which was apparent to an outside observer, and interpreted their attitude and behaviour as being appropriate in response to their environment. Thus patients with a psychotic depression might come to believe that the sins of the world were upon them, that their bowels were being eaten away by some progressive disease, or that they were bankrupt and a burden on society, when none of these things were in fact the case. The schizophrenic might come to believe that some group was persecuting him or that he had some special role in society even though reasoned argument could show that this was not so. Schizophrenia and the affective psychoses are two examples of psychotic illness.

In the neuroses (or psychoneuroses) insight is retained even in the severer forms of such conditions. Anxiety states, obsessional states and phobias would be examples of neuroses. These were considered milder conditions than psychoses at the time that such classification was being established.

Another term which we have already used is **affect**, in the sense of affective disorders or affective psychosis. The term **affect** refers to a continuing emotional or mood change, and is here applied to a pathological disturbance of mood or emotion. This is found, for example, in abnormal states of depression, or in mania or hypomania, where an abnormal state of elation occurs. Affect can, however, also be applied to mood changes associated with anxiety or with anger.

Three words which will crop up repeatedly throughout our book are **delusion**, **illusion** and **hallucination**. These are all symptoms which occur frequently in psychotic illness, and in other psychiatric states sometimes as well.

A **delusion** is a false belief held with conviction and contrary to the individual's upbringing and cultural background, and not amenable to reasoned argument. These qualifications are necessary to distinguish other types of false belief which would not be seen as delusional in this sense. Thus, the belief that lightning was a demonstration of the wrath of the gods and required the sacrifice of a sucking pig to prevent the crops failing might be appropriate in a primitive African village but would be delusional if held with conviction by an intelligent middle-aged businessman in a sophisticated Western society.

Similarly, superstitions—for example, that walking under a ladder or breaking a mirror may bring bad luck—would not be seen as delusional in this context. Fringe religious or political beliefs might be seen by non-believers as bizarre and illogical, but, if held by members of a group to which that individual subscribes, cannot be seen as evidence of a mental illness.

In some countries with repressive political systems, however, such beliefs have been used as evidence of mental illness in order to maintain a conforming attitude within that society. Sometimes the distinction can be a fine one, and evidence of psychiatric illness must depend not simply on the holding of false beliefs but on a wide range of symptoms which, when pieced together, show more definite evidence of thought disorder or mood change.

An **hallucination** is a false perception in the absence of an external stimulus. Thus the individual who hears a voice which no one else can hear seemingly coming from inside his head or from somewhere outside and nearby is said to be hallucinated.

Such perceptions are, of course, arising within this individual's central nervous system but are being perceived by the patient not as his own thoughts or memories but as in some way influenced from outside. The conscious brain is falsely placing these thoughts as if they were tracking in on the auditory nerve from the ear. Thus they are perceived as sounds.

Hallucinations may affect any sensory modality and not simply hearing. Visual hallucinations may be experienced, where the patient sees things that are not there, again the thought process perceiving something as if it is tracking in through the retina and optic nerve. Similarly, there may be hallucinations of smell, of taste or of touch.

An **illusion**, in contrast, is a mistaken or misinterpreted perception. Here, the individual perceives something through one of his senses but makes an error of perception in interpreting this data. For example, an individual who on a dark night sees the shadow of the movement of trees in the garden and is convinced that he has seen a man lurking in the bushes could be said to have been perceiving an illusion. The sleight of hand of the conjurer or magician is another common example of producing an illusion.

The term **paranoid** will crop up not infrequently in psychiatry. The derivative name **paranoia** has now come to refer to a group of conditions resembling schizophrenia in which a monosymptomatic delusional system may develop. Paranoid, however, has come to refer to abnormal suspiciousness, as seen in the suspicious nature of a paranoid personality and to a delusional degree in the ideas of persecution that may be seen in a paranoid type of schizophrenia.

The terms **psychopathy** and the 'psychopath' are used somewhat differently in different parts of the world. In the United States the former can be synonymous with a serious mental illness, but in Britain since the 1959 Mental Health Act the term has been defined and restricted to describe the severer type of personality disorder where there is persistently irresponsible and/or aggressive behaviour in an individual who lacks the ability to make close personal relationships and to learn properly from experience.

The 1959 Mental Health Act for medico-legal purposes defined four categories of illness, which are (1) mental illness, (2) subnormality, (3) severe subnormality and (4) psychopathy. Thus to describe behaviour as psychopathic is to refer to an individual who shows this type of temperament or personality.

Empathy is a term frequently used to describe relationships in psychotherapy. It refers to a mutual awareness of feeling; to a sympathetic understanding between two people which may develop in normal friendship or in the transference relationship that develops between patient and therapist.

Finally, let us look at the term **dementia** and distinguish between two important groups of people: the psychiatrically ill and the mentally retarded.

The term dementia when used correctly refers to a particular set of disease processes affecting the brain and producing deterioration of memory, orientation and intellectual function in an individual who has previously functioned at his own particular norm. Thus, to be demented or dementing refers to the intellectual change associated with the deterioration in function of the central nervous system.

The old term **amentia** used to be used to describe the mentally deficient or mentally retarded, that is to say an individual showing a subnormality of intelligence. The mentally retarded are not primarily mentally ill. They have had a maldevelopment of the brain from any of a wide variety of causes that may affect the growing foetus before birth, at birth or shortly after. Such a person's potential is never fulfilled, and unless something can be done to reverse this maldevelopment, which in most cases is not possible, they will remain retarded throughout their lives. They are in an entirely different category, therefore, and indeed are treated, should in-patient treatment be necessary, in different hospitals or hospital departments from the mentally ill.

The psychiatrically ill are individuals who have reached their full potential of development but in whom some condition or disease process has created a disturbance of function, dementia being one category of this total whole.

Further Reading

Clare, A. W., *Psychiatry in Dissent*, 2nd edn, Tavistock Publications, London, 1980.

Frankl, V. E., *New Dimensions in Psychiatry—A World Review*, Wiley, New York, 1975.

Haslam, M. T. (ed.), *Public Relations in Psychiatry*, Society of Clinical Psychiatrists, Clifton Hospital, York, 1978.

O'Gorman, C. O., *Modern Trends in Mental Health and Subnormality*, vol. 2, Butterworth, London, 1974.

'Recent Developments Series', *British Journal of Psychiatry*, 1978.

Sargent, W., and Slater, E., *Physical Methods of Treatment in Psychiatry*, Livingstone, Edinburgh, 1972

Sim, Myre, *A Guide to Psychiatry*, 3rd edn, Livingstone, Edinburgh, 1979.

Slater, E., and Roth, M., *A Textbook of Clinical Psychiatry*, 3rd edn, Bailliere, Tindall and Cassell, London, 1977.

Questions

1. What is psychiatry?
2. How do we distinguish psychiatrists, clinical psychologists and psychoanalysts?
3. What are hallucinations, delusions and illusions?
4. Where is your local psychiatric unit? How many beds has it? What is its annual admission rate? How many consultant staff has it and what other professional staff, are available?
5. Have you seen it? If you have the chance, go and visit. Does it have a 'League of Friends'?

2
General Concepts

We have discussed in some detail the distinction between psychiatrist and psychologist, and considered some definitions of general importance. We should now consider just who it is that the specialist in disorders of thinking, emotion and behaviour actually sees, and initially a discussion about the basic structure of psychiatry in Britain would not be amiss.

Health Service

The Health Service in Britain at present is still basically a tripartite structure: first, there is a branch of medicine known as general practice, which consists of the family doctor who deals with patients in the community and in their homes, forming the primary care team; next comes a public health sector dealt with by the community physician, which covers community health, preventive medicine, school health, and the statistics of epidemiology; and thirdly, there is the hospital service, in which there are consultants in various specialities—surgery, general medicine, gynaecology, psychiatry, skin diseases and so on. Working under the consultant will be resident or non-resident medical staff, mostly in training for these higher posts. In addition, there will be various ancillary services, such as physiotherapy, occupational therapy, social workers, etc. The consultant looks after the patients under his care in his particular hospital beds, and also sees out-patients at his clinics or, from time to time, at home at the request of the family doctor, if the latter wishes a consultation for a further opinion.

The hospital service is, therefore, divided into specialities, and, in general, these specialities are nursed in separate wards or in separate units, largely for administrative convenience. Many hospitals, particularly the newer district general hospitals, contain a psychiatric unit along with other specialities, where the short-term cases are dealt with exactly on the same lines as in any other branch of medicine. In addition, there are many hospitals devoted entirely to one speciality, such as obstetrics, orthopaedics, psychiatry or subnormality. The latter two subspecialities usually also remain separate from each other, since the problems of nursing, administrative care and treatment are by and large quite different for general psychiatric patients and the mentally retarded.

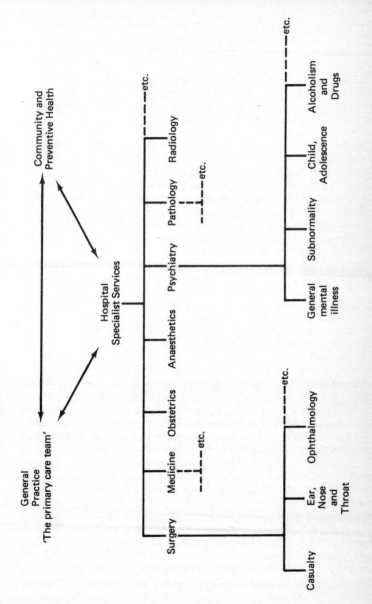

Fig. 3. Specialities in health care.

Size of Problem

If one considers the size of the problem in terms of the number of beds occupied by individual specialities, psychiatry is the largest speciality in the hospital service, since nearly 50 per cent of the beds occupied in hospitals in Britain are devoted to psychiatric problems. This is slightly misleading, however, because these figures relate to a legacy from pre-treatment and pre-health-service days when, around the turn of the century, many county mental hospitals were opened. These contained a large number of patients suffering from the long-term effects of schizophrenia, which was, until some 30 years ago, virtually an untreatable disease. This is no longer the case, but there remains a large residual group of patients who have been in hospital for many years. In terms of bed occupancy this group affects the figures considerably. There is, in addition, a large population of elderly people in hospital beds purely by reason of senile changes. Many of these patients are nursed in psychiatric beds because the condition from which they suffer is basically a disturbance of memory, and the disturbed behaviour that goes with this confusion. They are ambulent and are by and large better cared for by nurses with psychiatric training in facilities where they can be up and about and attending such things as occupational therapy. This is less easily organised in a hospital basically orientated to cater for physically infirm people, who may often be bedridden.

In fact, if one adds together the in-patient and the day-patient needs in the community the number of places required for psychiatry in the future is likely to be around 1 to $1\frac{1}{2}$ beds per 1,000 of the population. In addition, beds for a further 1 per 1,000 population will be required for problems of mental retardation or subnormality. The average length of stay in hospital for a new admission with a psychiatric illness is likely to be 4 to 6 weeks, so that each bed will be turned over some ten times in the year.

Type of Hospital Cases

Let us consider at this stage what kinds of patient are likely to be in psychiatric hospital beds (Table 1). It is customary to divide, for statistical purposes, the patients into short-stay, medium-stay and long-stay. Patients with acute short-term illnesses are likely to be in hospital for a period of less than 6 weeks. In the medium-stay category come patients who are likely to be in

Table 1. Composition of Psychiatric Practice.

In-patients	$\frac{1}{3}$ acute short-stay (mostly depression, neurosis, acute schizophrenia)
	$\frac{1}{3}$ psychogeriatrics (confusion in the elderly: dementing)
	$\frac{1}{3}$ long-stay (residual schizophrenia)
Out-patients:	$\frac{1}{4}$ in-patient follow-up (psychoses)
	$\frac{1}{4}$ neuroses ⎫ Not
	$\frac{1}{4}$ psychosexual ⎬ requiring
	$\frac{1}{4}$ personality disorders, alcoholism, psycho- ⎭ admission pathy, etc.

hospital for a period of months, perhaps up to six months. The long-stay category may possibly have been in hospital for a period of years.

Now it will be apparent that units in **district** general hospitals are likely to treat, by and large, the short-stay group because of the nature of their function. In contrast, those hospitals which specialise in psychiatry are likely to have short-stay admission wards as well as wards suitable for the medium- and longer-stay type of patient.

If we take a psychiatric hospital and consider the kind of patients that are likely to be seen there at present, we find that they fall into the following broad groups. The admission wards will occupy about one-third of the total beds, and will contain a preponderance of 'affective' disorders, principally **depression**. There will be some patients with **schizophrenic illnesses**, and a group with the severer versions of psychoneuroses, such as anxiety states and obsessional states. There will be a small number of patients with personality disorders and a small number, in all probability, with early dementias. Some 50 per cent of the patients will be there for the first time, and about 50 per cent may have had a previous admission to a psychiatric hospital at some stage in their lives before. The same is true of course of any hospital speciality: 50 per cent of surgical patients, for example, will have been in hospital before.

If one considers the rest of the hospital, however, including the longer-stay wards, one will find the general pattern is rather different. About a third of the patients will be elderly people suffering from dementing illnesses, these forming about half the long-stay group at present. Indeed some 50 per cent of the total hospital population will be in the over-65 age group.

The final third will be composed of longer-stay patients suffering from the residual after-effects of schizophrenic illnesses which were in the acute phase in the days before modern methods of treatment became available. These patients will be in the hospital more or less permanently, for a variety of reasons which will be considered in later chapters, and form the other large group of long-stay patients.

The psychiatric unit in the general hospital is likely to contain the same sort of patients as are found in the admission wards in a specialist psychiatric hospital. On the whole, for administrative reasons, the longer-stay patients, such as the residual schizophrenias and late dementias, will not be found there, as the facilities are usually not such that it can cope with this group. Thus it does not and cannot cater for the full range of psychiatric problems.

Four special hospitals are also maintained in England (Broadmoor, Rampton, Moss Side and Park Lane) and one in Scotland (Carstairs) for psychiatrically ill but dangerous or criminal patients.

There has been a considerable reduction in the number of hospital beds required for psychiatric patients in psychiatric hospitals over the last 10 years. This has been a result of the improved methods of treatment for schizophrenia, but it is unlikely that this trend will continue much further, since the problem now, as we have outlined above, is a different one.

In fact, the number of hospital beds required for psychiatric patients has decreased by some 30 per cent over the last 10 years. This does not imply, of course, a decrease in the total number of patients falling ill, but that patients now falling ill are in hospital for a much shorter time. Therefore, the turnover of patients in these beds is increased. The incidence of the severer psychiatric illnesses has not and is not likely to change, because of the nature of the aetiology of these diseases. Indeed, as prejudice decreases, the demand for hospital beds is likely to increase in one sense, since patients will more readily seek treatment at an earlier stage in their illness if they know that the chances of a cure are improved thereby.

Community Care

There has nevertheless been a movement in many countries, in particular some States in the United States of America, Italy and more recently in the United Kingdom, to close down the mental hospitals and develop community care programmes.

The advantage of this is that it removes the institutionalisation inherent in a system of institutional care, and provides a more homely atmosphere in hostels subsidised by the social services department or in other types of community residential care than could be provided in a large hospital.

At the same time there are challenges in this movement. The danger is that patients are discharged from hospital, that follow-up in the community proves to be inadequate and that the community proves not to be as caring as the more naive in the population might hope, and that as a result patients, in particular those with residual chronic schizophrenia or with major personality disturbances, may finish up receiving no care at all, and become lost to the system and sleep rough. Thus the clock could be turned back 250 years to the very reasons for the creation of the Vagrancy Act of 1744.

Another issue which is to be tackled by the reformers is the movement from a central base to a peripherally-based system which community care implies. On a central site it is possible to congregate services and social facilities and to provide staff who can cover a larger number of people, can be based in one place and can cover for each other during leave or sickness. Occupational therapy departments, social facilities, entertainment and a variety of supports can all be congregated in a mutually supportive manner.

In contrast, creating such detailed activities and social support systems for small peripheral units for 10 to 20 people scattered about a district has to rely much more on the support of local community facilities and these may or may not prove to be open to such disabled individuals. The cost of community support must mostly be borne by the poll tax, whereas the central system is provided through Government taxation. The provision of services such as pharmacy, medication, visiting medical and occupational therapy services and indeed even nursing can become a nightmare with 20 or so scattered units. The travelling time increases immensely and cover for leave and sickness is difficult. It is fairly easy to build up a centre of excellence but difficult to provide peripheries of excellence that might provide adequate training for doctors, nurses and other professionals who are learning the trade. Similarly there will be less peer support when workers are scattered throughout a district instead of congregated centrally and meeting over a cup of coffee in a morning.

The enthusiasts of centralism suggest that money would be better spent creating more homely and better-equipped central establishments, while the peripheralists are intent upon closing what they see as out-dated institutions, and replacing them not with a central facility but rather with a large number of small community hostels.

What appears to have happened in those areas where the system has been tried too enthusiastically and with insufficient forethought (for example Manhattan) is that the number of vagrants has vastly increased, the gaols have become fuller and disturbed people are much more frequently seen roaming the streets. Treatment and follow-up has proved extremely difficult to maintain. In Manhattan a large disused warehouse has had to be converted into what is in effect a doss house for those who have no roof over their heads and who have been discharged from the state mental hospital in the last few years.

In Rome a similar situation has developed as a result of the wholesale closure of the mental health services on an institutional basis some years ago by the then Government. A hostel has recently been provided in the Vatican on the orders of the Pope to provide for those homeless people who have nowhere to go. The vast majority are sufferers from the after-effects of schizophrenia or people with drug or alcohol problems who need more care than now can be provided.

In Britain the reformers do not appear to have taken much note of the problems in these other countries and are continuing to close mental hospitals at an increasingly rapid rate. Whether the social services provision in Britain will prove to be better than in the USA or Italy, and whether the community will prove to be any more caring is a very open question and the media is now looking carefully at the results in those areas where the policy has been put through. The whole issue remains an open question.

Out-patient Referrals

If one considers those patients who are seen in out-patient clinics, the picture is rather different. They can be divided into four groups as follows (Table 1). About 25 per cent are likely to be of the **psychotic group**—that is to say, patients with schizophrenia or severer depressive or other illnesses who have been in hospital and are being followed up on an out-patient basis afterwards. Another 25 per cent will consist of patients with **psychoneuroses**, principally anxiety states and depressive reactions, who do not require in-patient treatment but who will have been referred by the general practitioners for further opinion and treatment on an out-patient basis. The third 25 per cent will consist of **psychosexual disorders**, which include problems related to marital disharmony, to impotence and frigidity, and patients with problems of homosexuality or sexual deviation. This group forms an important section of out-patient work. The final 25 per cent will be composed of patients with **personality disorders**, many of the genuine kind, but also a fair sprinkling of 'old lags', malingerers and various people with social inadequacies who have been referred by their family doctor or by other departments in the hospital who may have got sick of their repeated attendance. This group should not be written off, as they often do receive considerable support from very simple regular psychotherapy at a clinic with an understanding doctor who has a little time to spend with them. It is doubtful, however, whether they come into the category of medical problems, and are rather the social dropouts of an increasingly complex society.

This then is the pattern that the average doctor practising psychiatry will see in his working day. There will be a sprinkling of emergencies, chiefly the acutely depressed with suicidal problems who may have attempted suicide, the occasional thought-disordered person who has made himself a public spectacle by some strange behaviour and got into the hands of the police, or occasionally a patient with epilepsy who, because of his illness, has developed disturbed behaviour. Most of the patients, however, will be seen on the basis of a waiting list, the appointments being made in advance.

The vast majority will be treated by physical methods, principally tablets or medicaments of some sort or another, with superficial supportive psychotherapy. The number of patients who require deeper psychotherapy, and indeed the number that the doctor will have time to see in this depth, will, in fact, be relatively few, so that the analyst's couch is not really a factor of any importance in normal psychiatric practice.

Normality: What is It?

A problem which commonly arises when discussing psychiatric illness is the question of normality. At what point does a symptom show evidence of a disease, and at what point is it merely a stress reaction in a normal personality? We should perhaps first consider the concept of normality itself.

When we apply this discussion to a concept such as height in the general population, we usually make a qualification by dividing average height into average male and average female height, acknowledging that there is a sex difference in this respect. If we then take a large group of individuals and measure them, we will discover that the average height for a group of English

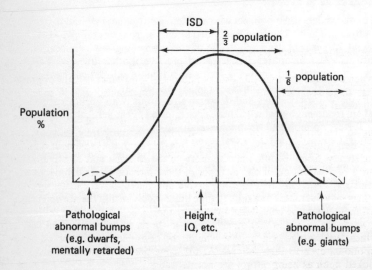

Fig. 4. The normal curve of distribution.

males is in the region of 5 ft 8 in. We derive this by adding together the heights of all the individuals tested and dividing this by their number. We shall find, however, that not everybody has a height of 5 ft 8 in., but rather that there is a variation between, say, 5 ft 6 in. and 5 ft 10 in. Some two-thirds of our sample will probably fall between this variation. A sixth will fall outside this variation by being higher, and a sixth will be lower than the majority. We thus say that this measure shows a **normal curve of distribution**. The fact that somebody is 5 ft 11 in. is in one sense abnormal, but is so merely as a statistical concept and does not mean that there is anything wrong with that individual or that he is in any way 'sick'.

Abnormalities in a Normal Curve of Distribution

If, however, one looks at the curve of distribution of height in the general population, one will find that the curve follows the normal pattern except at the extreme upper and lower ends of the range. Here the graph would show a little bump, which would refer to a group of people whose height was abnormal because of some disease process. There would be a very small bump at the top where people of 6 ft 10 in. or more might be found suffering from gigantism or acromegaly due to a disease affecting their pituitary gland. At the bottom end there would be a rather larger bump produced by the various pathological types of dwarfism. This would include various diagnoses from a failure of the development of the bones themselves, stunting of growth due to hormonal abnormalities, rickets, and some types of mental retardation—in particular mongolism, for mongols are usually of abnormally short stature. These groups will have only one thing in common, which is that their height is below the normal range and outside a normal curve of distribution. In this sense they show the same pathology regardless of the cause in the particular case.

Personality—Normal Ranges

When we relate this to psychiatric symptoms, it will at once become apparent that **there are variations in personality, in intelligence, and in mood or emotional stability, known as 'affect', among the general population.** Now these aspects of a person's total functioning may change temporarily according to the circumstances of the environment, or they may fluctuate for apparently internal reasons in some people despite the environment remaining steady. Some people may be more to the extreme end of our normal curve of distribution in one or other of these facets of their behaviour and thinking, some may be extremely stable and fluctuate very little, whereas others may fluctuate from time to time quite widely within the normal range. All these would be considered normal by the general population, although towards the extremes, i.e. outside the two-thirds of the population within which the average will lie, they might be considered eccentric or over-emotional even to their fellows. At the same time, this could be properly looked upon as being within the normal range.

At the extremes we are again likely to see changes in these aspects of functioning which go beyond the normal, and these include any diseases effecting emotion or the central nervous system in general, which by their nature are going to cause changes in thinking, mood or behaviour. Deciding on what is abnormal in such cases will be a matter of clinical judgement and experience, but will suggest to the doctor that some underlying pathology should be sought.

Intelligence

The same argument can be applied to intelligence. An intelligence score is usually derived from tests which examine various aspects of a person's intellectual functioning. Intelligence tests have been checked against a large sample of the normal population. A score will be produced. In adults it is customary to measure from the basis of **I.Q. (intelligence quotient)**, and in children it is usual to give a figure which describes the **mental age**. This can be converted to an I.Q. score by comparing it in a simple formula with the chronological age of the child. Thus I.Q. $= ma/ca \times 100$ where ma is the mental age and ca the chronological age of the child. Standard tests at present include the Wechsler Adult Intelligence Scale, a similar scale for children, the Stanford Binet Test and various others of simpler design, such as Raven's Matrices.

Average intelligence is by definition set at an I.Q. of 100. The normal population will show a score somewhere on either side of this figure. Two-thirds of the population will be expected to have an I.Q. between 80 and 120. A sixth of the population will be more highly intelligent, with an I.Q. of above 120. A sixth of the population will be less intelligent than the average, with

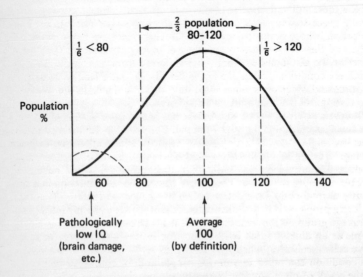

Fig. 5. The curve of distribution for intelligence.

an I.Q. below 80. It must be pointed out, however, that such people are still normal in the sense that we have described above. Their I.Q. is a chance result partly of their inheritance and partly of the influences of their early environment and upbringing.

The intelligence curve will follow a path of normal distribution, and at the top end there will be a small number of people who are exceptionally gifted. At the bottom end, however, we shall again find a bump in the graph as we did with height. These people will be of abnormally low intelligence, and the reasons for this would commonly be expected to be some sort of deficiency in brain function, which may be due to a wide variety of causes both inherited, acquired during the baby's 9 months within the womb, or at an early age following birth. For whatever reason, the brain has been prevented from reaching its normal full potential.

Mental Retardation—Amentia v. Dementia

These people would be described as suffering from **amentia, mental retardation or deficiency or subnormality**, whichever term happens to be in fashion.

Since the 1959 Mental Health Act was introduced, it has been customary for medico-legal purposes to divide the mentally retarded into two groups classified as **severely subnormal** and **subnormal**. In terms of I.Q. the 'severely subnormal' group would have an I.Q. of 50 or below and this would include most of those people who are patients in subnormality hospitals, often with other associated physical defects. The 'subnormal' group would have an I.Q. of between 50 and 70, and would include some who were at the bottom end of the normal curve of distribution and perhaps attending schools for the educationally subnormal, and, in addition, some who had suffered mild degrees of brain impairment.

Now these individuals are not suffering from mental illness, although their mental processes may be disturbed in other ways besides intelligence. They are people whose brains from birth or an early age have never developed fully, and they are not strictly speaking ill in any other sense. They must, therefore, be distinguished from those suffering from psychiatric illnesses, which are conditions, often like any other illness, but affecting thought or emotion, and which come on at some stage in the individual's life. We must also distinguish between amentia and dementia.

Dementia refers to a state where there has been a deterioration of intellectual function which was previously normal. For example, following a stroke a person might show a disturbance of memory and intellect due to brain damage. Testing of intelligence would obviously, in these circumstances, produce a result which was lower than that individual would have been capable of before the illness. Thus, there has been a new situation in a previously normal one. Some deterioration in intellectual function is normal in elderly people, and this is taken into account when measuring intelligence in this age group. At the same time, dementia is also quite common in elderly people as an illness caused by deterioration in the blood supply or in the nerve cells themselves, when it is known as **senile dementia**. Occasionally this condition can occur in younger people and, of course, dementia can be the result of other conditions in younger people, such as head injuries, infectious diseases affecting the brain, or a brain tumour. There is a wide variety of rare problems which could produce the end result of dementia; these will be discussed in the second part of the book.

Patients with a dementing illness will be nursed, in general, in a psychiatric ward, principally because their illness is such as to produce disturbances in thinking, emotion and behaviour. In addition, a nurse trained to deal with psychiatric problems is likely to be best fitted to handle such individuals, who will, by and large, require nursing when they are up and about during the day rather than bed-ridden.

It is usual to have separate hospitals to deal with the problems arising from subnormality as opposed to psychiatric or mental illness. This is because the problems are totally different, and the needs of the patients, and indeed the length of time that most of them will be in hospital, are totally different also. Hospitals for mental retardation that cope with problems of severe subnormality will be geared to the life-long care of many of the severer problems, and to the educational and social training of those who are somewhat better endowed.

In the psychiatric hospitals, while there will be a proportion of long-stay patients (principally the sufferers from schizophrenia who developed the illness in pre-treatment days and may still be there for partly social reasons) and those cases of dementia severe enough to need continuous nursing care, the majority of admissions and discharges will be those who are in hospital over a period of 4 to 6 weeks. They will be up and about during the day, engaged in occupational therapy activities and other remedial programmes. The routine will be geared much more towards treatment of their illness, and their intelligence will be the same as the general population.

In the same way as it has been found convenient in the past to develop special units—for example, for maternity work, for surgery, for general medicine and for children—this recognises that the needs of these different groups, in terms of their hospital care, will vary widely. Indeed, the nursing and medical skills required will also make some specialisation desirable, since here, too, the needs in training will vary widely. A maternity unit will be geared to delivering babies and to looking after the mother and baby in the immediate post-partum period. A surgical unit will be geared to operations. A psychiatric unit will require space more than anything else, particularly to allow patients during the day to lead as full a life as their illness allows. The beds will be used merely for sleeping in. The longer period of time in hospital compared with many general hospital cases will require that the patient has more space for clothing and such items. The nurses must be particularly trained in handling individuals who may be emotionally disturbed, and their role in nursing will be much more that of developing rapport with the patients and in this way assisting their recovery than in the sort of skills that might be needed on the labour ward.

Community

In the care of the elderly there has also been a trend in the last few years, a very laudable trend, to provide psychiatric care for those who need it nearer to the patient's home. To this end a range of facilities is being provided from the out-patient and day-patient facility in a local community unit for the elderly, where those individuals who are able to remain in their own homes or in a social services hostel or private hostel can attend for particular treatments or management during certain times of the week, through to the full in-patient care that may be needed by somebody with a more severe and prolonged dementia. These latter will still need full twenty-four hour nursing care to look after their particular needs, but the desirability of having such individuals adjacent to their familiar territory is clear. A degree of confusion from having to move will be diminished, and the opportunity for equally elderly relatives to visit and to maintain regular contact will be much improved. In the past many such patients have had to enter the local regional psychiatric hospital which may have been many miles from their familiar surroundings.

Limitations

Finally, therefore, let us review just what the doctor and his staff who specialise in psychiatry can and should do and also what they cannot and should not do.

There is a tendency on the part of the general public, and also often on the part of the Courts, to assume, on the one hand, that the psychiatrist is there to cure all ills, whether they be social, behavioural or medical. Now while his psychological training may well equip him to give some advice on the former two subjects, these are not matters which can properly be considered under the heading of treating ill people, which is what the doctor and the hospital staff are paid for. To attempt, therefore, to pontificate on these subjects leaves the doctor open to criticism from other groups who are in their own ways out to improve society. The psychiatrist has, to some extent, taken over the role of priest and confessor, but this is not, in fact, his job, except for those people who are attending him for reasons of psychiatric disturbance.

On the other hand, the general public tends to assume that once individuals have had a psychiatric illness, they are in some way permanently tarred with this brush. This is an example of schizophrenic thinking at its worst! The holding of two incompatible beliefs without seeing the incongruity of the situation is a symptom commonly found in this illness but unfortunately it is a pattern commonly shared by public attitudes. It must be remembered that **one in six women and one in nine men will enter a psychiatric hospital at some stage in their lives** (Table 2). This is not particularly startling. A much higher number of both sexes will enter a general hospital in their lifetime. Psychiatric illnesses are common, but most these days can be reasonably effectively alleviated, which is as much or often more than can be said for diseases in other medical fields. It is after all hardly the best cure for appendicitis to be able only to remove the offending organ from the body!

Table 2. Some facts and figures.

SIZE OF PROBLEM	(Approximate figures)
ENGLAND:	Approximate population 45,000,000
	Psychiatric in-patients 100,000
	Mentally retarded in-patients 60,000
	In local authority care 200,000

45% of all hospital beds are occupied by psychiatry (30% psychiatric illness; 15% mentally retarded). But only 11% of all consultants are psychiatrists. Only 22% of full-time nurses work in psychiatry. In hospitals for psychiatrically ill there is one consultant per 100 patients, and in hospitals for mentally retarded 1 to 500.

OUT-PATIENT ATTENDANCES

$1\frac{1}{2}$ million annually in England
New attendances 215,000

Patients in psychiatric beds 1950 = 145,000; in 1970 = 110,000 (England and Wales) but:
Total admissions 1950 = 60,000
                  1970 = 175,000

MEDIAN LENGTH OF STAY

1958   51 days
1968   33 days

Half the patients discharged had been in hospital less than a month, and nine out of ten less than 12 months. But 65% of in-patients in 1970 were of long-stay category.

MENTAL RETARDATION

1 child in every 100 born
60,000 in hospital
100,000 in local authority care.

WORKING DAYS LOST

40 million working days lost in Great Britain through psychiatric illness (DHSS, 1972); £45 million paid in sickness benefit.

Further Reading

Barton, R. W., *Institutional Neurosis* (3rd edn), Wright, Bristol, 1976.
Department of Health and Social Security, *Hospital Services for the Mentally Ill*, Circular HM(71)97, HMSO, London.
Department of Health and Social Security, *Services for Mental Illness Related to Old Age*, Circular HM(72)71, HMSO, London.
Early, D. F., and Nicholas, M., 'The Developing Scene. A Ten-Year Review of a Psychiatric Hospital Population', *British Medical Journal*, December 25, 1971.

Goffman, E., *Asylums, Essays on the Social Situation of Mental Patients and Other In Patients*, Penguin Books, Harmondsworth, 1970.

Mechanic, D., *Mental Health and Social Population* (2nd edn), Prentice Hall, Englewood Cliffs N.J., 1980.

Providing a comprehensive district psychiatric service for the adult mentally ill, Reports on Health and Social Subjects, No 8, HMSO, London, 1974.

Rakoff, V. M., *et al.*, *Psychiatric Diagnosis*, Brunner-Mozel, N.Y., 1977.

Stanton, A. H., and Schwartz, M. S., *The Mental Hospital*, Tavistock Publications, London, 1954.

Wing, J. K., and Hailey, A., *Evaluating a Community Psychiatric Service, The Camberwell Register, 1964–71*, Oxford University Press, London, 1972.

Questions

1. What is a normal curve of distribution?
2. How is the Health Service structured?
3. How is the Hospital Service subdivided?
4. How large is the psychiatric branch of the Health Service?
5. How do you distinguish psychiatric illness from mental retardation?
6. What is dementia? How many patients are likely to be over 65 years old?
7. What will be the difference between the in-patient and the out-patient psychiatric referrals?
8. What is the difference between amentia and dementia?
9. Where is your nearest mental retardation unit?
10. Where are the out-patient clinics for psychiatry? Is there an out-patient sub-normality clinic?
11. Does your local general hospital have a psychiatric unit?

3
Hospital Admission under the Mental Health Act 1983

The public tend to have a number of misconceptions with regard to referral for psychiatric treatment. Many people, when questioned on this point, believe that such referral or admission to a psychiatric unit will be different in some unspecified way from general hospital admission, and may see it as more threatening, despite the fact that they are likely to be up and about rather than remaining in bed, will have no fear of painful operative procedures, as may be the case in a surgical ward, and the type of uncomfortable or painful investigations that may come their way in general medical units will in psychiatry be at a minimum. Indeed, apart from the short-acting anaesthetic for electrical treatment, should this be needed, and the occasional blood test, admission to a psychiatric unit is a relatively stress-free affair.

The other anxiety which potential patients have about admission is that they will be with others who are worse than themselves and perhaps threatening or dangerous to them. As in any other branch of medicine, some patients will, of course, be more ill than others. Some will be at a stage of recovery and others will be but recently admitted. Equally, the patient with a varicose vein on the surgical ward may finish up next to a patient with cancer of the stomach. Both are in need of care and the less ill of the two can be thankful.

In practice, there is less likelihood of assault by one patient on another in a psychiatric unit than there is in walking the streets of our cities. Furthermore, unlike the streets in our cities, there are nurses available 24 hours of the day to help and look after people with emotional disturbances, and patients in that degree of distress would be in an observation bed. Unfortunately, these fears can be planted in the mind of the general public by films such as *One Flew Over the Cuckoo's Nest*, which, while it had undoubted artistic merit, portrayed a scene more accurate of an American state hospital in the pre-treatment days of the 1930s (which indeed was what the book was about) than anything remotely resembling modern psychiatric practice in Britain. The best way of allaying such fears is through education and by taking an interest in the psychiatric facilities in one's own area. Such education is the very purpose of this book.

Referrals to the psychiatrist, as to any other specialist in the Health Service, are channelled through the patient's general practitioner in the majority of cases. Occasionally, in emergency situations other agencies such as the social services or the police may be called in.

The initial interview will, of course, relate principally to those factors possibly relevant to the disturbances of mood, thinking or behaviour. Thus, a fuller social and family history will be necessary than with other branches of medicine, and, in contrast, one may get away with a less thorough physical examination. As will become clear in the second part of the book, however, a wide variety of physical conditions can produce psychiatric symptoms and a comprehensive physical examination will be essential at some point.

Again, as with other specialities, the general practitioner is seeking a second opinion when he refers the patient for an out-patient appointment. The psychiatrist assessing the case, who may be the consultant himself or one of his deputies, will provide his assessment and conclusions to the general practitioner, with advice as to what treatment should be provided. This may be all that is required, or the psychiatrist may take a patient on for further treatment on a regular out-patient basis or advise admission to hospital.

Reasons for Admission

There are only two reasons for admission to hospital. The first is to provide some form of treatment which cannot practically be given on an out-patient basis. In surgery, this would apply to all the more serious operations. In psychiatry, it usually will be required for patients undergoing electroplexy or perhaps some forms of behaviour therapy.

The second reason is to provide care. Some patients, because of the nature of their illness, may require 24-hour nursing care or at any event a degree of supervision and help until such time as they are well enough to resume their ordinary life at home or at work. To remove patients from their home or work environment for a time may be very helpful. In psychiatry, this is the usual reason for admission, but in general medicine or surgery it is also not infrequently the case—for instance, in elderly people with fractures, in those convalescing from surgery, or requiring closer observation in order to assess the amount of medication required, as in diabetes.

A total of 95 per cent of admissions to psychiatric units in British hospitals are on an informal basis, as is the case in any other hospital. There is, however, one big difference which singles out psychiatry from most other specialties and which accounts for the other 5 per cent. Because psychiatric conditions affect the function of the central nervous system and affect thought, emotion and behaviour, a small number of patients with severer forms of illness, such as may be found in the schizophrenic psychoses or in some manic-depressive conditions, will lose realisation of the fact of their disturbance and may become a danger to themselves or to others and be unaware that they require care.

Most reasonable societies are clear that under such circumstances somebody must act on behalf of such individuals and provide them with care, in a place of safety, until such time as they recover. This may on some occasions need to be done against the patient's will when acting in what one hopes to be their best interests. Civilised countries have, therefore, devised laws whereby this important step of removing a person's liberty for a period of time may be undertaken when the appropriate criteria are met.

These laws vary from country to country. They vary even between England and Scotland. Thus the criteria to be adopted and the measures built in to safeguard the patient's rights will vary in detail from place to place.

An enactment recognised worldwide as being a great advance in the care of the mentally ill came with the introduction in England of the 1959 Mental Health Act. While admittedly not perfect in all its aspects (and what law can be until it is tested?), this Act, along with the farsighted inclusion of psychiatry in the National Health Service Act of 1948, enabled a first-rate standard of care for every individual in the country to be provided free. Despite organisational troubles and staff shortages, the psychiatric services in Britain remain an example which most other countries would be hard-pressed to emulate.

The Mental Health Act 1983

Modern legal psychiatry in England dates from the Mental Health Act 1959. The 1959 act replaced a number of acts on the statute book which related to mental illness and to mental deficiency or retardation and before 1959 the two subjects were treated under different acts. Indeed only some 20 years before this time all patients admitted to psychiatric hospitals had to come into hospital on a magistrate's or County Sheriff's order. This system still operates in some of the States in America and in parts of the British Commonwealth.

The Mental Health Act of 1983 is an act to consolidate the law relating to disordered persons and replaces the 1959 act and the provisions of some other associated acts. It came into operation on 30 September 1983 and replaces the 1959 act and the mental health (hospital and guardianship) regulations of 1960.

The 1983 act is divided into ten parts and six schedules. The preamble gives the legal definition of mental illness, mental impairment and severe mental impairment and psychopathic disorder and interprets various aspects of the act.

Part Two is concerned with admission procedures and will concern us in this book since a proportion of patients may still need to be admitted to hospital under compulsory orders under the operation of the act.

Part Three of the act refers to the powers of the courts and the Home Secretary to detain, admit or transfer patients who are in custody as a result of the commission of a criminal act.

Part Four introduces a section on consent for treatment and within this part are a number of new concepts introduced in the 1983 act which enhance patients' rights and allow for independent opinions to be given in a case where compulsory detention has been required.

Part Five relates to the functions of mental health review tribunals which may hear such appeals against detention.

Part Six refers to the removal and return of patients within the different countries of the United Kingdom, while Part Eight introduces another new concept from the 1983 act, namely the Mental Health Act Commission and its function in giving second opinions on patients requiring compulsory treatment.

Part Seven refers to the management of property and the affairs of patients, the use of the court of protection and the powers of judges as to patients' property and affairs, while Part Nine refers to offences which may be committed which the act relates to such as the ill-treatment of patients, false statements and assisting patients to absent themselves without leave.

Finally, Part Ten is concerned with miscellaneous provisions as to the functions of managers, such matters as correspondence, the retaking of patients escaping from custody and members of parliament who may be suffering from mental illness.

Supplementary and finally within the Mental Health Act is Paragraph 149 which some might say sums up the whole business. Paragraph 149, Sub-section 4 states: 'Section 130(4) of the National Health Service Act 1977 which provides for the extension of that act to the Isles of Scilly shall have effect as if the references to that act included references to this act.'

Only certain parts of these acts need concern us. The legal definitions of mental disorders are worth quoting and knowing.

Mental disorder means mental illness, arrested or incomplete development of mind, psychopathic disorder and any other disorder or disability of mind and mentally disordered shall be construed accordingly.

Severe mental impairment means a state of arrested or incomplete development of mind which includes severe impairment of intelligence and social functioning and is associated with abnormal aggression or seriously irresponsible conduct on the part of the person concerned, and severely mentally impaired shall be construed accordingly.

Mental impairment means a state of arrested or incomplete development of mind not amounting to severe mental impairment which includes significant impairment of intelligence and social functioning and is associated with abnormal aggression or seriously irresponsible conduct on the part of the person concerned and mental impairment shall be construed accordingly.

Psychopathic disorder means that persistent disorder or disability of mind, whether or not including significant impairment of intelligence, which results in abnormal aggression or seriously irresponsible conduct on the part of the person concerned.

Part Two of the Mental Health Act

The nature of some psychiatric illnesses being that insight is lost and the patient becomes a danger to himself or to others for reasons of aggressive or suicidal behaviour, some provision must be made for the protection of these persons and for their care in order to protect them and society. Criminal law cannot be invoked for such people as they have not committed an offence, and indeed it seems to the author quite misplaced that the legal system in terms of sheriffs or magistrates should have any say in the compulsory detention of any individual who has not committed an offence since law officers have no background experience of psychiatric or medical problems.

Part Two of the act is concerned with regulations to safeguard the admission of such individuals and to allow for the proper possibility of care.

A patient cannot be detained in a hospital under the Mental Health Act against their wishes unless they are suffering from a mental illness, severe mental impairment, psychopathic disorder or mental impairment, and their mental disorder is of a nature or degree which makes it appropriate for them to receive medical treatment in a hospital. Furthermore, in the case of psychopathic disorder or mental impairment such treatment must be said to be likely to alleviate or prevent a deterioration of the condition, and finally it is necessary for the health or safety of the patient or for the protection of other persons that he should receive such treatment and it cannot be provided unless he is detained under this section.

In short, somebody can only be detained in hospital against their will if they are a danger to themselves or to other people by reason of being mentally disordered in one of the categories listed above.

The standard arrangement for such admission is that a recommendation is obtained both from a doctor who preferably has personal knowledge of the patient, which will usually mean the general practitioner, and someone who is recognised as a specialist in the treatment of mental illness, i.e. normally the consultant psychiatrist for that district. Based on these two recommendations an application must be made to the managers of the hospital either by a social worker recognised under the act as having specialist experience or by the patient's next of kin. While either party may make the application it is increasingly customary in the United Kingdom for the social worker to take on this role since it is often somewhat invidious for a nearest relative to be perceived as putting away one of their dear ones which may lead to subsequent problems in relationships within the family. Nevertheless, the family would normally have the power of veto and if a patient requires admission and the next of kin objects then there are various safeguards and additional procedures which need to be carried out before the patient can in fact be detained.

Under Section 2 of the act, therefore, a patient may be admitted to hospital and detained there for a period not exceeding 28 days beginning with the day on which he is admitted and shall not be detained after the expiration of that period unless before its expiration he has become liable to be detained by virtue of a second application order or direction under the further provisions of the act.

This in effect means that a patient can only stay in for 28 days unless Section 3 of the act, which is a treatment order as opposed to an assessment order, which is the official title of Section 2, has been applied. Treatment can of course be given under either of the acts, but for those patients who require a longer period of time in hospital and who have not made sufficient recovery after the 28 days for it to be appropriate for them to be made informal then Section 3 applies.

Under Section 3 the patient may be detained for treatment, but curiously in the 1983 act it is not until Paragraph 20 that we are told how long the authority may last. Here it states that a patient admitted to hospital in pursuance of an application for admission for treatment may be detained for a period not extending six months beginning on the day on which he was so admitted and shall not be detained or kept on for any longer period unless the authority for his detention is renewed under Section 20.

Other situations in which compulsory admission may be necessary are covered in later sections. The situation may arise where a patient in the community requires urgent admission to hospital, for example when caught in the act of trying to commit suicide and the necessary people and documents cannot be available at such short notice. In any case of urgent necessity under Section 4 of the act an application for admission may be made in respect of a patient in accordance with this provision by an emergency application being made by an approved social worker or the closest relative of the patient and one medical recommendation alone. The act allows the detention of the patient for a period of 72 hours from the time of admission to the hospital and allows for the completion of the second medical recommendation within this period of time, otherwise the detention order ceases to be valid and the patient becomes informal and may stay in hospital on an informal basis or take their discharge.

The vast majority of patients are in fact admitted to hospital on an informal basis and these sections only apply to a small number, perhaps 5–10 per cent of admissions.

Sometimes a patient who is already in hospital on an informal basis deteriorates in health and demands discharge when in fact in the opinion of the staff it is not safe for them to be discharged. Under these circumstances Section 5 allows for an application to be made for the patient to remain in hospital under the act, even though they are already an informal patient, and again this section allows a detention of 72 hours from the time of the furnishing of the report for the necessary documentation for Section 2 or Section 3 to be arranged.

A new introduction in the 1983 act is what is known as the nurse's six-hour holding power. If in the case of a patient who is receiving treatment as an in-patient it appears to the nurses that the patient is suffering from a mental disorder of such a degree that it is necessary that they be immediately restrained from leaving the hospital and it is not practical to secure immediate attendance of a practitioner for the purposes of furnishing a report under Sub-section 2 or 3 then the nurses may detain the patient on their own cognisance in the hospital for a period of six hours from the time when the fact was recorded or until the earlier arrival at the place where the patient is detained of a practitioner having power to furnish a report under one of the appropriate Mental Health Act sections.

In other words, the nurses can keep a patient who is a suicidal or homicidal risk in the hospital for a short time so that a doctor can be called to deal with the problem.

Finally, under Section 136 of the act, if a constable finds, in a place to which the public has access, a person who appears to be suffering from mental disorder and to be in immediate need of care or control the constable may, if he thinks it necessary to do so, in the interests of that person or for the protection of other persons, remove that person to a place of safety within the meaning of Section 135.

This means that a police constable can take such an individual found disturbed in a public place into a registered hospital, or can take them to a police station or some other designated place of safety so that they can be seen by a doctor and if necessary treatment under the act instituted. If the constable takes the patient to hospital then they may be detained for a period of 72 hours so that the provisions of Section 2 or 3 may be applied if in the opinion of the medical staff it is deemed necessary.

A patient who is detained in hospital may well, because of the nature of their illness, not appreciate the need for such treatment and may object. In order to protect such an individual from wrongful detention various safeguards have been built into the act whereby a patient may make an appeal.

The patient may initially appeal to the managers who are required to review the case and directly or indirectly the case should then be referred to the Mental Health Review Tribunal. The patient may have a right of appeal direct to the Mental Health Review Tribunal and this is covered under Part Five of the act. Each of the Regional Health Authorities is covered by a separate Mental Health Review Tribunal and there is a special one for Wales. (The 1983 act does not apply to Scotland or Northern Ireland.) Patients may apply if detained under Section 2 during the 14 days of detention to have their case reviewed or under Section 3 during the first three months of detention. If the patient has been reclassified at the end of six months for a further period of detention then they may again apply for review within the first 28 days and the nearest relative may also apply from being informed which they must be by the responsible medical officer.

The Mental Health Review Tribunal has a range of options in relation to any patient whose case they consider. They have the power to discharge from hospital or may recommend leave of absence, delay discharge or transfer. If their recommendation is not complied with they may reconvene. The tribunal must discharge a patient detained under Section 2 if they are satisfied that he is not then suffering from mental disorder to a nature or degree which warrants his detention in hospital for assessment or his detention is not justified in the interests of his health or safety or for the protection of others. Equally they must discharge any other Section 2 patient if they are satisfied that he is not suffering from one of the 44 categories of mental disorder of a nature or degree which makes hospital treatment appropriate or if his detention is not justified in the interests of his health or safety. Similar regulations apply to people detained under Section 3.

Part Three of the act refers to the detention of patients concerned in criminal proceedings or under sentence. This area is not of great concern in general psychiatry and is relatively rarely found. Nevertheless, a crown court or a magistrates court may remand an accused person to a hospital specified by the court for a report on his mental condition. If the court is satisfied on the evidence of a registered medical practitioner that there is reason to suggest that the accused person is suffering from mental illness, psychopathic disorder, severe mental impairment or mental impairment and the court is of the opinion that it would be impractical for a report on his mental condition to be made, if he were remanded on appeal, then the powers conferred on the court may be used.

A crown court may, instead of remanding an accused person in custody, remand him to a hospital specified by the court and the court can also make guardianship orders.

By and large, patients referred to hospital under a court order do not have rights of appeal as they do under the normal Mental Health Act detention sections unless they have been transferred to a hospital in England or Wales having previously been detained under the Mental Health Act's application in Scotland, the Channel Isles or the Isle of Man which have separate legislations.

Where a hospital order is made in respect of an offender by the crown court and the offence is of a sufficiently serious nature a restriction order under Section 41 can be applied. This may be without limit of time or during such period as may be specified by the court. Discharge under these circumstances can only be agreed if application is made to the Secretary of State, who has the final say as to whether the medical recommendations for discharge, if and when they are made, should be agreed.

Under Section 46 the Secretary of State may by warrant direct that any person who is required to be kept in custody during her Majesty's pleasure may be sent to a hospital as specified in the warrant. The hospital has the power to refuse the admission of such a patient if they feel they are not in a position to offer the necessary security.

The majority of present-day open psychiatric hospitals are not designed to care for those patients whom the law would classify as criminally insane and a number of special hospitals therefore exist and have been set up to cater for seriously disturbed patients who may be a danger to others. In England these are at Broadmoor Hospital, Rampton Hospital and Moss Side. But other secure units have more recently been set up such as Park Lane Hospital in Liverpool. The equivalent hospital in Scotland is the Carstairs State Hospital.

The moral dilemma here can be stated as follows. If a person is suffering from a disorder of brain function or mind, which by its nature makes them unaware that they are ill, should others who have experience in such illnesses take it upon themselves to treat the illness, acting as they hope in the best interest of the patient, even if the patient refuses to agree to treatment or to accept that it is necessary? To those who may be tempted to answer 'no' to that question one must pose an additional question. Should a doctor who knows that he can probably relieve suffering, cut short an illness and possibly save somebody's life or sanity, withold such help knowing that the patient is in no position to make a rational judgement, simply on the basis of some legal technicality with regard to consent?

The problem does not arise in other branches of medicine, whereby the patient is assumed to be capable of making a rational judgement. If I get an appendicitis and I refuse to have an operation despite the fact that it is explained to me that in so doing I am risking death from the complications then my advisors may grieve but would not feel it appropriate to force me to change my mind, but to take another extreme if I were bleeding and unconscious it would be assumed that if conscious I would accept help in stemming the bleeding. Therefore people act on my behalf. Should I require a blood transfusion and it is subsequently revealed that I belong to a religious group to which a blood transfusion is unacceptable then the doctors would not in such circumstances be accused of acting in bad faith.

It is, therefore, largely accepted by society that in the occasional cases where consent is not obtainable but where the patient is not capable of forming a rational judgement yet at the same time is in obvious need of help, that this may be given on the authority of the responsible medical officer or the consent of the nearest relative if this is possible, on the assumption that when the patient is restored to health he will be suitably grateful. Section 3 of the Mental Health Act gives the legal sanction for this process to be carried out and removes the fear of a court action for assault from those who have to make such a judgement.

The moral dilemma comes in those cases which are borderline or where methods of treatment which are controversial or could result in damaging side-effects might be employed. An example of a treatment of this kind would be a leucotomy operation. It would seem that the most satisfactory way of resolving this type of dilemma is to have such decisions made by experienced and well-trained practitioners with a strong code of ethics to back them. It is easy to say that in societies where this is not the case abuse could occur, and it is for this reason that the safeguards built into the Mental Health Act need to be carefully observed. An additional safeguard was therefore built into the 1983 Mental Health Act as a result of requests by various pressure groups, and this has resulted in the creation of the Mental Health Act Commission.

The Mental Health Act Commission

This body has been set up as a special health authority by the Secretary of State and like other health authorities it has to comply with directions from the Secretary of State but is otherwise independent in the performance of its functions and the advice it can offer. The Secretary of State for Social Services is responsible for making appointments to the Commission. The Commission includes lawyers, nurses, psychologists, social workers, psychiatrists and laymen roughly in equal numbers. Medical members of the commission have duties with regard to consents to treatment and under Section 120 are required to make arrangements for persons authorised by it to visit and interview in private, patients detained in hospital and mental nursing homes. The authorised persons must investigate any complaint which a detained patient thinks is not being dealt with satisfactorily by the hospital managers or any other complaint concerning the use of powers given by the act. The Commission can investigate a complaint made by an ex-patient which he does not feel has been satisfactorily dealt with by the managers as long as it relates to a period of detention under the act. Any person authorised by the Commission has the right of access to a detained patient and their records at any given time.

In particular, the medical members of the Mental Health Act Commission are required to interview a patient who is detained under the Act and who is required to have treatment but is currently refusing the same or is not capable of understanding the nature of such treatment.

This usually applies to the giving of medication on a long-term basis or to the use of electroplexy. Should the responsible medical officer in charge of such a patient recommend this type of treatment then he is required to obtain a second opinion from the Mental Health Act Commissioner who will visit the patient, interview him or her and interview a nurse and a non-medical, non-nurse person in addition, who has knowledge of the patient in order to ensure that the treatment proposed is justified and sensible.

The function of the Commission, therefore, should be to appoint medical practitioners for the purpose of the consent to treatment provisions under Paragraphs 192 and 196, to review treatment given only if a second opinion has been requested and to carry out the functions described under Section 120, i.e. the visiting of patients and investigations of complaints.

A Code of Practice has been produced by the Commission who are required to produce reports every two years.

The Commission's functions are quite separate from those of the Mental Health Review Tribunal which determine whether a patient should continue to be detained and meet at the request of the patient themselves. The Commission has no power to discharge a patient.

Part Six of the 1983 Mental Health Act is concerned with the removal and return of patients within the United Kingdom. This part of the act is necessary because different laws operate within Scotland, within Northern Ireland and within the Channel Isles and the Isle of Man where the English Mental Health Act does not appertain. The English Mental Health Act appertains in Wales where the legal system is now the same as in England.

Scotland, Northern Ireland, the States of Guernsey, States of Jersey and the Isle of Man each have their own legal systems and their own Mental Health Acts. While there are many similarities and the act in Scotland and Northern Ireland has recently been brought up to date there are critical differences which cannot be covered in depth in this book. The reader living in these countries, however, would do well to check on the legal differences which may be found. Certainly the sections referred to differ and in Scotland, for example, the length of time that these holding orders apply and the methods of detention vary to some degree with those found in England and Wales.

Thus should a patient be required to be moved from one country to another arrangements must be made so that the appropriate regulations have been transferred from one act to the other.

For example, under Section 80 of the Mental Health Act of 1983 for England and Wales, if it appears to the Secretary of State that it is in the interests of the patient to remove him or her to Scotland and that arrangements have been made for admitting this patient, the Secretary of State may authorise his removal and may give any necessary directions for his conveyance to his destination.

Sections are also concerned with the removal and transfer of aliens from Britain by which are meant those individuals normally living abroad. A particularly aposite section is Section 149, Sub-section 4 which refers to the National Health Service Act of 1977 which provides that anything referred to in the Mental Health Act of 1983 with regard to England and Wales shall also apply to the Isles of Scilly.

Part Seven of the act refers to the management of property and the affairs of patients. A particular concern here is the Court of Protection. The purpose of this part of the act is to safeguard the property or finances of people who may, through mental illness, be unable to handle their own affairs and might otherwise be open to exploitation.

Such problems are most likely to arise with a patient suffering from a psychotic illness such as schizophrenia or from a dementing illness where the memory and intellectual function may become impaired. This may therefore be a particular problem for the elderly and for such matters as the making of wills.

Legal documents should not be signed by a patient in a psychiatric hospital unless their validity has been accepted and witnessed by the medical officer responsible for the case. Relatives may sometimes find this regulation irksome but it does prevent unscrupulous people from taking advantage of someone who is ill and therefore is in the patient's best interests.

If patients wish someone else to handle their affairs and are in a state of mind competent enough to understand the nature of what they are doing and its significance (for example the state of their assets and the reasonable claims which relatives might have upon them), then they may sign a legal document, make a will or undertake financial transactions. They may grant a Power of Attorney to a friend or relative who can then sign cheques or carry out financial transactions on their behalf. If, however, a Power of Attorney has been granted before the patient's admission to hospital, it ceases to be valid from the time that the patient enters hospital. A new Power of Attorney can, however, be granted should the patient be fit enough to do so and wish it.

The problem comes when a patient is not fit enough to do so. If the individual is likely to be unwell for only a few weeks, then matters can usually wait. In longer-term problems however, particularly when sums of money are large, then the 'Court of Protection' exists to handle a patient's affairs and look after their interests.

Application may be made to the Court of Protection under the act by a solicitor acting for the patient or on the advice of a medical officer or social worker. The court having established that such an application is appropriate may then appoint some person as a receiver, often a near relative of the patient who is then answerable to the court for the proper execution of that patient's affairs. Thus bills can be paid, an allowance sufficient for the patients needs can be granted, and matters such as the maintenance and repair of property can be carried out as may be deemed appropriate. Without such a mechanism the spouse, son or daughter of the incapacitated patient might find that essential matters such as the payment of creditors could not be carried out. Should the patient recover sufficiently to be able to take over the handling of his affairs again such an order of the court can of course be rescinded.

The Lord Chancellor may nominate one or more judges of the supreme court to act for the purposes of this part of the act. The master of the Court of Protection takes an oath of allegiance and a judicial oath in the presence of the Lord Chancellor and the Lord Chancellor may nominate other officers of the Court of Protection for the purposes of this part of the act.

The Lord Chancellor also has a panel of Lord Chancellor's visitors of patients constituted in accordance with Section 102, which consists of a panel of medical visitors, a panel of legal visitors, and a panel of general visitors whose function it is to visit patients who are involved in Court of Protection orders and satisfy themselves that all is well.

Part Eight of the act is concerned with various aspects and functions of local authorities and the Secretary of State, the approval of social workers under the act and the provision of such matters as pocket money for patients. Part Nine deals with offences which may be committed by persons treating mentally ill patients, such as assisting a patient who is detained under the act to absent themselves from hospital without leave, illegal intercourse with a patient detained in hospital under the act, and matters concerned with the retaking of patients detained who have escaped from custody.

An interesting section is Section 141. Where a member of the House of Commons is authorised to be detained on the grounds that he is suffering from mental illness it is the duty of the court, authority or person on whose order or application and of any registered medical practitioner upon whose recommendation the detention was authorised to notify the Speaker of the House of Commons that the detention has occurred.

Where the Speaker receives a notification the Speaker should cause the member to whom the notification relates to be visited and examined by two registered medical practitioners appointed in accordance with the act, appointed by the President of the Royal College of Psychiatrists and they shall report to the Speaker of the House of Commons on the matter. Six months from the date of the report the Speaker can again cause the member to be visited, and if the second report concludes that the member continues to suffer from mental illness and remains detained then these reports are laid before the House of Commons and the seat of the member becomes vacant. This does not apply to a member of the House of Lords.

Further Reading

The Mental Health Act, 1983 HMSO, London.
The Mental Health Act, 1983 Memorandum on Parts 1–6, 8 and 10, Department of Health and Social Security, 1983, HM(W) 1912.
'Restoring Psychiatrically Disabled into the Community', *Lancet*, 11, 1963.
Stanton, A. H., and Schwartz, M. S., *The Mental Hospital*, Tavistock, London, 1954.

Questions

1. What are the reasons for admission to a hospital?
2. What percentage of patients in a psychiatric hospital are informal (i.e. not compulsorily admitted)?
3. What are the four categories under which compulsory admission can be initiated?
4. How can the affairs of a patient detained in hospital be handled?
5. What is the function of the Mental Health Review Tribunal?
6. What is the Mental Health Act Commission?

4
History of Psychiatry

The study of psychiatric illness will be found to go back many centuries. Hippocrates in 400 BC was laying down certain fundamental principles concerned with mental illness, and early Greek and Roman writings make reference to psychiatric symptomatology.

Susutra in the Indian subcontinent was also writing on the theme of psychiatry some hundred years previously. Cicero in the first century BC and Galen in AD 150 returned to the theme, though ideas on causation were, of course, products of the philosophies of their time. The Chinese of the Tang dynasties and Arabic writings at the time of Rhazes of Baghdad in the ninth century all contributed to ideas on conditions which would nowadays be described as depression, schizophrenia and perhaps hysteria.

In Britain the **Bethlem Hospital** was founded in 1247 and received psychiatric patients as part of its role from the year 1300. It was not until the eighteenth century, however, that psychiatry began to form itself into a proper discipline and some rational attempts at care and treatment were made along the lines of the discoveries which were taking place within the total framework of medicine and surgery.

Early Acts

Under the **Vagrancy Act of 1744** each parish was required to look after its own poor, and 'furiously and dangerously mad', who were to be 'locked up in a secure place as long as the madness shall continue'. Magistrates were required to sign the order for certification and such patients went to gaol or to Bridewells, and in the latter one did not have to pay for one's keep. A few were dealt with privately later at the Retreat in York and Cheadle Royal Hospital.

Before 1744 insanity in Britain had been very much mixed up with witchcraft. There was indeed very little choice of hospital care, which devolved upon the small private mad-houses which had begun to be set up in the seventeenth century, Bethlem Hospital in London, and a ward in the poorhouse at Bristol, where the Corporation of the Poor had been established in 1696.

In law at this time insane individuals were not distinguished from other vagrants, and it was not until 1714 that the first law was passed specifically for the control of those who were dangerously, psychiatrically ill. The Act of 1744 charged the parish with the expense of curing such a person during restraint.

A second hospital was opened for the care of the insane in Norwich in 1713. Guys' Hospital in London opened wards for lunatics in 1728, St Luke's hospital was built in 1751, and in the second half of the eighteenth century many of the larger provincial cities, including Newcastle, York, Manchester and Liverpool, established hospitals for the insane by public subscription.

Many of the establishments set up during the eighteenth century were custodial in nature, and considerable abuses of patients were perpetrated, sometimes in the name of treatment but sometimes simply for the entertainment of visitors who paid to watch the lunatics, or even perhaps in some cases to satisfy the sadistic impulses of some of the custodians. In the absence of any effective method of treatment in those days morale could not have been high, and it would be no surprise if a sense of defeatism pervaded any attempt at therapeutic innovation.

The nineteenth century saw the birth and growth of county asylums, and Parliament set up a committee to enquire 'into the state of criminal and pauper lunatics in England and Wales and of the laws relative thereto'. One factor of importance in the setting up of this committee had been an Act of Parliament of 1800 which had provided that persons who were found not guilty of serious criminal offences by reason of insanity should be kept in custody in some fit place, when in fact no such fit places had at that time been set up. The case in question was that of James Hadfield, who had attempted to murder the King and who was acquitted on grounds of insanity.

A result of the committee's report was the **Asylum Act of 1808**, which empowered every county to provide an asylum for the reception of pauper lunatics within its own boundaries. These asylums were to be paid for by the parish, and also at the time accepted criminal lunatics, until, in 1816, part of the Bethlem Hospital was developed to provide a state asylum. Broadmoor did not open until 1863.

Northamptonshire was the first county to develop what came to be the County Mental Hospital, and this opened in 1811. Stanley Royd Hospital at Wakefield followed in 1818, but by 1845 only eighteen counties had taken such action and the number of psychiatric patients requiring treatment at this time was estimated at more than 20,000.

Lord Shaftesbury was at this time a great reformer and his Act, the second **Asylum Act of 1845**, made the provision of such hospitals compulsory, whereas before it had been purely a permissive Act. Private mad-houses, however, continued to flourish. The **Mad House Act of 1828** had attempted to prevent abuses whereby sane people had been detained, often at the personal request of their families, as one method of removing a problem from their midst. Private patients could not thereafter be received into hospital without a certificate signed by two independent medical practitioners, nor paupers without an order signed by two magistrates or one of the clergy of the parish.

Also in 1845 the first full-scale **Board of Commissioners in Lunacy** was set up to supervise all institutions throughout the county. At the York Asylum an enquiry was held into abuses in patient care, and, indeed, before this commission, in 1796, William Tuke had founded the Retreat in York, a hospital intended for members of the Society of Friends and based strongly on Quaker precepts and patterns of living. This hospital rapidly obtained a reputation as a humane institution which set an example in subsequent decades in moral treatment by humane methods.

At the same time reformers such as Pinel in France had been developing humanitarian principles, and when R. G. Hill was appointed to the Lincoln Asylum in 1834, he set an example in abolishing methods of restraint which had until then been widely used to control psychotic behaviour, and showed that it was possible in a properly designed and well-staffed institution to avoid the need of recourse to such methods.

Other names that stand out in this reformist era are Connelly, the physician at Hanwell; and W. C. Hood, who took on the task of modernising the Bethlem Hospital.

As the nineteenth century progressed, however, the county mental hospitals became increasingly large and overcrowded. The scourges of psychiatry in this century remained by and large untreatable, and an accumulation of long-stay, disturbed psychotic patients produced a steadily increasing case-load, with little prospect of relief. A *History of Psychiatry* written by Lader and Alderidge quotes the Metropolitan Commissioners in Lunacy in their report of 1844 as follows: 'At Hanwell the two resident medical officers have between them nearly a thousand patients to attend and are required by the rules to see every patient twice a day. Each of these officers has an average of thirty persons on the sick list and about fifty on the extra diet list at any given time. Besides these duties they have to mix the medicines and keep the registers and diaries'. It was little wonder under such circumstances, with absurd under-staffing, that abuses were frequent and the therapeutic milieu very low. It is perhaps surprising, therefore, that, despite all this, in the latter part of the nineteenth century great advances started to be made.

The **Permissive Idiots Act of 1886** granted powers to local authorities to build additional hospitals principally for the treatment of the mentally retarded. Before this time there had been little differentiation between the mentally ill and those subnormal or mentally deficient. Then followed the **Lunacy Act of 1890**, and in 1913 the first **Mental Deficiency Act**, which laid down the four grades of mental deficiency, and after being amended in 1927 remained on the statutes until 1959.

In 1930 the **Mental Treatment Act** was introduced. This Act allowed concepts with regard to patient care in the light of new knowledge to be updated, and for the first time created a category of 'voluntary patient'. Before this all the admissions to county mental hospitals had been on the basis of compulsory orders under the old Act, and required a magistrate's signature. Out-patient clinics were at this time also first given official sanction, and local authorities were given powers for after-care.

An event whose importance cannot be over-emphasised was the result of a white paper in 1944 which led to the 1946 **National Health Service Act**. Initially, the psychiatric hospitals were not to be included in the powers of this Act, but a far-sighted decision enabled Aneurin Bevan to introduce a full National Health Service with psychiatric services included. Before this, psychiatric hospitals were paid for either out of county rates or public subscription, and there is little doubt that the immense strides that have been made in the last 30 years in psychiatry have in no small measure been helped by the national funding of such hospitals allowing the creation of standards equivalent to those seen in general hospitals, and the introduction of a sensible staffing structure for doctors, nurses and ancillary professions such as clinical psychology and occupational therapy.

The Mental Health Act 1959

Next came another great milestone with the introduction in 1959 of the Mental Health Act. The principal advantage of this new Act was that it created a situation within the psychiatric hospital whereby the vast majority of patients could be admitted informally—that is to say, with the same status as in any other hospital ward and with no legal restriction, therefore, on their liberty. Modern methods of treatment had made such restrictions unnecessary in the great majority of cases, and the law had been out of step. More than 90 per cent of admissions could now enter hospital on this basis, and the remainder were granted a more logical type of admission procedure with built-in safeguards against abuse.

The 1959 Act brought together again mental retardation and mental illness, and all previous Acts referring to both subjects were repealed. Four new categories of patient were designated for purposes of administering the Act—namely, **mental illness, psychopathy** (which replaced the old definition of moral imbecile in the Mental Deficiency Act), and two categories of mental retardation designated **subnormality** and **severe subnormality**, which replaced the old categories of idiot, imbecile and moron, terms which had become abusive in everyday parlance.

The Mental Health Act 1983

Over the 25 years that the 1959 Act was in operation a number of problems were noted with regard to its workings. Furthermore, the expectations of the public also changed and attitudes towards responsibility, towards individual freedoms and patients' rights all changed. Pressure groups developed and felt that the safeguards contained within the 1959 Act with regard to consent to treatment and with regard to appeal under the detention sections required revision.

A movement also took place, particularly in the United States and pursued largely by such organisations as the scientologists, to look into the effectiveness and desirability of electroplexy as a treatment. These pressure groups managed to persuade a number of sponsors of the 1983 Bill as it went through Parliament to built into the Act the necessity for second opinions to be obtained before such treatments were carried out and this led to the development of the Mental Health Act Commission and a number of other safeguards which were built into the detention sections. These have been discussed in more detail in Chapter 3. The term mental illness remains undefined, and the four categories under which various types of detention can be applied are now renamed as mental illness, mental impairment, severe mental impairment and psychopathic disorder. The definition of psychopathic disorder has been revised from the 1959 Act and refers now to 'whether or not including significant impairment of intelligence' rather than 'subnormality of intelligence'. As in the 1959 Act psychopathic disorder must be a persistent disorder or disability, in other words there must have been signs that disorder has existed for a considerable time before a patient can be classified as having a psychopathic disorder, and it must result in abnormally aggressive or seriously irresponsible conduct if detention is to be applied and to be legal. Furthermore, with regard to treatability of the condition this is no longer mentioned, but the effect of Sections 3, 37 and 47 are that those with psychopathic disorder, or indeed with mental impairment cannot be compulsorily admitted to hospital for treatment unless it can be stated that medical treatment is likely to alleviate or prevent a deterioration in their condition. This proviso is more stringent than the inclusion of the words 'requires or is susceptible to treatment' in the definition of psychopathic disorder or subnormality of the 1959 Act.

Under Paragraph 16 of the 1983 Mental Health Act Memorandum from the DHSS it is noted that patients may not be dealt with under the Act as suffering from mental disorder purely by reason of promiscuity, other immoral conduct, sexual deviance or dependence on alcohol or drugs. This means there are no grounds for detaining a person in hospital because of alcohol or drug abuse alone though it is recognised that alcohol or drug abuse can be accompanied by, or associated with, a mental disorder arising from, or suspected to arise from, alcohol or drug dependence, or withdrawal of the same, should admission be required for this purpose.

Diagnostic Criteria

In the early days of the setting-up of county mental hospitals the ability to diagnose and distinguish between different types of psychiatric disorder were primitive and haphazard. Furthermore, in the last 150 years considerable changes have been seen in the incidence of certain types of psychiatric problem, which reflect in terms of in-patient care the advances that have been made in treatment.

The pioneer of classification was **Kraepelin**, who, towards the end of the nineteenth century, delineated the psychoses from neuroses and subdivided the former into **dementia praecox**, the old term for schizophrenia, and the **manic depressive psychoses**. Up to this time dementia had formed a very large part of psychiatric in-patient work, but it was an amorphous mass of conditions poorly delineated, and it had not been possible at this time to distinguish the various causes. One must remember that no X-rays were available. The microscope was not able to distinguish infective agents with any certainty, and it was not possible to grow bacteria in culture media. Even such instruments as the stethoscope were in relatively primitive form.

Dementia was the name given to a group of conditions where an intellectual deterioration occurred with disturbance of memory and general disintegration of personality and social functioning. *Dementia praecox* was simply one subgroup, which tended to have its onset in adolescence but progressed steadily over the years to the type of deterioration outlined above. We now know, of course, that dementia praecox is not a true dementia at all but a pseudo-dementia, the result of the late effects of the schizophrenic process. In the nineteenth century, however, this had not been recognised.

In the early nineteenth century two great scourges also classified under the dementias swelled the ranks of psychiatric beds. One was known as **dementia paralytica** or 'general paralysis of the insane', and the other was the alcoholic dementia which came to be known as **Korsakoff's psychosis**. Both these conditions produced a true dementia, the former due to the late stages of a syphilitic infection and the latter due to damage to the central nervous system by the toxic effect of poisoning and vitamin deficiency from the malabsorption of the vitamin B group which tended to go with it.

Dementia Paralytica

Though it was recognised that dementias could be subdivided and that some typical features tended to occur within these subgroups, causation was still a matter of guesswork. Syphilis is said to have been introduced to Europe by the sailors on the ships of Columbus returning from the Americas. It had swept Europe and reached epidemic proportions in the seventeenth century. The early stages of the disease were recognised as coming from sexual contact, but the delayed effect of syphilis, resulting from long-standing chronic and unrecognised infection, may not become apparent for 20 years or more from the initial contact. Thus, until the causative organism had been recognised in the central nervous system, spinal column or the greater vessels in the heart, where they tended to lodge, the connection was not apparent.

The first description of *dementia paralytica* is attributed to Haslam in 1798. He worked as an apothecary at the Bethlem Hospital and had noted the typical symptoms of the disease, at first thought to be due to psychological causes. It was not until 1913, however, that Noguchi and Moore demonstrated organisms in the central nervous system of *Treponema Pallidum* in these patients at post-mortem.

More will be said about this in Chapter 16. Suffice it to say that this discovery was of immense importance to psychiatry. At this time 20 per cent of admissions to psychiatric hospitals suffered from *dementia paralytica*. The discovery of the association with syphilis, and the development of treatments which could kill the organism, brought psychiatry back into the mainstream of medicine at a stroke. Suddenly a large group of otherwise incurable cases could be effectively treated, and a new sense of hope and enthusiasm was instilled into those working in the psychiatric field.

Now only some two per cent of cases of dementia prove to have this diagnosis. Ehrlich in 1910 had established the effectiveness of neoarsphenamine in the treatment of *dementia paralytica* even before the causative organism had been proven. In 1917 Wagner von Jauregg noted that *dementia paralytica* was much less frequent in countries where malaria was endemic. He suggested that the inoculation of such patients with malaria might be effective in controlling the extension of the *dementia paralytica*. This proved to be the case, although the treatment was not, of course, without hazard, since malaria itself could be a serious illness. This ingenious idea, however, did restore many people to health who would otherwise have remained chronic patients and gradually progressed to a vegetable existence. It subsequently proved that the effectiveness of this treatment related to the high fever induced by the malaria, this raising of temperature being sufficient to kill the *treponema* which was infecting the central nervous system.

This provides another interesting example of a treatment which has been developed and proved of immense benefit to mankind even though the initial understanding of its mechanisms was ill-understood. Once the mechanism was understood, other methods of inducing hyperthermia were able to supplant malarial therapy, and this remained a reasonably effective method of treatment until the advent of penicillin in the 1940s rendered it unnecessary.

The other great scourge of the eighteenth and nineteenth centuries, alcoholism, is still with us. The long-term effects of alcohol will be discussed in Chapter 14, but damage to the central nervous system from the toxic effect and from a disturbance of vitamin B metabolism, which often goes with it, has been recognised for many years. It has been estimated that there are some 350,000 alcoholics in the British Isles. About a tenth of these receive treatment. A smaller number produce, if unchecked, an eventual dementing condition, one type of which is Korsakoff's psychosis. This is another type of dementia, which in the late nineteenth century was teased out from the general mass with this diagnostic label.

Another scourge which affected psychiatric hospital admissions early in the twentieth century resulted from a viral condition, namely **encephalitis lethargica**, which swept many parts of the world at the end of the First World War. It was the damaging result to the central nervous system, with the ensuing dementia or subnormality of intelligence, which largely led to the 1927 amendment to the Mental Deficiency Act.

The Psychoses

The two other main contributors to psychiatric hospitals were, on the one hand, *dementia praecox*, and, on the other, the manic depressive psychoses as delineated by Kraepelin. The cause of these conditions was unknown and treatment had been of very little effect. Some generally acting sedatives were available, but had no directly curative properties and in some cases carried with them the danger of addiction. Opium and its derivatives were the main preparations available until the end of the nineteenth century.

In the mid-nineteenth century, however, a new drug came on to the market in the form of **bromide**, which had been introduced in the treatment of epilepsy, and this became widely used as a sedative. Unfortunately, the effect of large doses of bromide was to induce its own hazards. A condition known as bromism, which induced mental sluggishness, confusion, and a skin rash, was commonly seen if the type of dosage necessary to control the disturbed behaviour of psychotic patients was used.

Other drugs, such as chloral, were followed in the early 1900s by the barbiturates, which have been extremely widely used over the last 50 years. Their use in epilepsy and in quick-acting anaesthetics is still invaluable, but their general sedative effect, while making them valuable as hypnotics, can rapidly lead to dependence, which has again limited the usefulness of this group of drugs.

The first drug treatment shown to be effective for depressive states was that of **amphetamine**. Synthesised in the 1920s, this combated fatigue and induced a sense of well-being. Amphetamines were widely used in that decade to relieve depressive symptoms, and also as slimming tablets, since they suppressed appetite. Certain dangers, however, rapidly became apparent in that addiction to the drug could occur and a psychotic state not unlike schizophrenia could be induced in some cases. This has led to some interesting research into the causation of schizophrenia, but the effect on depressive states was short-lived, and eventual withdrawal of the drug often left the patient worse off than before. Thus its use is now very limited, principally to the treatment of narcolepsy, a condition of abnormal sleepiness where amphetamine, because of its property of inducing wakefulness, can be helpful.

Until 1930, therefore, the treatment of illness remained at a primitive level. Apart from the advances in the treatment of such conditions as *dementia paralytica*, all that could be done for the psychoses, which formed the bulk of the hospital in-patient population by this stage, was to sedate and to provide nursing care until such time as it was hoped the condition would burn itself out. The next decade, however, was to see dramatic advances in the treatment of these major psychiatric illnesses.

The observation that epileptic fits in patients suffering from psychotic illness appeared to produce at least temporary remission in some cases led to the theory that if an epileptic seizure could be artificially induced in psychotic patients, this might have some restorative function. This was further reinforced by an observation, which in fact proved erroneous, that schizophrenia was rarely found associated with the condition of epilepsy.

In the late 1920s early attempts at inducing generalised seizure discharges in the central nervous system had been attempted by Meduna, who had also observed that carbon dioxide inhalation could be effective in the relief of anxiety and agitation not only in psychotics but in those with anxiety states. The experimental work with **convulsive therapy**, as it came to be called, showed considerable promise, and a number of acutely ill patients were enabled to be discharged. It was noted, however, that depressive psychoses appeared to respond more effectively than did schizophrenia. These early attempts at inducing seizures artificially made use of the injection of substances such as camphor, but there was considerable hazard, since the strength and duration of the fit were unpredictable.

Sakel in 1933 in Vienna was achieving even better results with the administration of **insulin**. This drug had been developed for treatment of diabetes and was shown to induce coma if given in higher dosage. An effect of insulin-induced hypoglycaemic coma is to produce just the same type of seizure discharge in the central nervous system. The treatment was widely used for newly admitted schizophrenics, and hospitals throughout the world rapidly followed this practice, noting the dramatic results which had resulted from the work in Vienna.

Meanwhile, Meduna had introduced cardiazol in 1934, and Cerletti and Bini in the late 1930s developed the use of electrical stimulation to induce the seizure discharge. This was a considerable advance in terms of the safety of the procedure and appeared even more effective, particularly in the affective or depressive psychoses. So important has been this development to psychiatry that Chapter 8 is entirely devoted to **electroplexy**, as the treatment came to be called.

Another dramatic advance in treatment was the introduction by Egas Moniz of **brain surgery** in the alleviation of psychotic and severe obsessional symptoms. His leucotomy operation was first developed in 1936 in Portugal, and was found to be effective in chronic unremitting depressive states, severe obsessional states and some cases of schizophrenia. The early operations, however, induced a degree of personality change which, while acceptable in the relief it gave to otherwise chronically hospitalised patients, was too marked to be of value in the less severely afflicted. The procedure had been developed as a result of noting the changes in behaviour and personality which could accrue from damage to the nervous system such as might follow injury, and, by experimental work. Such operations were used perhaps over-enthusiastically by their pioneers, but, markedly modified, they have enabled many patients previously destined for a life-time in the mental hospital to return to the community or lead a more normal, fuller life.

Moniz originated cerebral angiography and in 1949 received a Nobel prize. The leucotomy operation was developed by Freeman in the United States in 1942, and subsequently considerable sophistication in the type of surgical procedure has clarified the indications for the operation and made the results more satisfactory. However, modern methods of drug treatment and behaviour therapy have made these indications much less frequent than was the case 40 years ago. This topic, of great historical importance, is referred to in more depth in Chapter 9.

Drug Therapy

Some 10 years after the great decade of advancement in physical treatment of the 1930s, the ability to treat psychotic and neurotic illness with medication began to appear. The 1950s could be said to be the decade of advancement of drug therapy, and this led the way to dramatic improvements in mental hospital care.

An 'open-door' policy could now be developed. Locked wards could gradually be discarded and the high railings surrounding the 'airing courts' taken down. The 'old school' worried that the longer-term patients might all run away. In fact, rather sadly, many of them were so institutionalised that they continued to walk round the same old patch in the airing court regardless of the fact that the boundaries had been removed.

An expansion of day care and out-patient facilities and a general attitude of mind which encouraged the therapeutic milieu spread throughout the world. Only those who have worked in psychiatric units in both the pre-1940 and post-1940 years can realise the difference which these new methods of treatment made.

The Major Tranquillisers

The original phenothiazine molecule from which the majority of drugs used in the treatment of schizophrenia have been derived was in fact synthesised in 1883, in the laboratory, but was first used in medicine in 1934 as, of all

Table 3. A timetable of psychiatry.

	400 BC	Hippocrates, Susutra
	100 BC	Cicero
	AD 900	Rhazes
	1300	Bethlem takes psychiatric patients
	1700	Norwich Hospital, 1713
		Vagrancy Act, 1744
Opium		
		The Retreat, York. Tuke, 1796
	1800	Haslam (1798) describes *dementia paralytica*
		Asylum Act, 1808. County asylums
Bromide		
		Asylum Act, 1845. Board of Commissioners in Lunacy
		Broadmoor, 1863
		Kraepelin, the classifier
		Permissive Idiots Act, 1886
	1900	Lunacy Act, 1890
		Freud and Pavlov
		Mental Deficiency Act, 1913
		Wagner von Jauregg, 1917
Amphetamine		Mental Deficiency Act, 1927—*Encephalitis lethargica*
		Mental Treatment Act, 1930
		Meduna. Seizure discharge therapy
		Sakel, 1933. Insulin coma therapy
		Cerletti and Bini. Electroplexy
		Moniz. Leucotomy, 1936
	1950	Mental Health Act, 1959
Chlorpromazine		1950 phenothiazines
Anti-depressants		1957 mono-amine oxidase inhibitors
		1957 Imipramine
Tranquillisers		1960 Chlordiazepoxide

things, an anti-helminthic against worm diseases. Some derivatives of the basic molecule were also useful as urinary antiseptics and insecticides, and one derivative, promethazine, showed itself to be useful in allergy and as a sedative. It was used initially to potentiate anaesthesia.

Arising out of further work on this molecule the chemical **chlorpromazine** was synthesised, and proved to be effective in inducing tranquillity without the level of sedation older drugs had produced. Its anti-psychotic effect in treating the thought disorder, delusional ideas and hallucinations of schizophrenic breakdown were soon realised, and by the early 1950s the drug was available and proving highly effective in controlling psychotic behaviour. This drug is of immense historical value, leading as it did to many of the reforms that were made possible in the disturbed wards of that time. By 1960 more than 50 million patients throughout the world had been able to benefit from the control of their symptoms by this drug.

As with all prototypes, however, improvements can always be made. The early phenothiazines, and in particular those like chlorpromazine with an aliphatic side chain in the molecule, were found to have some serious disadvantages in terms of side-effects. In particular, chlorpromazine produced an irritating photosensitivity, which was the reason that most long-stay patients in this decade were required to wear wide-brimmed hats when sitting in the sunshine! This, plus occasional development of jaundice, lowering of blood pressure and some sedative action, made it by no means a perfect remedy. Moreover, those parts of the brain concerned with dopamine metabolism (and which are deficient in Parkinson's disease) seemed to be affected and damaged by the drug, so that long-term side-effects in terms of abnormal movements known as *tardive dyskinesia*, chorea and parkinsonism could be seen.

A search was, therefore, made in the years that followed for safer drugs and for those which would be more potent and effective in smaller dosage. Many improvements have indeed been made and many drugs are now marketed (see Chapter 7). The most recent advance in the last decade has been the development of long-acting delayed-release injections of some of these products, which have meant that patients do not need to take regular daily oral medication, and that doctors equally can be sure that the medication is being taken in adequate quantity.

Anti-depressants

A similar story can be told of the development of anti-depressant medication. Apart from amphetamine, which has been discussed, two major groups of drugs found to be effective in some depressive states were developed in the 1950s. These were the mono-amine oxidase inhibitor drugs, MAOI for short, and the tricyclic anti-depressants, effective in affective psychoses and chemically related in their molecular structure to the phenothiazines used in schizophrenia.

Again, the original tricyclic molecule iminodibenzyl had been synthesised in 1898, but it was not until the late 1940s that these drugs were investigated for their anti-allergic activity. The first to be synthesised and tested in depressive states was Imipramine, and this was introduced into psychiatry as an effective anti-depressant in 1957.

The side-effects of these early preparations made it necessary to search for safer and more effective compounds, and a wide variety of derivatives from these original compounds has become available in the last 20 years. Rapidity of action, freedom of side-effects and greater potency are the rationale for introducing new products.

The other major group, the MAOI drugs, derived from isoniazid, were synthesised in 1951 as part of a search for anti-tuberculous agents. It was noted that some patients being treated for tuberculosis with these compounds, which were effective in killing tubercle bacilli, also felt an euphoriant effect. Subsequently, less toxic compounds, such as phenelzine, were introduced, and their efficacy was again established in 1957. These drugs have proved effective principally in depression associated with psycho-neurotic states and in phobic anxiety.

The development of drugs effective in controlling anxiety has gone through a similar process. Initially, sedatives were used, and our story has brought us up to the development of barbiturates used extensively in the earlier part of the twentieth century. Many other drugs, derivatives of the higher alcohols such as Meprobamate, were in use by the early 1950s, but the main group of tranquillisers now available are the **benzodiazepines**. These were first synthesised in Poland in the mid-1930s by Sternbach, but the archetype of this group, chlordiazepoxide, was not effectively marketed until 1960. Since then a wide variety of similar products has become available, and their safety has resulted in their replacing virtually all the older anxiolytic compounds.

With the development of drugs effective in controlling schizophrenia, treatment which could quickly clear up the majority of affective or depressive psychoses, and the development of safe anxiolytics, the way was clear for psychiatric hospitals to integrate much more closely with the general hospital. In the last ten years, therefore, the movement has been towards building psychiatric units within the new district general hospitals and gradually running down the older and more isolated of the larger mental hospitals. A big increase in day hospital care and out-patient therapy has resulted, and with the introduction of the National Health Service facilities, these are in theory available to all, subject to supply being able to meet demand. Lengths of stay in psychiatric units are now down to an average of five weeks, and although readmission may be required for some patients, as indeed it is in general hospitals for a wide variety of conditions, the chronic long-stay patient is now increasingly less in evidence.

All these are hopeful signs. It has to be admitted that within the Health Service physical methods of treatment, and in particular the prescription of medication, has tended to be the only practical method, though probably also the most successful, because of the time available for each individual case. Most National Health Service psychiatrists have far too large a case-load, and are responsible to a community catchment area of some 60,000 individuals rather than to the particular group on their current list, as in private practice. Thus, those patients with neurotic illness who may be desirous or in need of psychotherapeutic techniques can become relatively neglected. Nevertheless, advances in this aspect of psychiatry have also been made during the last century. It is fair to say, however, that their area of effectiveness has contracted with the development of simpler methods of treatment, which appear to give equally good if not better results. There is neither point nor practicality in spending hours talking with somebody if relief of their symptoms can be effected through the simple taking of an anxiolytic for a period of time.

Nevertheless, at the same time that psychiatric hospitals were developing and progress was being made in physical methods of treatment and drug therapy, the psychotherapeutic techniques developed for the out-patient treatment of neuroses had not been standing still.

Psychotherapy

Psychological theory is no doubt as old as humanity. Texts are available from ancient Greek, Roman and Sanskrit writings, and operations on the cranial vault are known to have taken place in ancient Egyptian times.

At the end of the nineteenth century two workers were studying different aspects of psychological function from quite different viewpoints. Both were to have great influence on the subsequent development of this subject. In Russia, Pavlov was investigating the role of conditioned reflexes in learning, and developing theories on the influence of the environment in controlling the emotional state of animals and how it affected their learning processes.

This has led to the growth of learning theory, as developed by Clarke and many other workers in more recent times, and to a method of treatment widely used in dealing with anxiety known as **behaviour therapy**. At the same time, **Sigmund Freud** was developing his theories, which led to the creation of the school of thought and type of psychotherapy known as psychoanalysis.

Sigmund Freud was a neurologist born in Freiberg in Moravia. He studied medicine in Vienna and in 1885 he went to Paris to study under Charcot. Charcot had learnt the art of hypnotism as developed by Messmer, and Freud was impressed by the possibilities of this technique in treating hysterical symptoms in some of his patients. To be a successful hypno-therapist, however, requires a technique best developed by certain personalities, and Freud found this line of treatment not always easy to apply. He developed instead a technique known as 'free association'.

In 1896 Freud produced a work entitled *The Interpretation of Dreams*, which has remained a classic and makes fascinating reading. It was the result of Freud's self-analysis, which he made during correspondence with Fliess, a physician in Berlin.

From 1920 Freud shifted his main emphasis from the study of instinctual drives to a study of the ego—that part of the thought processes which is in consciousness and related to the outside world. Freud developed a moral psychology, an analysis of the control of the antisocial or asocial natural instinctive drives. His theories have been modified with time but have held much sway in analytical treatment in the USA. **Melanie Klein** developed Freud's ideas in the analysis of childhood neurotic problems, and his early theories have been adapted by such practitioners as Fairbairn, Winnicott and Guntrip in recent years. A fuller development of both the theories of psychoanalysis and behaviour therapy are to be found in *Psychology Made Simple*.

Two major off-shoots of orthodox psychoanalytical thinking developed during Freud's life-time. **Carl Jung**, an early associate of Freud, developed an analytical psychology which introduced some rather mystical and philosophical ideas, embracing his theory of the collective unconscious. A small number of Jungian analysts practise in Great Britain and more in the United States. **Alfred Adler** also developed analytical theory in his system of individual psychology, which has made famous the notions of the inferiority complex and the ideal self.

Psychoanalysis has not obtained widespread acceptance in Great Britain. A full analysis is very time-consuming, lasting as it does over a period of some two years with attendances once or twice a week. This type of luxury is not available through the Health Service except as part of some teaching-hospital commitments, and taken privately is extremely costly. It is, therefore, a treatment for the few and for the rich, and has little practical place in routine Health Service practice in the treatment of the majority of conditions which hospital doctors will see. The results are difficult to assess and in terms of symptom relief in the neuroses are probably little better than the natural remission rate and less rapidly effective than more conventional methods. The psychoanalyst would, of course, argue that in his treatment the whole self is being considered, and that a greater understanding and self-awareness by the patient is the aim.

Psychoanalysis has, in the author's view, no place in the treatment of pyschoses nor dementias. It is in dealing with the younger personality problems and neuroses that psychotherapy in general has its major function, and psychoanalysis can be seen to be an extension of this, using one particular theoretical formulation.

Nevertheless, Freud's theories have had tremendous implications in the study of neurotic symptomatology in the interpretation of dreams and in the realisation of the importance of sexual feelings and aggressive impulses in human motivation. Its contribution, therefore, to psychotherapeutic techniques, and the understanding of the mentally ill person has been immense.

Further Reading

Freud, S., *The Standard Edition of the Complete Works of Sigmund Freud*, Hogarth Press, London, 1966.
Hare, E. H., 'The Origin and Spread of Dementia Paralytica', *Journal of Mental Science*, 105, 1959.
Lader, M. H., *A History of Psychiatry*, SKF Publication, 1979.
Mental Health Act, 1959.
Mental Treatment Act, 1930.

Questions

1. What has been the significance of *dementia paralytica* to psychiatry?
2. What have been the major landmarks in the development of physical methods of treatment?
3. When was your local psychiatric hospital built?
4. Where was the local Bridewell?

Much information can be obtained from the local library on such matters. You should also attempt to look at the Mental Health Act, at the Vagrancy Act quoted in this chapter, and at Shaftesbury's Act, which were all historical landmarks at a political level.

5
Causation

In this chapter we shall be considering the reasons why people develop psychiatric illnesses, and looking at the type of research which is being carried out.

Labelling

It is fashionable among some groups at present to suggest that what is meant by psychiatric illness in medical terms is a myth. The medical model, whatever that may mean, is talked of in somewhat disparaging terms, and some groups have tended to look upon psychiatric illness as purely the product of the social environment of the individual. They imply that here only is the key to psychopathology. We should look at this problem, therefore, with these points in mind, and sift the evidence available.

The purpose of classifying symptoms into individual syndromes or disease entities is two-fold. First, it is a guideline for research and in identifying methods of possible treatment, and this can only be done rationally if a cohesive group can be identified. Second, it will give guidelines to the therapist as to the probable outcome and course, known as **prognosis**.

If we take the example of the diabetic, we might find that before the development of tests to identify sugar in the urine, an individual would visit the doctor complaining of feeling unwell, loss of weight, increased thirst and a number of rather non-specific symptoms. The doctor would notice that over a course of time some of this group of patients did badly in that they became more and more debilitated, finally lapsing into coma, with death usually occurring soon afterwards. When the possibility of identifying sugar in the urine of such patients became a practical proposition, it would be noted that of patients presenting to the doctor this sort of history sugar would be found in the urine of a certain number of them. Because of the course which these symptoms took in this group of people, it was convenient to identify them by a label, calling them diabetics, and to seek the cause and the possible methods of treating this disorder. In the course of time it would further become established that in such patients the pancreatic gland was deficient in its production of insulin. A rational method of treatment then becomes possible—namely, the giving of insulin to such patients.

Before this discovery no rational treatment for the disease would be known, and the line of treatment might perhaps be to restrict sugar intake in such people. Indeed, this would have met with some degree of success. However, without such a test for sugar in the urine, any attempt at treatment would depend purely on the results of trial and error. If some accident of fate had shown that a low sugar diet was beneficial to some patients who saw the doctor complaining of malaise, weight loss and excessive thirst, then this would provide a successful method of treatment at the time, even though the cause and effect relationship would still be unknown. The same type of circumstances applied, for example, to malaria when treated by quinine.

Now let us take as an example the condition known as **schizophrenia**. What is the justification for considering this an entity in its own right? First, we must define the meaning of our term, and this we will do by stating that it is a condition where certain groups of symptoms are found to be present—namely, a **disorder of thinking** characterised by **delusional ideas** and **hallucinatory experiences**, usually of voices of a characteristic type, the patient appearing to perceive them as coming from outside. There is an associated **incongruity of emotional response**, and this takes place within a context of clear consciousness.

Now it may be that such symptoms could be produced by a variety of factors, of which the environment might conceivably be one. Nevertheless, for convenience, we identify patients presenting with such symptoms and give them a label in order to try to identify a cohesive group. We find, in fact, that the condition has a distribution of approximately 1 per cent of the population: that is to say, in a community of 100,000 people one would anticipate that 1,000 of them would have suffered or be suffering from schizophrenia at any given time. Thus, this group of symptoms is fairly common—as common, for example, as appendicitis.

Now allowing for some variation in health facilities and for differing views as to what constitutes such a group when there are as yet no objective tests to verify such an opinion, we find, nevertheless, that the incidence of this syndrome in a population holds good more or less throughout the world. It does not appear to be influenced by political dogma, by religious beliefs, or by the type of community or family structure which exists in any of the groups studied. The incidence is not affected by the social class of the parents of such individuals, and it is not affected by intelligence. The individual symptoms and delusional ideas may vary with the cultural background of the patient, but the condition itself remains remarkably constant. This suggests that the quality of the environment and the type of upbringing a child can expect in a given community make remarkably little difference to the total incidence of the condition.

Furthermore, if a group of individuals suffering from such a condition is taken and all their close relatives are assessed, the incidence of the condition in this group of relatives will be found to be higher than it is in a matched control group. In the former case the incidence will probably be around 12 to 15 per cent of those interviewed, whereas in the control group it will remain at approximately 1 per cent—that is to say, the same as the general population.

If individuals suffering from the condition who have a twin brother or sister are taken and examined as a group, it will be found that the incidence is much higher in identical twins than in non-identical twins. In other words, where the genetic material in the twins is likely to be extremely similar, having developed from the same egg cell, if one of these twins develops schizophrenia, the chances are high of the other twin also developing the disease at some stage. If, on the other hand, the twins are non-identical—when they develop from a different egg and are, therefore, genetically no more related than other brothers and sisters—then the incidence of schizophrenia in the twin of an affected person is no higher than it is among ordinary brothers and sisters: higher than the general population but not as high as in the identical twins. Finally, if, as has been done, identical twins who have been reared together are compared with identical twins who, for various reasons, have been reared apart through adoption or some similar reason, and those out of this group where one has developed schizophrenia are examined, it is found that the incidence of schizophrenia in the identical twin is just as common whether the twins are reared together or whether they have been reared apart.

Now the above research findings have great significance in establishing the possible cause of any kind of condition. It implies an inherited factor. A familial incidence of a disease would be found, for example, if that disease were infectious, but in such a case the incidence in close relatives would be the same whether they were twins or not, and the difference between identical and non-identical twins would be non-existent. Furthermore, the infectious disease would be caught by those living with the infected person and not by those reared apart. This type of epidemiological research is very important in identifying the cause of a wide variety of diseases, not only in psychiatry, and extensive research of this kind is at present going on, although it will be appreciated that it requires a large community survey in order to obtain sufficient numbers to make the study valid.

Aetiological Factors

What are the factors in general which can cause diseases in human beings? The commonest factors can be grouped as follows:

1. *Infection.*
2. *Trauma* (as in a broken leg).
3. *Abnormal growth* in tissues, such as is found in cancer.
4. *Wear and tear*, such as occurs in rheumatism and in some senile conditions.
5. *Inflammatory conditions* due to allergic response and autoimmune mechanisms, such as is found in asthma and some kinds of rheumatism.
6. *Toxic processes* from poisoning by chemicals.
7. *Genetic abnormalities*, often due to some inherited disability, as is found in some kinds of subnormality and in haemophilia, etc.
8. *Biochemical disturbances*, where the body produces incorrect proportions of certain enzymes or fails to produce them, again often associated with a genetically determined malfunction.
9. *Endocrine and hormonal disturbances*, where the gland is producing too much, too little or the wrong sort of hormone, as in thyrotoxicosis.
10. *Environmental disturbances*. These can produce a wide variety of problems. For example, the child who never gets any sunlight may develop

rickets for purely environmental reasons, although the disturbance in the body is the result of vitamin D deficiency; or children brought up emotionally deprived may develop the inability to form satisfactory personal relationships when they get older through lack of normal mothering. A child's intelligence might be stunted for similar reasons. Both the early environment of the individual must be considered, and the present environment, which may act as a trigger to illness in a predisposed individual.

One could add to this list, but the reader will have grasped the gist of the argument. A variety of possible causes must be considered, and without the background facts concerning incidence false conclusions can easily be drawn.

The other main function of diagnosis—that is, to give guidelines as to treatment and outcome—may also be considered with these points in mind. The outlook in an untreated case of what we are describing as schizophrenia is poor in 70 to 80 per cent of cases, for the progress of the condition leads to an ultimate deterioration into a cabbage-like withdrawal, which state gave rise to the original description of schizophrenia as *dementia praecox*. The personality deteriorates to an extent which makes the individual socially unacceptable, often unpredictable and possibly violent in response to delusional ideas and auditory hallucinations. To this used to be added the effects of long-term institutional care, which, in the overcrowded conditions that often existed, caused a further deterioration of personality. However, to blame the end results of a schizophrenic illness on the effects of institutional care alone is to overlook the fact that the same end result is seen in various societies who treat their mentally ill in various ways. The advent of medication which can control, to some extent, the thought disorder found in such conditions has allowed these individuals to be treated much more successfully and humanely, in that their symptoms are relieved sufficiently for society to be able to accept them again in its midst. Before such treatment was available, the prospect of discharge and the use of open wards and active social rehabilitation while in the hospital were impossible.

Returning to the theme of this chapter—to consider the possible causation of psychiatric disturbances—we must look, then, at the **epidemiology** of the conditions, the possible environmental factors either in the present environment or in the early history which may be relevant, and examine the possible biochemical or other internal disturbances which might be predicted to produce changes in emotion and the thought processes if they were malfunctioning. If this can be related to rational methods of treatment to alter such metabolic disturbances, should they be found to exist, then we should be at the same stage of treatment as exists for diabetes at present. All these possibilities must be considered in the context of any condition where the cause is not clearly known.

Treatment may then be designed to relieve symptoms, to correct the basic fault, to prevent the occurrence of symptoms in people who might be identifiable as likely to get the condition (known as **prophylaxis**), or to modify the environment of those who are suffering from such a condition in such a way as to allow them to lead maximally effective lives. Exactly the same can be said for many conditions in medicine. Thus the patient with bronchitis requires treatment for the disorder in the chest, advice as to life style, controlling smoking and such factors as may influence the condition, modification of his work routine and advice on the psychological implications of this; and finally the community as a whole can be made aware of the possible causes of chronic bronchitis so that prevention may be attempted.

Where then do these thoughts lead us when looking at conditions affecting thought, emotion and behaviour? Major schools of thought have influenced psychiatric thinking over the past century. One of the earliest breakthroughs within psychiatry was the recognition that *dementia paralytica*, originally simply one of a large amorphous group of dementias but accounting for some 20 per cent of admissions to psychiatric hospitals at the turn of the century, was indeed an infectious process, being the late manifestation of previously contracted syphilis. The recognition of an infective agent led to the possibility of treatment through both prevention and through destroying the causative organism once it had infected the body.

No evidence of an infective agent has been found, however, in the major psychoses or neuroses, nor in the other degenerative condition of old age, senile dementia. In this latter condition, however, there is clear evidence of a metabolic disturbance, which may perhaps soon yield to research.

Within the psychoses and neuroses, argument has long raged between those who see these disease processes as internally derived, with genetic factors and a probable underlying biochemical disturbance, and the environmentalists, who see such conditions as the result of a disturbance of interpersonal relationships and the individual's adaptation to his environment and society. This latter line has tended to be taken by those whose interest has been sociological. Both sides have tended to ignore the evidence produced by the other, and to concentrate on their own line of research.

Strong evidence has been adduced for the presence of internal factors with genetic malfunction in the areas traditionally described as psychotic, namely schizophrenia, mania and depression. The genetic factors do not, however, seem to show a clear-cut dominant or recessive inheritance, as is found in some diseases, but, nevertheless, the type of studies using sibling and twin cohorts, as described earlier in the chapter, have been confirmed for schizophrenia by a wide variety of researchers. The inherited factor between monozygotic twins is around 50 per cent and for dizygotic twins around 15 per cent concordance.

A variety of adoption studies show biological factors to be more important than rearing. All the evidence, therefore, suggests that what is inherited is not the certainty of developing schizophrenia but rather a vulnerability to it. The twin studies in particular show that environmental factors must be necessary for the expression of this vulnerability in at least half the cases, since concordance in monozygotic twins is not 100 per cent.

With regard to the inherited models the possibility can exist of a single gene, two interacting genes, a polygenic and heterogeneous type of inheritance. Two locus models have more recently been suggested by Böök, who proposes a dominant gene affecting mono-amine oxidase activity, with a recessive gene affecting dopamine beta-hydroxylase.

In affective psychoses the major contribution of genetics in the last 20 years has been the validation of the division of affective disorders into unipolar and bipolar depressions. (In the latter both depressive and manic episodes occur.) The risk is higher for relatives of the bipolar disease as opposed to the unipolar. The percentage morbidity risk of bipolar probands, averaging the various research studies published, is somewhere in the region of 15 per cent, and the percentage morbidity risk in relatives of unipolar probands is only some 7 per cent. The same has held for twin studies, where for monozygotic twins the rate has been 72 per cent and 40 per cent respectively, and for dizygotic twins 14 per cent and 11 per cent respectively.

The increased incidence in females of affective disorder suggests the possibility that the X sex chromosome is the area where linkage occurs. This seems more likely in the bipolar than the unipolar disease. In the bipolar disease there is evidence of linkage with some types of colour blindness.

The probability is that such genetic factors would manifest themselves through a biochemical or metabolic disorder within the central nervous system in those affected. Thus, much research has been devoted to identifying possible biochemical disturbances. These have related particularly to theories of a disturbance in the transmitter agents, which allow impulses to pass from one neurone to another and which are chemically a variety of mono-amines. There is certainly considerable evidence that this may be the case. Mono-amines particularly suspect seem likely to be dopamine, acetylcholine, and serotonin, and other catacalamines may also enter into it.

From different points of view, both the analytically orientated and sociologically minded researchers have explored the type of environmental circumstances that may be important in acting as a trigger in setting off the disease in those predisposed to show it. In this respect one must concentrate on two areas—namely, the early environment, i.e. the sort of factors that may affect the stability of the nervous system of the growing child, such as relationship disturbances, deprivation phenomena and the like; and, secondly, the influence of the current environment on triggering off an attack. Some promising research has been published in both these areas. The interested reader is recommended to read more deeply into this through the list of further reading at the end of the chapter.

The Professor of Psychology at York University, Professor Venables, has demonstrated the presence of physiological abnormalities (in particular with such measurements as skin conduction recovery times and pupil reactions) in patients suffering from psychotic illness, and, in some cases, among their relatives. Since these disturbances depend on changes in mono-amine activity, i.e. transmitter agents, this is further evidence for such a biochemical disturbance. Furthermore, Venables has been able to do prospective studies on at-risk groups, and has identified such changes in some children who are now being followed up to assess whether in due course signs of the disease will develop. An association with minimal brain damage at or around birth has also been postulated.

The neuroses have always been the province of the environmentalists. Freud's theories were primarily concerned with the development of neurosis through the development of the id, ego and super-ego, and the use by the subconscious of defence mechanisms which come into play with the failure of the resolution of the Oedipus complex. Behaviourists have also seen the neuroses as environmentally determined, basing their ideas on the original work of Pavlov, Sherington, Hull, Clark and many others, who have pointed to the influence of learning and conditioning in the development of maladaptive behaviour responses. These theories have had much influence on the type of therapy adopted in attempts to alleviate neurotic behaviour patterns.

Even so, there must at a cellular level be a chemical mediation of activity in those parts of the central nervous system that control emotional levels, arousal, anger and so on. One can, therefore, postulate that within the limbic lobe (that part of the brain producing this emotional response) there will be some alteration in activity of the transmitter agents, though this may be secondary to reactions which have occurred in response to the external environment. Nevertheless, the effectiveness of tranquillisers which act on this part of the brain shows that some chemical control of behaviour is possible in order to relieve unnecessary anxiety, and it would still seem possible to speculate that an endogenous or internally arising disturbance in this part of the central nervous system might be responsible for at least some of those conditions labelled psychoneuroses. We shall look later in this chapter at the biochemical evidence for this. But let us now look briefly at the type of research which is at present being carried out in psychiatry.

Research into Schizophrenia

Biochemical research has centred around efforts to isolate the presumed chemical abnormalities which seem likely to occur, particularly in schizophrenia, certain types of depression and in manic states. Changes have been found in enzyme production and transport in schizophrenia, and abnormal amines have been found in the urine and cerebrospinal fluid of some patients suffering from this group of disorders. Purified extracts from these products have been shown to cause behaviour disturbances in animal experiments— for example, when injected into rats—whereas a controlled specimen of normal urine or cerebrospinal fluid does not produce this effect. The same situation has been found in humans. Investigations have been carried out into those drugs, principally **stimulants** and **hallucinogenic drugs** such as **LSD** and **mescaline**, which can provoke conditions which appear very similar to schizophrenic illness in some individuals who take them. Most of these drugs are mono-amines, with a chemistry similar in many respects to the amines in the cells of the central nervous system which are necessary for the proper function of the nerve cells and ganglia associated with thinking and emotion in the brain.

The botany of hallucinogenic drugs makes a fascinating study in itself. By far the largest group comes from plants found in Central America. Most are extracted in the natural state from certain cactuses and some kinds of toadstool, though they can be found in other plants such as coleus and in the leaves of some vines. Extracts of many of these plants have been used in religious rituals, and been known for over 1,000 years. Some, such as mescaline, are used in drinks and are extracted from peyotl. The products obtained are usually derivatives of mescaline, psilocybin or lysergic acid. Some of these can now be made in the laboratory.

An intriguing aspect of the botany of such substances is that in the impure form, as used by the native peoples of Central America, different types of plant, presumably with a slightly different chemical structure, can produce very different kinds of hallucinatory experience. Some, for instance, produce the effect of voices, where an individual's thoughts seem to be externalised and he perceives them as something divorced from himself, coming from outside, speaking to him. Sometimes a thought echo is produced and the native peoples believe they can commune with the spirits in this way. These symptoms are very similar to those found in schizophrenia. Yet other plants produce visual hallucinations, and the drug-taker may perceive visions of the little people. It would be nice to think that such plants grow in Ireland, but in fact this is not the case! An interesting aspect is the subtle difference in the type of hallucinatory response, which does not depend so much on the individual taking the substance as on the particular type of infusion or extract consumed. Similarly, stimulant drugs such as amphetamine, or dexedrine (which has been used in this country in the past as a slimming tablet and anti-depressant), can be shown in susceptible people to induce a psychotic state indistinguishable from a schizophrenic breakdown.

Other experiments on the metabolism of schizophrenia have been inconclusive but to take just one further example, **melatonin**, a hormone found in the pineal gland in the brain and normally concerned with pigment metabolism, has been shown to be abnormal in some cases of schizophrenia, and the use of drugs such as penicillamine to reduce the abnormal by-products has resulted in some improvement in symptoms. Other evidence comes from diseases which are known to be inherited enzyme disturbances, such as **homocystinuria**, where a psychotic state very similar to schizophrenia may be found, and where a disturbance of mono-amines in the central nervous system is known to occur.

Finally, it has been shown that certain groups of drugs used in the treatment of schizophrenia, principally the group known as phenothiazines, are themselves allied to mono-amines and appear to act by altering the metabolism of these natural substances. Furthermore, their use in patients suffering from schizophrenia is to control the symptoms of thought disorder, delusional ideas, and hallucinatory experiences from which such people suffer.

Research into Affective Illness

Turning now to manic and depressive illnesses, those known as the **affective psychoses**, biochemical research again, though not conclusive, is very suggestive of underlying biochemical disturbance. Here, two things in particular have been noted. First, it was shown that certain drugs, principally **reserpine**, used in the treatment of high blood pressure, appeared to act by depleting certain nerves of the amines required for proper nerve cell activity to take place. These drugs caused, in some people, the onset of a depressive state. Furthermore, it was shown that drugs known as **mono-amine oxidase inhibitors** (MAOI for short), used initially in the treatment of tuberculosis, appeared to cause a state of elation. These drugs act by preventing the breakdown of mono-amines at the cell junction, and from this discovery a group of drugs which were successful in treating some depressive states was developed. Another group of drugs that was subsequently developed was known as **tricyclic anti-depressants**, because of their chemical structure, which, in a slightly different way, also caused an increase in mono-amines at the cell synapse. This group has proved very effective in treating other types of depressive state. Thus we have a situation where depression appears to occur with a depletion of certain types of amines, and relief of the depression can be effected by increasing them or preventing their breakdown in the cell.

The second disorder identified in affective illness is an **alteration in the normal levels of electrolytes** such as sodium, potassium, and chloride between the inside and the outside of the nerve cell. Normally there is a certain balance between these ions, but in both the manic and depressive phases of cyclical manic-depressive disorders disturbances in these chemicals, and in the total quantity of water distributed between the inside and the outside of the cell membrane, have been found. These changes in such cyclical illnesses can be shown to pre-date the alterations in the emotional state of the individual. A fascinating discovery in this respect has been that lithium, a chemical element similar to sodium but inactive in the body, is very effective in controlling such mood swings in this group of patients. It appears to act by replacing sodium, molecule for molecule, in the nerve cell. Since the level of sodium appears to be too high in manic-depressive illnesses, and the lithium, by replacing it with an inert substance, in effect lowers the total sodium level, there would appear to be a strong possibility of a relationship between this alteration and the relief of the disturbed emotional symptoms.

Research into Neuroses

Finally, in this review of biochemical possibilities, let us look at the neuroses, where **anxiety** is the characteristic abnormal symptom. This group of disorders has traditionally been the province of those analytically minded psychiatrists who look upon the early environment as an all-important factor in causation. In many cases this may be true, but in a certain group of patients, typified by the onset of acute anxiety symptoms pervading the whole of their life-style and apparently coming on out of the blue from time to time without an obvious trigger precipitant, some interesting findings have emerged.

For example, if such individuals are given an intra-venous infusion of salt solution (such as might happen after an operation or following, for example, a severe burn), then their response is quite normal. Similarly, if a sugar solution is given, there is no abnormal response. If, however, such individuals are given a lactate solution (which again is a solution commonly used in intra-venous transfusions but which has slight differences in that it alters the acidity of the cell and thus the activity of the cell membrane), then such people develop an acute anxiety state. This can be turned on and off, as it were, by controlling the infusion of lactate, and still works in this manner even if the study is done completely blind, so that neither the doctor nor the patient knows which of the particular infusions is being given at the time. They still respond in this way to lactate and not to the others. A normal group of the population, however, without a history of anxiety, when subjected to such a routine, do not develop an anxiety reaction with lactate or with glucose or salt solution. What this means is not yet clear, and has led to a number of theories being propounded, but certainly it seems unlikely that it can be explained on the basis of the early environment of that patient as a child.

Following this discovery, it has been noted for many years that one method of relieving an anxiety attack in a controlled hospital setting has been to inhale carbon dioxide. This idea was originally developed by Meduna (who also first developed electrical treatment in the control of depression) and has been carefully written up as one method of anxiety relief, though not all that successful and now little used as other treatments have proved more effective. Nevertheless, the inhalation of carbon dioxide does relieve anxiety in certain cases, at least on a temporary basis, and it is interesting to note that the chemical changes resulting from an inhalation of carbon dioxide are exactly opposite to those produced by an intra-venous infusion of lactate. Research has shown that there appears to be a connection between the two, and that those patients who can have anxiety attacks induced by lactate will also respond by relief of symptoms if carbon dioxide inhalation is given.

We have considered, therefore, two major lines of research useful in psychiatric problems—namely, genetic research aimed at identifying inherited factors and biochemical research aimed at identifying abnormal function in the tissues in the central nervous system.

The lack of any gross pathological change in the cells and the lack of an identifiable infective process in schizophrenia, depression and anxiety states makes infection as a line of research seem unfruitful. But that one must look for such things in initial research is borne out by the experience with *dementia paralytica* mentioned earlier, which proved to be a long-term effect of syphilis.

Personality Disorders—Environmental Influences

We are left with a large number of cases often seen by the psychiatrist where disturbed personality, often associated with neurotic symptoms, is predominant. It is in these cases that the influence of environment seems to be most important.

A study of the environment must fall into two parts—the **early environment**, which individuals experienced in their formative years, and the **present environment**, the stresses of which may be causing or contributing to the symptoms seen. A consideration of the early environment will usually of necessity be retrospective—that is to say, the information will be gathered some years after the events took place—and reliance must be placed on parents and close relatives to give information about early history. This leads to certain problems which can affect the reliability of the information.

An alternative is to do a prospective population survey, where a group of individuals is taken at birth and followed through for 20 or 30 years if necessary. If the survey is large enough, a proportion of the group will be expected to develop various kinds of illness, and an attempt can then be made to relate the early findings with the subsequent symptoms. This type of study has been particularly rewarding in producing evidence that the emotionally deprived child may more commonly develop a personality disorder of characteristic type in adolescence.

This sort of study of the environment, to be valid, must not depend simply on an untested theory, whether it be analytical or behavioural in orientation, but on statistical evidence pointing towards associations which suggest a cause and effect relationship. This requires a knowledge of statistical method, which now forms a prominent part of the training both of doctors in general and of psychiatrists in particular. The usual need is to find a relationship or correlation between two items—such as a separation experience in childhood and later development of psychiatric symptoms—which exists significantly more commonly than would be expected by chance. It has, for example, been shown that certain types of depressive states occurring in adults appear to be associated more strongly with the death of a parent during childhood than one would expect from the death rate in the general population. One cannot conclude a cause and effect in this manner, but at least an association can be identified and from this a possible cause may be sought.

What sort of areas are likely to prove fruitful when examining the possible influence of environment?

In the early environment factors affecting growth and intelligence, the possibility of damage of minor degrees to the central nervous system during the perils of birth, and other physical or disease factors, may be present. The young child is developing relationships initially with its mother, and later with the father and siblings, other relatives, friends and people in the outside world. The proper development of any of these processes can be marred by deprivation, by loss through death or other reasons for departure, or by some internal deficiency in the child's makeup which prevents him from making full use of these relationship experiences. Thus internal or inherited and external or acquired factors may mingle inextricably. There is evidence to suggest that the central nervous system may not develop effectively under these adverse conditions, and this can be shown at microscopic level in the degree of development of interconnections between the neurones themselves within the brain through the branching of the dendrites. Absence of adequate stimulation to the growing organism slows down the development of such intimate interconnections.

Ethologists' work on imprinting (critical phases in development when learning can occur) and on bonding, as shown in many animal species, is quite likely to be relevant in humans, though to some extent masked by other factors.

In the present or immediate past environment major disruptions to one's security may well reactivate some of these earlier deficiencies, and lead to the development of neuroses or even psychosis in the more vulnerable. We can postulate a level of vulnerability or proneness to certain diseases, and link this to trigger events in the environment which may have special relevance to that individual. Thus financial insecurity, emotional insecurity with spouse, children or parents, or even political or religious changes in one's life-style may all need to be considered. Sometimes it may not be one major disastrous event but rather an accumulation of disturbances which become the final straw that breaks the camel's back. To tease out these individual factors is the main problem of this type of research.

Unfortunately, in the individual case, many of these ideas are of little value either in predicting outcome or in establishing the most appropriate treatment. For schizophrenia and affective disorders the type of tests we have mentioned are still research procedures, of little value to the clinician in a routine out-patient clinic. They may prove to have value in the future, but, at present, diagnosis must be made on the basis of clinical judgement. This demands experience that takes some years to acquire, since to spot, for example, the early signs of thought disorder requires a long familiarity with the condition and cannot really be learnt by textbooks or lectures alone, nor can it usually be identified in other than gross forms by objective psychological testing.

What is important, however, in the patient who presents to a psychiatrist with a disorder of thinking, emotion or behaviour is that causes in the field of general medicine should not be missed, for, as we have emphasised, many general medical conditions, particularly those affecting the endocrine glands but many others besides, can present disturbances of this kind. Unless a few screening tests and a general examination are made, mistakes can occur and totally inappropriate treatment may be started. It is for this reason, among others, that it is essential anybody attempting to treat psychiatric illness should have a thorough background of general medicine before specialising. This fact is sometimes not appreciated. While it is true to say that some 20 per cent of patients presenting to their doctor have, at least in part, psychiatric symptoms, it is also true to say that some 20 per cent of patients presenting to the psychiatrist prove to have associated general medical conditions.

The patient visiting the clinic or entering the psychiatric unit will, therefore, be subjected to a full physical examination, and will in addition most likely have a few screening tests, which can be followed up should they prove abnormal. It is usual to test the blood for evidence of anaemia, since certain types of anaemia may commonly present with psychiatric symptoms. Investigations of the kidney and liver function, and, particularly in those presenting with anxiety, tests of thyroid gland function, may be desirable. A routine urine test is usually also performed, for that will exclude diabetes and some other types of kidney disorder.

These sorts of test and a number of others are particularly important in the more elderly person, in anybody who shows evidence of confusion or disturbance of memory, and in those where abnormal physical signs have been noticed on examination. In these cases one or two further blood tests may be required, and, in addition, an X-ray of the chest and skull is usually considered wise. Certain other neurological tests, such as an electro-encephalogram (EEG) or brain scan, may also be required. The EEG is an estimate of brain activity rather like the electro-cardiogram in heart disease, and will identify epilepsy and some degenerative conditions affecting brain function. All these tests are painless.

Further Reading

Barrett, J. E., *Stress and Mental Disorder*, Raven, N.Y., 1979.

Everitt, B., 'An attempt at validation of traditional psychiatric syndromes by cluster analysis', *British Journal of Psychiatry*, 119, 399, 1971.

Jaspers, K., *The Synthesis of Disease Entities in General Psychopathology*, Manchester University Press, Manchester, 1963.

Popper, K., *The Logic of Scientific Discovery*, Hutchinson, London, 1968.

Reverley, A., 'The genetic contribution to the functional psychoses', *British Journal of Hospital medicine*, 242, 1980.

Slater, E., and Cowie, V., *The Genetics of Mental Disorders*, Oxford University Press, 1971.

Wied, D. de, *Hormones and the Brain*, M.T.P. Publishers, Lancaster, England, 1980.

Questions

1. What are the advantages of classification in disease?
2. How does one investigate a possible genetic factor in the cause of a disease?
3. What biochemical factors seem to be relevant in the psychoses?
4. What justification is there for including personality disorders in the concept of disease?

6
Treatment

General Concepts

In this chapter we shall be discussing the general principles of treatment of those conditions which are usually considered to be the psychiatrist's province.

It is perhaps pertinent at the outset to consider just what the doctor is attempting to do when a patient visits him complaining of certain symptoms. The individual who attends is, by and large, **wishing for permanent relief from such symptoms**. The doctor is aware that in achieving this he must ideally **discover the cause** of such symptoms and, having done so, **restore whatever has gone wrong to full, normal functioning**. This is an ideal and is in practice usually unlikely to be achieved in full. This generalisation applies almost without exception, regardless of the type of malfunction or disease process, and regardless of the area.

The specialty of psychiatry has tended to be criticised on two counts. First, it is expected by the client and relatives that it should be able to cure everything. Psychiatrists' comments have tended, in recent years, to be sought by solicitors and many other groups on a variety of problems, often social or even political in nature, for which they are not trained as experts. The fact that the psychiatrist has on occasions been willing to comment as an individual, and that his comments have been given expert weight, have not helped his specialty. At the other extreme, it is a common criticism among his colleagues in other branches of medicine that he cures nothing, and that his treatment is by and large merely palliative.

Let us examine in brief, therefore, the record of other specialties in this regard. The surgeon presented with an inflamed appendix will remove it. In so doing, he relieves the symptoms and restores the body, in effect, to its normal functioning, though he does not, of course, restore the appendix to normal functioning. Fortunately, this does not seem to matter. In other surgical procedures, however, the removal of a part certainly does matter, and there are often residual effects. Thus, in pronouncing a cure the surgeon is using the word in a rather special sense.

If we look at general medicine, we find that in the last 30 years great advances have been made in the treatment of infectious diseases caused by bacteria. Penicillin and the antibiotics in general kill many bacteria and, as a result, such conditions as pneumonia, septicaemia and even the great scourges such as bubonic plague could be cured. General physicians have gone further and have been able, by means of immunisation programmes, to prevent even the development of such diseases in the first place.

If we turn, however, to almost all the other diseases in the textbook, we find a different story. For the most part, symptom relief is the best that can be accomplished. This may, indeed, maintain the patient for a long time in a good state of health and allow the body to undergo natural recovery. But the doctor is aiding the body in this process rather than supplying the cure. Obvious examples come to mind. In diabetes the pancreas for some reason ceases to produce a proper insulin supply. This affects many of the body's processes and, in particular, the levels of sugar in the blood. The doctor can treat this condition by, for example, supplying insulin to a person by means of daily injections, thus making up for the body's deficiency and allowing the patient to lead a relatively normal life. This is not cure, but is useful palliation. The patient is on his injections for life or until somebody invents some better method.

In rheumatism, cortisone and pain-relievers can be given. In pernicious anaemia, vitamin injections can be given but need to go on for life. In duodenal ulcer, a diet can be advised; and in high blood pressure, drugs can be given to lower it again. In all these, however, palliation is the key, since the underlying process which caused the condition in the first place is usually unknown, and the body is certainly not able to be restored to its original normal function.

How do we fare, therefore, in the treatment of those conditions which produce disturbances of thinking, emotion or behaviour? The **depressive illnesses** can usually be cleared up fairly quickly with modern drugs or electroplexy. Since the illness is self-limiting, this usually allows normal restoration of function, and unless the patient is unlucky and subsequently has a recurrence, that is the end of the matter. **Schizophrenia** probably ranks with diabetes as being controllable to a large degree by present medication, but the individual will need to continue it for a long time. In the other large group of in-patient problems, the **dementias**, some can be corrected, but for the majority there is no cure, and palliative treatment to give comfort to the elderly person so afflicted is all that can be arranged.

Many treatments are available for **anxiety states**, ranging from simple symptom relief by means of suitable medication to more radical attempts to alter the underlying neurotic process by means of psychotherapy or behaviour therapy techniques. Psychotherapeutic procedures become even more valid in those where the disturbance is basically of personality structure, and it is in this area that psychiatry overlaps with those who attempt to modify the individual's social problems in the community.

This process of assessment and diagnosis, and from this a planned programme of treatment, begins at the first interview. This may be in the out-patient department at the local hospital, or at the patient's home at the request of the family doctor wishing for a second opinion, or in the hospital itself if there has been need for urgent admission arranged direct by the family doctor in the community. The problem will be pieced together from information given by the patients themselves, from the letter by the family doctor, from relatives, and possibly from a social history provided through the social services department in appropriate cases.

In-patient or Out-patient?

The first decision that must be made is whether the person consulting the psychiatrist should be advised that treatment on an out-patient basis is satisfactory or whether admission to hospital would be preferable.

The **reasons for hospital admission** are really two-fold in any kind of problem. The individual may require a type of treatment which is not practically administered in the community. For example, it would be essential for someone with appendicitis to enter hospital, since the only available treatment is removal of the appendix, an operative procedure which requires facilities only the hospital can provide for a smooth recovery.

The second reason for admission, more often appropriate in psychiatry than in other branches of medicine, is for the **care** of the individual in terms of ensuring his safety and welfare until he is reasonably recovered. Being in hospital allows for 24 hour nursing care, the ready availability of medical staff at all times, and the opportunity to observe and look after individuals at a time when they may, as a result of their illness, be unable to do this for themselves without considerable stress.

If we take a severe depressive state as an example, it will be apparent that these two principles may operate. For example, the patient may be sufficiently deeply depressed for electrical treatment to be advised. This procedure is usually rapidly effective but requires an anaesthetic, and it is much better for the patient to be in hospital during a course of such treatment. Secondly, is the degree of depression such for there to be any risk of a suicidal attempt? If there is any doubt in people's minds on this point, then both doctor and relatives will rest easier in the knowledge that the sick person is being looked after by properly trained people until he recovers.

The vast majority of people will enter hospital reasonably happily if the need is made clear to them. Occasionally in illnesses affecting thinking or emotion the individual does not appreciate that there is such a need, and refuses admission, even though it is apparent to those around him that it is essential for his safety or possibly for the safety of others. Under such circumstances in Britain the 1983 Mental Health Act allows doctors to recommend admission on an order, with the application made by the nearest relative, or member of the social services department if the former is inappropriate (see Chapter 3). This allows for the occasional situation where, because of disturbances in a person's thinking or mood, someone must act for the time being on his behalf. This sometimes applies where there is a recognised suicidal risk or in the occasional case where there may have been a threat to other people's safety, as a result of disturbed and unpredictable behaviour on the part of someone who is ill.

Having established whether out-patient or in-patient treatment is appropriate, and made the diagnosis, consideration must be given to what types of therapy are likely to be most effective. General considerations must be taken into account: whether an out-patient should be advised to stay off work, whether an in-patient requires to be in bed or can be up and about, whether patients require 24 hour observation or can be safely left to occupational therapy or similar departments during the day, and so on.

The **type of therapy available**, in more specific terms in the treatment of psychiatric problems, can be considered under the following broad headings:

1. Drugs.
2. Physical methods of treatment, such as electroplexy.
3. Psychotherapy.
4. Behaviour modification, using such aids as relaxation, hypnosis or abreaction.

In the rest of this chapter we shall consider some of the general principles behind each of these groups.

Drug Therapy or Medication

We shall first consider the question of drug therapy. While by no means necessarily the most important aspect of treatment, it is, in fact, through the aid of medication to relieve various symptoms that the majority of patients are likely to benefit. Whatever the virtues or otherwise of a technique such as psychoanalysis, in practical terms it cannot be available to the vast majority of people with emotional problems, and whether one likes it or not, the palliation of symptoms by treatment with medication is likely to be the most satisfactory method for the great majority of those who visit their doctor.

A word of explanation should be given with regard to the word 'drugs'. Some people seem to equate 'drug' with 'drug of addiction' or 'dangerous drug', and envisage something which is habit-forming, potentially dangerous and used and abused by the addiction-prone subculture in the population. This is, of course, not the case. Any preparation which is taken into the body other than as a food, and which has some measurable effect on bodily function, is a drug. This applies as much to aspirin, to insulin, to tea or coffee in some circumstances, as it does to any of the preparations to be described. Indeed, the stimulant effect of the chemicals in tea or coffee are much more habit-forming than most of the drugs used in everyday medicine.

Drugs used in psychiatry can be divided into groups which deal largely with particular types of symptoms found in the various syndromes to be described. The first group is a large number of products concerned with the relief of anxiety and these are described as **anxiolytics**. Secondly, there are those products used in the treatment of depressive symptoms which fall naturally into two types—**tricyclic anti-depressants and mono-amine oxidase inhibitors**—corresponding to the two main types of depressive syndromes which are seen. Thirdly, there are those drugs (**neuroleptics**) which modify the thought disorder commonly found in schizophrenia and occasionally in other syndromes. These drugs mostly come from a group known as **phenothiazines** and other similar related compounds. Fourthly, there are **anti-convulsant** drugs used in the treatment of epilepsy and some behaviour disorders. Finally, there are sedatives, which are used to sedate either for sleep disturbance or for the very agitated individual. We shall take these groups in turn. (See Table 4.)

Anxiolytics

Medication to relieve anxiety has existed for very many years, but has until relatively recently been of the sedative group—that is to say, its effect has

Table 4. Drugs used in psychiatry.

---

1 *ANXIOLYTICS*
   Alcohol, barbiturates, etc.
   Benzodiazepines (e.g. chlordiazepoxide, oxazepam, diazepam)
2 *ANTI-DEPRESSANTS*
   Amphetamine (obsolete)
   Mono-amine oxidase inhibitors (MAOI) (e.g. phenelzine, tranylcypramine)
   Tricyclic anti-depressants (e.g. imipramine amitryptiline, tetracyclic drugs and
   other derivatives (such as mianserin, nomifensine, viloxazine)
   Lithium
3 *NEUROLEPTICS*
   Reserpine (obsolete)
   Phenothiazines
      1 Aliphatic side chain
      2 Piperidine side chain
      3 Piperazine side chain
   Thioxanthines (e.g. flupenthixol)
   Butyrophenones (e.g. haloperidol)
   Pimozide
4 *ANTI-CONVULSANTS*
5 *SEDATIVES*

---

been not simply on that part of the brain (principally the limbic lobe) which is concerned with emotional levels, but has tended to depress the function of the whole of the nervous system and, in particular, the cerebral cortex. The result of this will tend to be to induce a state of poorer concentration and some drowsiness, which slows thinking and is detrimental to the individual's everyday life. General sedatives, therefore, are by no means ideal, and research workers have gone to some lengths to develop products which will act more specifically on the over-active areas.

Examples of the older sedative anxiolytics include alcohol, bromide, paraldehyde and such groups of drugs as the barbiturates. By and large, however, in the treatment of anxiety such groups have been superseded by newer products known as the **benzodiazepines**.

The benzodiazepines were first developed some 30 years ago, and the original product, which has stood the test of time, was **chlordiazepoxide**. The advantage of this group of drugs is that their action is principally on the limbic lobe, and in particular on such nuclei as the amygdaloid nucleus and the hippocampus, which are nuclei in the base of the brain that are concerned with emotional response. The effect of chlordiazepoxide appears to be specifically to inhibit the abnormal anxiety response while providing very little general sedation to the rest of the central nervous system. This group of products is now very widely used in the relief of symptoms where anxiety predominates, and is probably almost as popular as is aspirin for the relief of pain.

Many newer benzodiazepines have been developed, principally either because they have fewer side-effects than the early products or are more potent in smaller dosage. Some seem to be particularly good for certain types of problem, but by and large their properties are all very similar. They include **oxazepam**, **diazepam**, **lorazepam** and **medazepam**. Some have been developed particularly to help those people with initial insomnia, where tension prevents the person from getting off to sleep. These include such products as **nitrazepam**, **flurazepam**, and **temazepam**.

Although benzodiazepines have been very widely used, and indeed over used, the reasons for this have been largely their remarkable safety record in comparison with other anxiety relieving drugs such as barbiturates, alcohol, and related drugs and indeed in terms of safety, or rather the lack of it, nicotine.

Nevertheless, it has been recognised in recent years that the benzodiazepines themselves are capable of inducing dependence, and the withdrawal effects when discontinuing such drugs, should patients have been on them for some length of time, can be quite dramatic in a small number of cases and certainly for many people as difficult to get off as alcohol or nicotine might be. It is necessary, however, in view of much adverse publicity in the last two or three years to recognise that the majority of people do not find difficulty in coming off these drugs, particularly if they are only used for relatively short-term management of acute anxiety or insomnia, and that much of the adverse publicity has been a rather histrionic over-reaction. There is very little evidence that those patients who do become dependent on benzodiazepines and take them long term come to any great harm, certainly they come to no greater harm than the long-term users of alcohol, nicotine, barbiturates or indeed many other commonly used medicaments.

For a patient, of a general practitioner, to be worried that they are taking 5 mgm of diazepam or 1 mgm of lorazepam daily but not seemingly to be over-concerned at the 20 cigarettes they smoke a day or the half a bottle of gin per week they consume is completely illogical. Furthermore, if the patient does discontinue benzodiazepine anxiolytics one must think about what they might care to use instead for the control of their states of tension. This is not to say that other methods of treating tension in the long term by behavioural means, hypnotherapy or similar methods of inducing the ability to relax are not preferable. Certainly it is now recommended that benzodiazepines should only be used for short-term management of acute episodes and that they should not be continued for longer than six weeks at a time. As far as night sedation is concerned it is preferable for such drugs to be used intermittently, rather than every night so that a habit does not develop.

A considerable volume of interesting research has emanated from the Psychopathological Research Unit at Leeds and papers by Dr Ian Hindmerch, a research psychologist in charge of this unit, have shown that reaction times (important in car driving and the operation of machinery etc.) vary the day after having taken benzodiazepines for night sedation. This relates to the way in which the benzodiazepine is broken down in the body and whether the metabolite continues to be active in an anxiolytic. Similarly, the half life of the drug may be relevant, and the type of binding which the drug has to the GABA and other binding sites within the central nervous system. Thus it can be shown that some drugs are considerably more dependent making than others within this group. It would appear that the safest for night sedation are probably lormetazepam, triazolam, and temazepam since they are the least likely to produce a hangover effect and to produce dependency. In long-term use lorazepam and the diazepam group and their derivatives seem more of a problem. Nitrazepam seems to produce more of a hangover effect than the others quoted above despite its popularity and flurazepam also produces problems.

Anti-depressants

The second group of products are those drugs useful in the treatment of depressive symptoms. As will be seen in subsequent chapters, depression is a symptom rather than a disease. Indeed, a number of disease processes and reactive states may produce depressive symptoms. They may be found in reactions to stress among more vulnerable personalities. They may be found as a natural reaction to bereavement. They may be found as a concomitant of other diseases, both physical and psychiatric, but particularly in association with post-operative states and in disturbances of electrolyte balance in the body, and in response to some drugs—for example, those used in the treatment of high blood pressure.

Finally, depression may be found in the condition known as **endogenous** or **psychotic depression**. This appears to be an illness in its own right, of biochemical or hormonal type, which occurs particularly commonly around the menopause in women and after pregnancy, but is common in both sexes.

MAOI Drugs

The first group of anti-depressants to be developed, again some 30 years ago, were the MAOI or mono-amine oxidase inhibitor group of drugs. This rather long name describes the method of action of the group, which works by inhibiting the enzymes which normally break down mono-amines in the body and, in particular, at the synapses in the central nervous system. As we have learnt, the mono-amines are a very important group of chemicals in nerve-cell function. The result of blocking the MAO enzymes is to allow a build-up of amines at the nerve-cell ending. This presumably produces a more efficient functioning of the disturbed part, but although the mode of action seems fairly clear, at this stage the underlying reason for the fault which seems to go along with such depressive states is as yet unresolved.

As we have said, this group was developed more or less by accident. Initially, similar drugs were being used in the treatment of tuberculosis for their anti-tuberculous activity. It was noticed that in some the depressed mood, which went along with their tuberculosis, was much improved while on the particular drugs, and from this a consideration of their possible use in depression led to much research to enhance the anti-depressant effect while removing some of the toxic side-effects that tended to occur in the more powerful anti-tuberculous type of preparation.

The first drug of this group to make any impact was **phenelzine**. These drugs seem particularly effective in those depressive states which exist in association with anxiety, or are reactive to environmental stress in a neurotic personality. Apart from one or two minor side-effects, which those people who are extra-sensitive to the drug may experience (and indeed any drug worth taking, aspirin included, gives some people side-effects), there is **one main snag about this group of preparations**. Even the newer ones on the market require the individual who is taking them to maintain certain **dietary restrictions**. The reason is that the mono-amines contained in the normal foods that we eat are, because of the way in which the MAOI drugs act, not broken down on absorption as quickly as normal. This matters with only one mono-amine, namely **tyramine**, which is related to drugs used to raise blood pressure. If the product accumulates in the body after a large meal, then a temporary rise in blood pressure may cause the patient to have quite unpleasant side-effects in the shape of headaches. While this reaction does not affect everybody on the drugs (in fact, only about one in fifty), people must be warned to avoid tyramine-containing foodstuffs. These are principally cheeses and concentrated meat extracts such as Bovril and Marmite. Broad beans tend to contain a high level, and so does green banana chutney. Finally, some types of wine (Chianti is one) contain tyramine, so that the patient is well advised to keep off alcohol.

These restrictions are somewhat irksome, and unless the individual is finding marked benefit from the drugs after a reasonable period of time on a proper dosage, he might as well discontinue it. In some people, however, the results are so successful that they are happy to be maintained on these products long enough to allow the underlying problem time to resolve itself. This often means a period of something like 18 months.

Tricyclic Anti-depressants

The other major group of drugs used in the treatment of depression was developed a little later. The action is again on mono-amines at the nerve-cell junction in the central nervous system, but their mode of action is slightly different, apparently releasing larger quantities of mono-amines rather than inhibiting the enzyme. These drugs, of which **imipramine** was the earliest, form a group known as tricyclic anti-depressants because of the type of chemical structure by which they are made up. They do not present the same problem with regard to dietary restrictions, and have been found to be particularly effective in those cases which previously would only respond to electrical treatment—namely, the depressive illness of endogenous type. They are not particularly effective for the depressive reactions associated with anxiety in neurotic personalities. The development within this group of a wide variety of newer preparations, some with a stimulant and some with a sedative property, has meant a considerable revolution in the treatment of depressive illnesses, which can now often be controlled on an out-patient basis. Because the depth of the depression does not become so great, electrical treatment can often be avoided. Such illnesses may affect some 2 per cent of the population, and the development of an easy method of treatment is, therefore, of considerable benefit. Medication must often be maintained for many months, however. New derivatives are the tetracyclics, and latterly fluoxetine, fluvoxamine, trazadone and amoxazine.

Fortunately or otherwise the safety regulations under the Committee for the Safety of Drugs are now much more stringent than they were a quarter of a century ago. This does mean, however, that old and well-tried remedies that have been on the market for many years, but which may be quite toxic and dangerous in overdoseage remain available while newer drugs which show very rare but occasionally hazardous side-effects may be removed by the Committee even though it is apparent that these drugs are safer than some of the older ones, such as chlorpromazine, imipramine and amitriptyline. Thus in the last two or three years zimelidine has gone, despite it being an extremely useful member of a new group of serotonin uptake inhibitors which act more specifically on certain areas in the central nervous system which seem relevant to depressive illness and which therefore produce many less of the more generalised side-effects which were troublesome with the older drugs.

Interestingly viloxazine, which has a high incidence of nausea as its main side-effect has remained on the list, largely one might suspect because virtually nobody seems to use it. However, many new anti-depressants are currently being developed along the line of specific serotonin uptake inhibitors, and those available on the British market are currently fluvoxamine and fluoxetine, both of which avoid the anti-cholinergic side-effects such as dry mouth, constipation and blurred vision, but do sometimes produce nausea as their main side-effect. Nevertheless, they have been proven to be very effective not only in depressive illness, but in panic states and obsessional compulsive neuroses.

Before the development of such anti-depressants a group of stimulant drugs known as **amphetamines** were used for a time. These drugs, commonly referred to as 'pep pills', had a stimulant action on the central nervous system rather like that of drinking tea or coffee but much more powerful. Cannabis smoking has similarly been used medically for its euphoriant effect. The snag of these preparations is principally that when they wear off the individual feels worse than ever, and they are not in any way getting at the underlying biochemical or psychological causes. Furthermore, the amphetamines are potentially addictive, and a small number of people develop an acute toxic psychosis, not unlike that found in schizophrenia, as a consequence of being on them. Because of these dangers, they have now ceased to be used in the treatment of depression, since the newer preparations do not have these dangers and are more effective.

The amphetamines are, nevertheless, an interesting group of products, since their similarity to mono-amines which operate in central nervous system function, and their tendency to cause schizophrenia-like psychoses, have led to some interesting research.

Lithium

One final drug, lithium, must be mentioned in the treatment of depressive states. This substance has been known for many years. It is similar to sodium and has been used as a salt substitute. It is inert in the body and, therefore, does not ionise in the way that sodium and potassium do; in consequence, it has no effect on the electrical activity of the cell. As has been noted, the intra-cellular levels of sodium are raised in some depressive states and lithium will replace sodium, molecule for molecule, thus in effect reducing the abnormally high sodium content of the cell. This appears to be effective in preventing the symptoms of illness, and if taken over a long period of time, can be greatly beneficial in those patients subject to recurrent cyclical mood swings. These have not in the past responded well to other medication, and in those for whom lithium is effective the improvement is dramatic.

Neuroleptics

The third major group of drugs to be considered are those which are effective in the treatment of thought disorder and the behaviour disturbance associated commonly with schizophrenia and some manic states.

Two substances which were noted to be effective in this field became available in the 1940s. The first was **reserpine**, a derivative of products initially used to lower blood pressure but which were found to have an anti-psychotic effect. It is interesting from a research point of view that reserpine has a tendency to cause depressive states in those susceptible to them. The other product was **chlorpromazine**, the first of a group of drugs known as phenothiazines.

The side-effects of the former group have made it impractical for continued use, but research with phenothiazines has led to a wide range of products which have been remarkably successful in relieving the symptoms found in schizophrenia. Again there is a biochemical basis for this, which appears to be related to the transport and metabolism of mono-amines in the central nervous system. The presence of phenothiazines in the metabolic pathways seems in some way, as yet unknown, to correct this disturbance.

Phenothiazine drugs are of three basic types, according to the chemical structure which they enjoy. These three groups go by the name of the **aliphatic**, **piperidine**, and **piperazine** groups, because of the type of side chain the molecule possesses. Chlorpromazine belongs to the aliphatic group, and, although still widely used, has really too many potential side-effects to make it ideal for long-term treatment. It tends to over-sedate, and has a major drawback in that it produces an excessive sunburn reaction when people are exposed to sunlight. In addition, it can from time to time produce liver toxicity, with jaundice and one or two other rarer complications, which all in all make it of value only for settling the acutely disturbed person on a short-term basis. Promazine is a milder product which is composed of the basic molecule.

The other two groups have produced a much wider range of usage.

The **piperidine** group has no really serious side-effects, and contains the most commonly used **thioridazine** and **pericyazine**. The only snag in this group is their slight tendency to make women plump, a fault they share with some of the anti-depressants, but they can be useful in the treatment of anorexia (loss of appetite).

The **piperazine** group has a number of frequently used preparations, of which **trifluoperazine** and **fluphenazine** are examples. The main side-effects of nuisance value are their tendency to cause a stiffening of the muscles in some people, and restlessness, but these can usually be relieved by taking other medication. A greater advance in the treatment of schizophrenic conditions has been the development of **delayed-release long-acting preparations** in this group, which can be given by a **monthly intra-muscular injection**. This has created much better control of the condition in a smaller and, therefore, less toxic dosage, and has allowed many cases of long standing to return to leading much more normal lives.

Related to the phenothiazines are two other groups of products of great value in the control of schizophrenia and mania. These are the **thioxanthines** and the **butyrophenones**.

The **thioxanthines** have been particularly valuable in dealing with the later effects of schizophrenia, where a residual loss of drive and flattening of emotional response is commonly found. Some members of this group are also produced as a long-acting injection.

The **butyrophenones** have proved particularly useful in two fields. First, they help to control the over-activity and psychotic elation found in mania, and, secondly, they seem to have been of value in dealing with paranoid symptoms found in schizophrenias of late middle age.

The phenothiazines and allied products have also been used, in much smaller dosage, for controlling agitation and anxiety associated with other conditions, such as depression.

For those sufficiently interested to go into the chemical and molecular structure of the various compounds described there is a fascinating field for speculation and research into the interrelationships between psychotic illnesses and the metabolic pathways involved.

Various drugs used for dealing with the dementias and other organic states, including epilepsy, will be described in the relevant chapters. The use of sedatives for anything other than assisting sleep is now rarely of value. Benzodiazepines are commonly used for those with initial insomnia, and the tricyclic anti-depressants taken before retiring often help those people with an early waking problem, which is common in depressive states. It is important when dealing with insomnia to attempt to discover the underlying reasons for this problem, and potentially habit-forming products such as barbiturates and methaqualone should be avoided except as a last resort, or for the short-term management of the more acutely disturbed individual.

Physical Methods of Treatment

We now turn to physical methods of treatment used in the field of psychiatry. In effect, this means modified electrical convulsive therapy ('electroplexy'), certain physical abreactive techniques, electrical relaxation through the use of 'Somlec', and the occasional use of a modified leucotomy operation.

Convulsive therapy was first introduced by **Meduna**, who used a camphor injection to induce convulsions in 1933. Later another substance, cardiazol, was used, and about the same time **Sakel** in Vienna introduced insulin coma therapy. This worked on the same principle. The lowering of the blood sugar by giving insulin eventually induced a generalised electrical discharge in the central nervous system. These types of treatment in the thirties revolutionised the outlook in psychotic illnesses, but they had basic snags. The severity and length of fits was hard to predict, and the treatment was not without risk. **Cerletti** and **Bini** in 1938, however, developed a procedure of inducing this generalised electrical discharge through introducing a small electric current across the forehead, and from this developed the modern electro-convulsive therapy (ECT).

In the early stages this treatment had to be given with the patient initially conscious, and must have been rather unpleasant and frightening, but with the advent of quick-acting anaesthetics given by injection, and muscle relaxants to prevent the muscular convulsions usually associated with an epileptiform kind of fit, the procedure has become much more pleasant. It can even, on occasions, be given to an out-patient.

The individuals receive an injection which puts them rapidly to sleep, just as they would perhaps at the dentist or in minor surgery. The electroplexy is then given, and in a matter of five minutes or so the patient comes round from the anaesthetic and can shortly be sitting up and having a cup of tea. Side-effects are minimal, usually some slight headache or muscle stiffness for a short while, and sometimes some confusion, which generally wears off quite quickly. The treatment is extremely safe, there being virtually no contra-indications other than those associated with anaesthetics, such as severe heart disease or chest disease, but the main contra-indication is the presence of dementing conditions.

The mode of action of convulsive therapy has been the subject of considerable research. There is no doubt of its extreme effectiveness in psychotic illness. It appears to reverse some of the biochemical changes found in depressive states. The effect of a firing-off of the nerve cells may correct the faults in the cell membrane and thus restore the electrolyte balance, or it may allow release of mono-amines that have been blocked. It is also possible that it disrupts response patterns that have developed between the limbic lobe and the frontal cortex. The fact that these theories are not proven in no way detracts from the value of the treatment, which has been a life-saver in cases which were potential suicides now for over 30 years. Usually a course of two or three treatments is given weekly, to a total of somewhere between four and eight. The patient is usually put concurrently on appropriate medication, which he then continues for some months as an out-patient. The value of the treatment lies in the speed of recovery, and to those who feel that a bit of electricity through the forehead is in some way a rather primitive procedure I would again suggest that the treatment of appendicitis by cutting out the offending part is in no way preferable! The use of electroplexy will be considered in further detail in Chapter 8, since it has occupied such an important phase in psychiatric history.

The use of **insulin coma treatment** virtually went out of use some ten years ago, but a method of treatment known as **modified insulin** is still used for people with marked weight loss, as a means of stimulating the appetite and building them up again. Insulin is given but is followed by a large meal after a suitable period of time, instead of allowing the patient to lapse into a comatose state.

The operation of **leucotomy**, which some 30 years ago had a considerable vogue, is now rarely used. It had been known for thousands of years that damage to the frontal cortex in the brain could cause changes in personality. **Moniz** in Portugal, however, published a paper in 1936 on the beneficial effects which could be obtained by dividing certain of the nerve tracts which run from the area of the limbic lobe to the frontal cortex. Division of these tracts in suitable people produced an improvement in mood and behaviour, with a relief of agitation and tension. The operation was used with some success on chronic depressive states, obsessional states and in some disturbed cases of schizophrenia. Indeed, the operation was over-used by enthusiastic preponents, and the original type of operation, known as the 'standard leucotomy', had some side-effects in terms of personality change which were disadvantageous to the patient. Nevertheless, it did allow many otherwise chronically hospitalised patients to return to the community. A modified operation has now become the usual procedure, and in experienced hands can give great benefit to the intractable type of case.

The indications for leucotomy are now much more carefully delineated, and the operation is relatively rarely used, having been replaced in many cases by newer methods of treatment which give as good results without the risks. The main indications are now those cases of chronic depression which do not make a satisfactory permanent response to anti-depressants or electrical treatment, and in severe obsessional states where the obsessional behaviour is ruining the individual's life and has not been controlled by other methods of treatment. This will be discussed later in more depth in Chapter 9.

So far we have discussed those physical methods of treatment suitable for the psychotic illnesses, principally depressive and schizophrenic in character. The **neuroses**, where anxiety is the predominant symptom of affective change, have been looked upon as the main province of psychotherapeutic techniques. Drugs, however, have been used extensively in the relief of anxiety, as has been mentioned earlier, and certain physical methods of treatment have been combined with the psychotherapeutic approach in order to try a short-cut to recovery in what can otherwise be a rather long drawn out therapeutic programme.

While hypnosis cannot be considered as a physical method of treatment, attempts to induce the same degree of suggestibility by the injection of drugs or the inhalation of gases which alter consciousness, such as ether, carbon dioxide, or thiopentone and amphetamine intravenously, have been made. More recently the development in Europe of an electrically operated inductor of relaxation through a small stimulus to the forebrain has also been developed and proved successful. These are all designed to relieve tension, and will now be described in some further detail.

Ether was first used to allow the patient to express repressed material of an emotionally charged kind. This treatment was first used on soldiers who had suffered severely frightening experiences in battle, and had reacted with an hysterical amnesia known as shell-shock. It was found that if such a patient inhaled ether, this allowed a release of inhibitions and the patient was able to recall and relive such emotionally charged material. The handling of such an abreaction and the subsequent security the patient was able to feel allowed the tension to be dissipated and much of the anxiety to be relieved. Some startlingly good results were found in such battle neuroses, but the treatment is by no means so effective in the ordinary anxiety states of everyday life, principally because there is usually not such an accummulation of anxiety-provoking material which has been repressed. Indeed, as we have said, it is probable that in many cases of anxiety states a biochemical over-activity in the limbic lobe is likely to be the cause rather than external trigger situations.

Nevertheless, many phobic states where an individual becomes fearful of a particular situation do seem to have an environmental origin, and can thus be treated by behaviour-therapy orientated methods.

The use of ether has been superseded by quick-acting drugs which can be given by injection, such as **thiopentone** (a barbiturate) and **methedrine**. A high concentration of carbon dioxide has also been used as an abreactive inhalant. Many workers have found that, although the abreactive side of this treatment is not of great significance in most anxiety states, the relaxing effect can be of value in the same way as can hypnosis in allowing the patient to contemplate anxiety-provoking matters while in a state of relaxation and of increased suggestibility. This can be utilised to improve the patient's confidence after coming round from whatever procedure is adopted. Doctors have had some success in treating phobic anxiety states by a combination of drug-induced relaxation or hypnosis with behaviour therapy methods to relieve phobic symptoms.

Somlec is an extension of this physically induced relaxation procedure, and again it is not used for abreactive purposes but for inducing a state of calmness in the individual over a period of perhaps an hour or so. It can also be used for helping people with certain types of insomnia, where, under hospital supervision, the patient can relearn natural sleep. Some of these methods can be used in group situations, and are a useful adjunct to psychotherapy or to anxiety-relieving drugs.

Relaxation Techniques

Let us now devote a little space to a consideration of relaxation procedures induced directly by the therapist, and to hypnosis. These methods of treatment are, as it were, in between psychotherapy itself and the physical methods of treatment. Most people will be familiar with such relaxation procedures as are commonly used in ante-natal clinics and in yoga. Whatever method is used, the basic principle is the same—namely, to obtain calmness and control over oneself and one's body functions. These procedures can have considerable benefit in those with neurotic personalities and in sufferers from long-standing mild anxiety.

The relaxation procedures usually consist of teaching the patient to relax muscle groups, taking each group in turn, and gradually putting the whole together so that the patient finishes up being able to adopt readily a complete relaxation of all their musculature. This technique usually takes a few sessions to learn, and it can then be utilised as an anxiety-relieving procedure by the individual at home when necessary, or in the clinic as part of a desensitisation programme to phobic symptoms.

Hypnosis is merely an extension of this technique whereby the patient enters into a more deeply relaxed state, in which hyper-suggestibility can be used to produce, in suitable subjects, post-hypnotic suggestion and again relief of anxiety symptoms. Many people have a rather unrealistic attitude to hypnosis, however. The procedure is fairly time-consuming and not readily available under the Health Service, partly due to lack of training in the techniques but also to the time generally available for each individual. However, group techniques can be used. In fact, hypnosis is probably more used by doctors who are not practising psychiatry than by those who do. It is used in dentistry, in preparing people for childbirth, and by anaesthetists for a variety of reasons.

Its use in psychiatry is relatively limited. It is of no value in the psychotic illnesses of schizophrenia, depression and mania. It is of no value for treating the other large group of hospital patients, those with dementia. Its main value lies in some of the neurotic conditions, though other techniques such as thiopentone injections may be often as effective and quicker to use. Furthermore, only a limited number of people are capable of reaching the deep trance state necessary for post-hypnotic suggestion, though the majority can reach a light level of hypnosis suitable for desensitisation techniques. Finally, the therapist himself needs to be practised and confident in hypnotic procedures if he is to have a reasonable measure of success. The likelihood of all these combinations being present in a suitable case are not, therefore, all that high. Its use in removing vices such as dependency on cigarettes, alcohol or other harmful delights is limited, and physical methods of treatment adopting behaviour therapy techniques are likely to be more successful if not as pleasant to the patient. Hypnotherapy and hypnoanalysis, however, form an interesting technique currently enjoying a surge of interest.

Psychotherapy

Finally, we look briefly at the **psychotherapies**. Some mention has been made of these procedures in earlier chapters. They range from **superficial psychotherapeutic counselling** techniques, where an attempt is merely made to talk through a patient's problems (in this sense such procedures are utilised by a wide variety of workers in the social and medical and paramedical fields) to **deep psychotherapy**, usually of analytical orientation, such as is practised by **psychoanalysts.** One might also include under the general heading of psychotherapy those techniques more recently introduced which are based on learning therapy and are generally known as **behaviour therapies**.

Whatever the therapist's theoretical orientation, there are certain principles which exist in any psychotherapeutic situation. There is a certain special relationship between patient and therapist which results from the process of interaction between the two. The relationship is special in that, although it is impersonal and does not or should not conflict with the personal relationships of either patient or therapist, once they leave the four walls of the clinic, it can, nevertheless, often produce a marked emotional dependence in the patient which needs to be worked through. The analytical school describe this process as **transference**, and attribute it to the concept that patients imbue the therapist with the emotional attitudes they have had to important people in their own lives, in particular parents, during their formative years. Thus the therapist has transferred on to him or her the emotional attributes of the patients' own parent figures or other dominant people in their emotional lives. This transference may be positive and so assist in the therapy, but a negative transference may develop, where feelings of dislike for the therapist can be seen and have to be worked through. Counter-transference may also be seen, where the therapist's own feelings and reactions towards the patient may need analysing.

Therapists with a non-analytical orientation may well feel that some of the Freudian ideas on transference can be taken to extreme, and that the emotional intimacy which can develop can simply be explained by the dependency of the person confessing on the one hearing his confession. In some circumstances a simple attraction of one person for another of a more straightforward kind is all that is present.

Regardless, however, of the theoretical interpretations, the implications of such a relationship require some maturity and experience in the therapist, and the handling of a transference calls for considerable strength of personality. Such relationships must be worked through, and it is this process which seems to be the key to the beneficial effects seen in deeper psychotherapy. The number of sessions required to achieve such a result, however, and the length of time which patient and therapist must, therefore, spend together, may be considerable, and there are problems in obtaining the required time in ordinary Health Service practice. Thus, the therapist must be carefully selective in whom he takes on, and one must emphasise that while a large percentage of the population might benefit from psychotherapy, not only in psychiatric practice but in all walks of life and experience, those who will derive considerable benefits are relatively few, and are usually younger people with milder neurotic personality disturbances. To obtain treatment outside the Health Service can be very expensive. More of psychotherapy will be discussed in Chapter 7.

Behaviour Therapy

Alongside and to a large extent in competition with psychotherapy of the analytical school there has appeared in the last 20 or 30 years an increasing number of behaviour therapists, whose ideas with regard to effecting symptomatic improvements of a patient's life-style are based on learning theory concepts rather than analytical ones. In practical terms, these concepts have usually been applied to behaviour modification of individuals with antisocial problems, to the treatment of neuroses, particularly of phobic kind, and to training procedures for the mentally retarded or long-stay residual schizophrenic patients in hospital who need to relearn social habits.

Most of these procedures are based on 'stimulus response' theories. The cooperation of the patient is essential. Conditioning occurs as the result of an individual's response to a potentially need-satisfying stimulus. Two common types of problem where such treatment may be used will be stated briefly as examples.

Take a simple example of a child who has become frightened of dogs, perhaps through being bitten. This fear may have generalised to all four-legged creatures and the child has developed a severe fear response. The parents are likely to respond in such a situation by those very principles which behaviour therapy will adopt, though perhaps in a less sophisticated form. They may well buy the child a fluffy dog toy, and they may go on from there to buy the child a puppy, at the same time calming its fears by suitable reassurance or some fear-relieving procedure, which, with children, is often the giving of a reward, such as sweets. Thus the child will gradually be reintroduced to the fear-provoking stimulus, but the fear engendered will be much smaller than it would be if he or she were suddenly confronted with a large Alsatian.

The principles underlying this are that the child has learned that dogs are fear-provoking creatures, and he attempts to avoid such fear by removing himself from the stimulus whenever possible. His expression of fear may well assist him in getting away from such a response, since, for example, by screaming he will cause the offending dog to be removed from his presence. If this fear-response can be associated with something which has the opposite effect, and is fear-relieving or relaxing, and if the latter response can be made stronger than the fear-inducing one, then in theory and indeed in practice the fear response will gradually be extinguished and the relaxation will replace it.

Thus, the principle must be that the fear-inducing response must be presented to the patient as its smallest, with the fear-relieving reward made strong enough to overcome this initial fear. If, for example, a patient had a great fear of thunderstorms, it might be possible first to present this fear to him in his imagination only, and then perhaps with a tape-recording of a thunderstorm played very softly, gradually increasing in intensity, and, if it were practical, finishing up with the real thing. None of these steps are presented to the patient until his fear of the first stage in the procedure has been overcome, and each stage is treated in this way so that a hierarchy of responses is set up.

The fear-relieving response which is going to be associated with the anxiety-provoking situation can be of a variety of types. Relaxation techniques or hypnosis can be used, as described earlier, as can drug-induced relaxation procedures, such as thiopentone. Simple rewards such as sweets would not normally be effective with adults, but some adult equivalent can be utilised in appropriate circumstances. Some of the successes found in psychotherapy may well be due to the anxiety-relieving effect of a stable therapeutic relationship.

The opposite process can be employed to destroy a habit which is immediately enjoyable or satisfying but which is anti-social or dangerous to one's health. This might apply to alcoholism, dependency on cigarettes or sleeping tablets, or to sexual deviances, where the individual obtains immediate gratification but perhaps in a socially unacceptable form that can lead to legal or other complications. The idea here is to associate an unpleasant response with a normally gratifying one in order to extinguish the gratifying response. In this case the unpleasant response would need to be stronger than the habit-forming one.

This type of treatment was first used on alcoholics, by the induction of vomiting. A drink would be provided and a vomiting-inducing injection given to the patient at the appropriate moment, so that the response to quaffing his favourite ale was an immediate feeling of nausea. This association would eventually produce an aversion to alcohol and discourage the patient's habit. The success of such a procedure depended very much upon the timing, and on the patient being prepared to avoid the consumption of alcohol during the treatment period except under treatment conditions. This usually meant admission to hospital. The cooperation of the patient in such treatment, which was slightly hazardous to health and certainly unpleasant, was very necessary, and those who administered the treatment did not exactly find it pleasant either.

A refinement of this process, therefore, was the development of electrical aversion therapy, whereby the individual was wired up to a rather more powerful edition of the child's shock-box toy so that a shock, sufficiently strong to be unpleasant without being dangerous, could be administered to the patient, or the patient could administer it to himself, at the appropriate moment, in the forearm, a finger or any convenient area. Thus if, as an example, we take the individual who wishes to give up smoking, one would devise a scheme whereby, under controlled conditions, each time he lit a cigarette and put it to his mouth he would receive an aversive response, which in time would condition him to dislike the results of lighting up.

This procedure may sound, put as baldly as this, a little naive. However, the method has worked successfully with a variety of conditions, and one can see how the same principles could, for example, be applied to fetishism, transvestism, gambling on fruit machines, or such problems as deviant sexual desire for children.

The procedure of using imagery as opposed to reality is in fact successful, probably because it is the excitement of the anticipation of an act which is largely the driving force which perpetuates the habit. Again, much depends on the willingness and cooperation of the patient, and one should emphasise that aversion therapy is only practical in someone who is prepared to co-operate in a treatment programme and appreciate its purpose.

Some people have argued that there is something ethically distasteful about applying pain to an individual in order to cure a bad habit. It is difficult entirely to see the logic of such an argument, since the cooperation of the patient will always be required, although some might say that the pressures on the individual from society were those which drove them to seek a cure. Nevertheless, the infliction of pain in itself is no reason for discontinuing a treatment which is effective. To do so would be to ban all dentists. It is up to society to decide the ethics under which individuals should be able to operate, and few people would deny that something which is injurious to another, such as paedophilia, is worth attempting to eradicate.

The use of reward techniques for habit training in mentally retarded individuals and for the longer-stay group of the psychiatric hospital population, usually those with a residual schizophrenic defect state, characterised by loss of drive and apathy, has also shown some good results. The system is simply that of establishing desirable patterns of behaviour by rewarding in some appropriate manner each time the individual produces such a response, and by ignoring any other response in that situation. One can build up patterns of response which allow the individual to make more effective social contacts, and in due course, it is hoped, resume a more normal existence. To this end ward units may be run on what is known as a 'token economy' system, where, instead of rewarding simply with sweets, cigarettes or something similar, tokens can be given and the individual can exchange them for goods at a shop. In this way a concept of money can be built up, and the individual can learn the value of a reward even when there is a delay in receiving it.

These behavioural techniques, based on learning theory, have been modified and elaborated and for more detail the reader is referred to specialised textbooks. The main underlying principles however, are: (*a*) **reciprocal inhibition** techniques where gradual reintroduction of graded anxiety-provoking experiences is introduced; (*b*) **implosion therapy**, where the patient is exposed to a massive over-presentation of the anxiety-provoking experience and works through the panic in a no-escape situation; and (*c*) **aversion therapy**, where an aversive result is introduced into the stimulus response system.

This completes what can only be a brief résumé of those currently accepted methods of treatment which have been proved by experience to be effective. For a fuller account of some of the individual methods of treatment the reader is referred to the standard textbooks available on the subject, and to the chapters in Part 2 of this book. In particular, the use of rehabilitative procedures, such as industrial therapy and occupational therapy, for the longer-stay patient will be considered in Chapter 10.

Further Reading

Bremner, C., *An Elementary Textbook of Psychoanalysis*, International Universities Press, New York, 1973.

Hersen, R., *et al.*, *Progress in Behaviour Modification*, Academic Press, New York, 1975.

Pritchard, M. J. 'Prognosis of schizophrenia before and after pharmacotherapy', *British Journal of Psychiatry*, 113, 1345, 1967.

Rogers, C. R., *Client Centred Therapy*, Houghton-Mifflin, Boston, 1951.

Scott, D. L., *Modern Hospital Hypnosis*, Lloyd Doker, London, 1974.

Small, L., *The Briefer Psychotherapies*, Brunner-Mozel, New York, 1979.

Walker, N., *A Short History of Psychotherapy*, Routledge and Kegan Paul, London, 1957.

Wing, J. K., *The Industrial Rehabilitation of Long-Stay Schizophrenic Patients*, Medical Research Council Memorandum No. 42, HMSO, London, 1964.

Wolpe, J., *The Practice of Behaviour Therapy*, Pergamon, Oxford, 1969.

Questions

1. What are the principal reasons for a patient to be admitted to hospital?
2. What general groups of medication are found of value in psychiatric treatment?
3. Why does dietary restriction need to be advised with MAOI drugs?
4. What were the disadvantages of amphetamines?
5. What groups of drugs are useful in schizophrenia?
6. How has abreactive treatment developed and what is its usefulness?
7. What are the principles upon which behaviour therapy is based?

7
Psychotherapy

In this chapter we shall be discussing in more depth what was mentioned briefly under the general chapter on treatment. The psychotherapies are many people's stereotype of what psychiatry is all about. Psychotherapy is the talking cure. It is the attempt to influence people's thinking, behaviour and emotion by means of working on their mental mechanism, sorting out their repressions, teaching them new ways of coping. It embraces a wide variety of techniques from orthodox psychoanalysis through to behaviour therapy. Whatever the theory, however, it assumes a condition in the client or patient caused by early and previous experiences, fed by current tensions, and capable of being alleviated by the therapist's influence.

It is, however, necessary to put psychotherapy in some perspective in terms of our book. Psychotherapy seems most effective for those people with neurotic personalities resulting in problems in coping with their everyday living. It is one method of treating neuroses. Some types of therapy will be a rather time-consuming way of treating these neuroses and for this reason and for financial ones may be unrealistic for many people. It is not easy to do controlled trials which will prove the efficacy of psychotherapy, which is inevitably a somewhat subjective form of treatment. The same criticism can be levelled at psychotherapy, therefore, as has been levelled at electroplexy—namely, that there are few controlled trials which have proven its efficacy.

Nevertheless, the dynamics of psychotherapy are an essential part of the interview techniques which any psychiatrist must acquire, and although psychotherapy in its purer form may be relatively infrequently practised within the National Health Service, its basic skills are essential to an understanding of most neurotic conditions.

Recalling our earlier remarks on the type of patient likely to appear in a psychiatric unit, however, it must be said that the 30 per cent of patients who will be suffering from dementing illnesses, commonly in the elderly, while they may benefit from sensible ward routine and from the supportive counselling which every human should be capable of giving to another, psychotherapy proper would usually be inappropriate. The same argument applies for 30 per cent or so of the longer-stay patients with schizophrenia. Programmes of rehabilitation may well incorporate ideas from analytical or behavioural therapy but there is no evidence that psychotherapy is of proven value in the psychoses, chronic or acute. The same, therefore, applies to the 30 per cent of patients admitted to the acute short-stay wards (the bulk of these will be suffering from endogenous depressive states where psychotherapy may be frankly contra-indicated) and to the acute patients suffering from schizophrenia who, because of their psychosis, would be unreachable by such techniques anyway. Thus, relatively few of the in-patients are likely to receive or benefit appreciably from psychotherapeutic techniques apart from the rehabilitative group work which we have mentioned above.

Psychotherapy, therefore, is more a treatment for the out-patient and the psychotherapy clinic, and the specialist psychotherapist within the medical team may find that a relatively small part of his work will be allocated to in-patients. Nevertheless, it is an area of particular interest because of the theoretical models on which it is based and it does form the fourth specialist area within the Royal College of Psychiatrists and within the examination for the membership.

Talk crops up from time to time about trying to limit the use of psychotherapy to individuals with recognised training. Psychotherapy is practised by non-medically qualified practitioners to an extent far greater perhaps than most other therapeutic modules. The absence of any current need for a licence allows any individual to set up as a psychotherapist and it behoves the patient or client who is seeking help from such people to make proper enquiry about their training qualification and ethics before embarking on what may be an expensive series of consultations with somebody whose background knowledge may in fact be extremely inadequate with limited experience. Psychotherapy is a tool which, in proper hands, can be effectively used but in the hands of amateurs is just as dangerous as the wrong prescribing of medication. Many fringe groups with their own somewhat 'way-out' ideas have recognised the financial pickings to be made from the public's gullibility. In the bigger cities, therefore, many groups have been set up practising varied therapeutic skills—some no doubt excellent, and some dubious in the extreme. That they attract customers is perhaps an indictment upon the Health Service that it fails to provide a proper and adequate facility for this human need. At the same time, such therapy groups can be seen more within the context of human personality problems and their solution seen more within the realm of religion, politics and self-expression than within the realm of treatment in the medical model or indeed any other model designed to provide therapy for a genuine dysfunction.

With these preliminary remarks, therefore, let us look at the psychotherapeutic treatment modules which are available and to what usefulness they seem mainly able to be put.

Jaspers has defined psychotherapy as follows: 'Psychotherapy is the name given to all those methods of treatment that affect both psyche and body by measures which proceed via the psyche. The cooperation of the patient is always required. Psychotherapy has application to those who suffer from the many types of personality disorder and to all who feel ill and suffer from a psychic state, and almost without exception to physical illnesses which so often are overlaid with neurotic symptoms and with which the personality must inwardly come to terms. In all these instances we have in our possession the following means of influencing the psyche: (1) suggestion; (2) cathartic measures; (3) methods of practice, training and re-education; and (4) methods that address themselves to personality.'

Jaspers draws attention to an important point—namely, that psychotherapy will probably be of more use to somebody who has just suffered a heart attack or has become aware that they have cancer than it will to the patient with an endogenous depression or schizophrenia. At its supportive counselling level, there are probably few of us who could not derive some benefit from a gentle stranger, trained in psychotherapy, in whom we could confide and on whom we might perhaps depend. The only people who will not benefit from such a therapy are those who, because of illness, are out of touch with reality and are unable to respond to such an approach. Most of these individuals are in psychiatric hospitals.

Types of Psychotherapy

Psychotherapy is commonly divided into three levels of intensity. Psychotherapy 1 is the level of interaction between patient and therapist which all medical and nursing staff should achieve as part of the developing sensitivity and empathy with others for which their training equips them. This superficial supportive psychotherapy may be called counselling or guidance or a variety of names by groups who see themselves outside of the medical model of disease. It is universally useful and is practised by marriage guidance counsellors, Samaritans, priests, social workers, psychologists and all staff who have anything to do with patient or client care.

Psychotherapy 2 implies a degree of skill which necessitates some special training. Here the client is not given only supportive counselling, advice and suggestion but their underlying motivations may be explored, their opportunities for change in life-style discussed and some insight acquired into the underlying mental mechanisms which are relevant to the neurotic process.

Psychotherapy 3 is a specialist procedure only likely to be acquired by those who complete a course of analytical psychotherapeutic training through the Institute of Psychoanalysis, which gives training in Freudian theory, or through one of the other schools of psychotherapy. At this level of psychotherapy the patient will expect long-term treatment which will unearth repressed and hidden motivations; treatment will regress the patient back to the origins of his neurotic state and deal with the subconscious mechanisms which it is believed are causing his conscious disturbances.

Such therapy is based on analytical theory. A new school of therapy known as **behaviour therapy** has also developed alongside this more traditional work and arises out of the theories of Pavlov, Hull, Clark, and more recent workers who see behaviour as determined by the learning of responses which in the neurotic may be maladaptive and which become self-perpetuating. In such a case, the relief of a symptom may be the relief of disease. These arguments have been rehearsed in *Psychology Made Simple*. A variety of treatment modules is now available based on these differing theories which leads to differences in emphasis with regard to the type of therapy provided.

Psychotherapy may be utilised in a variety of situations. Individual therapy deals with the patient on a one-to-one relationship with the therapist, and if it is Psychotherapy 3, will involve the interpretation of transference relationships which will develop. Therapy may also be planned on a group basis using psychodynamic principles but treating a group of people with similar neurotic problems. Psychodrama and such techniques may be used and a transactional analysis type of approach maintained.

Similarly, **family therapy** may employ some psychodynamic concepts where the disharmony of a whole family can be treated by the therapist meeting with the family as a whole all at the same time.

Hypnotherapy may be utilised to provide psychotherapy of the analytical type and short-cuts to regression and the uncovering of repressed traumatic emotional material may be made.

Marital therapy, treating particularly the psychosexual problems which couples may find, may use psychodynamic or behavioural principles. A number of groups run usually outside of the Health Service have used somewhat differing principles such as encounter groups and Reichian or other types of cognitive therapy.

Psychotherapy of the analytical type is based on certain features considered to operate in the psychodynamics of human beings. Firstly, they adopt various defence mechanisms in order to avoid mental pain or conflict or to control an unacceptable impulse. These mechanisms may be almost wholly conscious or may be so totally unconscious that they are only revealed by years of psychotherapy. The end product of these mechanisms is often a form of maladaptive behaviour or a neurotic symptom. Often this symptom has an expressive as well as a defensive function and may well have damaging consequences for everyone, not least for the individual in whom the mechanism is occurring. Although individuals may be well aware of these self-destructive consequences the forces involved are so strong that they are usually powerless to control them. A vicious circle can be set up between the individual and his environment. One of the main tasks of the therapist, therefore, is to analyse in his own mind and then to interpret to the patient the end product of these mechanisms in terms of the devices adopted for avoiding mental pain, i.e. the defence, the feared consequences of expressing these feelings, the anxiety, and thirdly the nature of the hidden feelings themselves.

Transference

Transference is a fundamental concept. Whenever a patient speaks he may be unwittingly making a communication about his relation to the person he is with, i.e. the therapist, or his feelings about the therapeutic situation. Patients often tend to develop intense feelings about the therapist and very frequently such feelings really belong to someone in the patient's past from whom they have been transferred—hence the word 'transference'. This word has gradually become more loosely used for any feelings that the patient may have about the therapist. It is in the working through of these emotional responses that much of the benefit of psychoanalytical therapy may be seen. Benefits result from bringing the hidden feelings into consciousness and being able to express them.

Thus the qualities needed by the therapist dealing with such work are not only that of the underlying theoretical knowledge but the ability to handle maturely human emotions and to allow patients to work through the transference relationship in such a way that they benefit and mature from it and that it is a growing experience rather than yet another destructive one.

David Malan in his book on individual psychotherapy discusses the origins of transference, pointing out that the original observations were made by Joseph Breuer, a Viennese physician who pre-dated Freud. Freud, however, developed the concept into a useful therapeutic tool and the analyst would now say that although there may be successful therapies that do not involve any interpretation of the transference these must be the exception rather than the rule. Every therapist must be prepared to recognise the transference the moment it arises, to accept it uncritically, to interpret it to the patient when appropriate, to perceive the relation in which it originated and to interpret this to the patient as well.

Individual Psychotherapy

Individual psychotherapy within the Health Service will be carried out by therapists from a variety of backgrounds and training. It will principally be used for out-patients suffering from neurotic states and personality problems which make it difficult for them to come to terms with their lifestyle and with others. But psychotherapy at stages 1 and 2 is what most people will receive and it will be inevitably restricted in the amount of time available. Short-cuts must therefore have to be experimented with and used.

The consultant psychiatrist himself or one of his trained deputy staff may carry out such therapy or it may be handed over to a paramedical colleague such as a clinical psychologist whose orientation is commonly behavioural, or to a member of the social work or nursing teams probably under supervision from the consultant who will discuss the case at a team meeting from time to time. Specialist analytical psychotherapy may be available from a psychiatrist employed specifically as a psychotherapist within the area in which the hospital functions. Usually, however, such specialists are only available on a limited basis at regional centres—for instance, in the university department—where much of their time is engaged in the teaching role. Since analytical therapy may involve the patient in weekly attendance for upwards of two years and is not readily available within the Health Service, short-cuts have had to be sought. For the majority of patients with neuroses it remains the case that physical methods of treatment in the shape of medication or short-term behavioural counselling, or treatment such as Somlec, will be what is available, practical, and indeed, in very many cases, all that is necessary. For the others, attempts to utilise better the therapeutic time available has led to the development of other methods of therapy where more than one patient may perhaps be treated at the same time.

Group Therapy

Group therapy along with abreactive treatments and the widening scope of other psychotherapeutic techniques had its origin in the First World War. A pioneer was William Trotter, a neuro-surgeon, who published a treatise on the herd instinct in peace and war. McDougall in the 1920s further elaborated the concept of groups with the organised and disorganised group idea. Indeed, Freud himself in 1921 was involved with group psychotherapy and stated that it did not make sense to consider the individual psychologically except in relation to other individuals, so that in a way all psychotherapy is essentially group psychotherapy!

Kaplan and Sadock's book on group psychotherapy provides further insights into these early ideas.

Group psychotherapy must utilise quite different techniques by the therapist compared with the individual relationship. The group provides its own dynamic force and group interactions are the areas which the therapist will need to try to interpret. The therapist acts as a catalyst and controller of the group but allows its own dynamics to form. Thus he takes a relatively passive part as a superficial onlooker, though the way in which the group moves must be subtly determined. Groups are usually composed of some eight individuals whose problems are sufficiently similar to make the group cohesive.

Groups may be open or closed. The supportive counselling group that functions at psychotherapy 1 may operate on a ward basis and allow appropriate individuals on that ward to join it while they are in the hospital. It can be supportive and directive and may be run by any member of the ward team. Particular interest groups may be developed, for example, in the handling of alcoholics or people with sexual deviancy problems or drug addicts.

The more formal closed group operates at psychotherapy 2 and is usually more appropriate for the out-patient. It will meet at weekly intervals, probably over a period of six months or more, and the composition of the group will remain the same so far as possible throughout that time. Thus a much more intense group experience will develop in which mutual trust and confidence between the members must be maintained. It must be a rule that anything raised within the group must be with the individual's consent and must remain confidential to it. This sort of cohesion takes some time to develop.

Such groups are primarily psychotherapeutic and the techniques are based on Freudian or related disciplines, or may be handled by those with behavioural training.

Another area where group therapy has been employed is in the encounter group, where **psychodrama** or various forms of acting-out behaviour may be encouraged and physical contact utilising touch of a non-sexual kind, or utilising massage techniques, may be usefully employed. Again these are normally groups run for out-patients, closed in character, and perhaps involving weekend commitments. People with personality inadequacies or psychosexual problems may find such groups particularly helpful in releasing inhibition.

Psychodrama

Psychodrama is a particular group therapetic technique which employs what is in essence play-acting, with one of the participants or the whole group acting out roles which they have found it difficult to cope with in normal life. This can also be done on an individual basis as in assertive therapy, where the patient and therapist engage in role playing so that the patient can learn to handle situations in a more appropriately assertive manner and avoid the maladaptive responses which he or she has adopted previously.

Moreno is credited with having pioneered psychodrama. It was he who coined the term 'acting out' some 45 years ago and which has come into popular usage. While for the analyst acting out can be seen as a resistance, for Moreno it represents a therapeutic manoeuvre which may be particularly useful in certain types of personality neurosis. Out of psychodrama have been developed the encounter groups and Gestalt therapy, transactional analysis and many behavioural techniques.

A wide variety of group techniques is now employed. Analytic group psychotherapy on Freudian lines conducts its treatment in a transference climate. Transference and resistance phenomena are analysed and the group equivalent of free association and dream analysis are employed and interpreted. Careful attention must be given to choosing the group in order that it may be workable.

Other analytic groups may employ the theoretical concepts of the Adlerian school, or follow the methods of Jung, Sullivan, or Horney.

Behaviour therapy in groups encompasses a broad range of short-term procedures which employ desensitisation and assertive training processes. Initially employed principally for phobic patients, such procedures can be used for psychosexual disorders and other more generalised anxiety states. Conditioning is employed based on modern learning theory. Success in behavioural therapy is measured by the number of maladaptive habits that can be eliminated. The group needs to be homogeneous and will cover probably some dozen to twenty sessions. Discussion, role-playing and modelling and psychodrama techniques may all be used with this theoretical model.

Gestalt Therapy

Gestalt therapy, derived from work by Perls, is a technique designed to help people come to terms with their emotions and attitudes by a group method which involves rules and games. The games represent a commentary on social behaviour and patients are asked to act out feelings or express them in fantasy, the primary function not being interpretive.

The goals of the Gestalt therapist are to promote feelings and prevent their avoidance, and to help the participants, therefore, function in a more integrated way. It is often good for the patient with a low level of drive but for some patients the degree of exposure to other people in the group may be something with which they cannot cope, so that unless such groups are run by highly skilled therapists much harm can be done to those inappropriately placed in such a group.

Bioenergetics

Bioenergetic group procedures are another variety of therapy often practised in non-medical and non-psychiatric circles and derive from the work of Alexander Lowen. Techniques employed include massage, breathing exercises and body posturing, and much tactile experience within and between group members. The participants are taught simple ways of easing tension, the goal being to facilitate personality change through the activation of healing forces. Many of these types of therapy are tied up with theoretical constructs coming from Eastern philosophies and, in particular, the Taoist philosophies, having something in common with the theoretical constructs of acupuncture.

Similar techniques are employed in many other encounter groups where emotions are challenged in an immediate and dramatically direct manner. Feminist groups have developed therapeutic techniques for non-orgasmic women which employ group encounter work and the exploration of the individual's sexuality. In Western countries the employment of such techniques within male groups would probably infringe fairly deep-seated male taboos.

Transactional analysis

Transactional analysis is a psychotherapy technique in use since 1954 and developed by Berne. Berne's theory of personality divided the behaviour of persons into distinct ego states which he defines as coherent systems of feeling and behaviour patterns. The division of the ego into child and adult is followed by an additional ego state, the parent. These become the basic concepts for a structural analysis. For the purposes of group treatment a person's behaviour is best understood if examined in terms of ego states, and the behaviour of two or more persons is best understood in terms of transactions, a transaction being a stimulus and a response between two specific ego states.

This theoretical concept and the treatment derived from it has led to many popular off-shoots of role-playing games.

So far as group therapy by transactional analysis is concerned the group is heterogenous and there is no selection. The treatment contract is an acceptable answer to the question: 'How will you know and how will we know when you get what you are coming to the group for?' The answer to this question is worked over in the presence of all group members, which allows each member of the group to sort out the vast number of transactions that take place during a group session and to focus on the stimuli and responses they consider relevant.

In the author's view transactional analysis has been a particularly interesting development in group therapy. The opportunity to obtain satisfactory training and experience is, however, limited and many workers are in effect self-taught. Again it is as well for the potential client, therefore, to know some background of the therapist before entering treatment.

Cognitive Therapy

Another more general theory applicable to psychotherapy has been that of cognitive therapy developed by Beck. The general concept is that poor early experiences lead to the formation of dysfunctional assumptions. Negative disturbed thinking may show as perceptual errors, descriptive errors, inferential errors or evaluative errors. Examples of these might be: 'I am always awkward in company', 'I am inadequate', 'It's all my fault', 'Everyone is fed up with me' or 'I can't help behaving the way I do', 'I'm awful', 'If that happened it would be awful'.

The characteristics of this type of therapy when applied to individuals or groups is that there is a brief and time-limited number of sessions, of say 20. The technique is based on a therapeutic relationship with active collaboration and is problem-orientated. Sessions are structured and directive with a cognitive model of emotional disorders and educational model of treatment. Homework and setting goals are essential features. Roleplaying and assertive training and other procedures may be adopted within the group. Staging of the process within therapy would be firstly to target problems and relieve distress, then to look at behavioural deficits using perhaps a weekly activity schedule to sort out how things are going. Life's problems are looked at later and finally the possibility of prevention of further dysfunctions is taken up.

Family Therapy

Family therapy in this country has been developed by John Howells. It is a system of theory and practice of psychiatry where the family is taken as the unit to be evaluated and treated. The family is the patient. The sick individual, whatever the age, is taken to be the index of a sick family and attention moves from the individual to the family. The general aim is to accept a sick disordered family and to produce a healthy, coordinated family. This system applies to the programme of referral, the elucidation of symptoms, description of the circumstances and treatment. Thus husband, wife, parent, child all are included within the therapeutic process and within the treatment sessions. Treatment depends upon developing empathy, understanding and mutual confidence within the whole family unit. Howells summarises the aim of therapy using a technique which he describes as venexparential psychotherapy: 'Adults come into the present family after suffering an adverse experience in their own preceding families. This adverse experience must be reversed in both parents to effect a harmonious family climate, so that its epitomes going forth to succeeding families will make a healthy psychic contribution to those families. The adverse process can be ameliorated by three main approaches; (1) venexperential psychotherapy, (2) vector therapy, and (3) the creation of a salutiferous society. The three approaches are complimentary and should be used together.'

Venexperential psychotherapy consists of the use of a new beneficial experience. With vector therapy the change of forces produces a new beneficial experience and corrects disadvantageous ones. A vector denotes a quantity which has direction: vector therapy thus readjusts the pattern of the emotional forces within the life space to bring improvement to the individual family within the life space. 'Salutiferous' refers to the promotion of health as it extends from the family into society.

Behavioural Psychotherapy

It is beyond the scope of this book to detail in depth the large varieties of behavioural therapy which have been derived from learning theory. Behaviour therapy aims to modify current symptoms and focusses attention on their behavioural manifestations in terms of observable responses. In therapy it is not alway seen as necessary to unravel the origin of symptoms. Treatment is particularly useful in individuals with anxiety neuroses, particularly of phobic type. Hierarchies of anxiety-provoking situations carefully graded can be worked through in a training programme, allowing the gradual development of confidence as the patient learns to overcome anxiety in each situation in turn. As is described elsewhere in this book, behavioural therapy may also utilise aversion techniques for removing habits which are immediately gratifying but in the long term damaging to the individual. Behavioural principles may also be used in the treatment of psychosexual problems, and the sensate focus treatment also described elsewhere is one example of this. Behavioural treatments have been particularly the field of the clinical psychologist and many well controlled trials have established its efficacy, particularly in the areas mentioned above. Principles of behaviour modification may also be used in the training of the mentally handicapped and in the long-term rehabilitation of the chronic psychotic.

We have seen then in this chapter that psychotherapy, using the term in its broadest sense, has a wide application. More specific techniques which require a special training additional to that required by most psychiatrists or psychologists may have very limited availability, certainly within the National Health Service. Principles of psychotherapeutic techniques, however, are required and are utilised within everyday individual or group treatments.

The usefulness of more specific types of psychotherapy must be weighed against the time involved both for the patient and therapist, its comparitive effectiveness and, if obtained privately, the cost. These treatments are mostly of use for the neuroses and personality problems. It is not easy to provide controlled trials which will prove the efficacy of some types of psychotherapy against other perhaps more straightforward treatments. There is no virtue in embarking upon a time-consuming and possibly expensive series of sessions unless it can be shown that this has some substantial benefit in long-term results over other simpler and more cost effective treatments.

It must be recognised in this context that the majority of neuroses of acute onset do, in fact, go into a natural remission. If follow-up is made of a group of such patients then at the end of six months a fair proportion will have made a spontaneous recovery. At the end of two years some 70 per cent of patients will have recovered from the problem with which they presented to the psychiatrist in the first place. The longer follow-up the more the numbers of patients who have recovered will be. Thus, any treatment that cannot claim better than a 70 per cent recovery rate at the end of 12 months may have no more value than the straight passage of time. Treatment, therefore, must aim either at effecting some more permanent change in personality which prevents subsequent relapse or recurrence, or must alleviate symptoms and suffering at a more rapid rate than the natural passage of time would be expected to do. This is as true in physical medicine as it is in psychiatry. Thus the patient with an acute anxiety state may be satisfactorily and very simply treated by the provision of anxiolytics, or tranquillisers, for a limited period of time in the same way as an aspirin may be used to treat a headache.

To compete within these concepts, therefore, psychotherapy must convince the practitioner that it will either effect some more permanent beneficial change or that it will alleviate suffering more quickly than would simple reassurance and the provision of some physical method of treatment. Unfortunately, for the supporters of psychotherapy, the more specific types of deep psychotherapy have not really been proven to do either of these with markedly measureable effect. There is no doubt, however, that the patient may benefit from the interaction with a therapist and that the support which this can give may be the most important factor determining who should be offered what is a relatively scarce treatment module.

Further Reading

Freud, S., *Three Essays on the Theory of sexuality*, Standard Edition, Vol. 7, Hogarth Press, London, 1905.

Horny, Karen, *Neurosis and Human Growth*, Routledge and Kegan Paul, London, 1951.

Howells, J. G., *Principles of Family Psychiatry*, Pitman Medical, London, 1975.

Jaspers, K., *The Nature of Psychotherapy*, Manchester University Press, Manchester, 1964.

Kaplan, H. I., and Sadock, B. J., *Comprehensive Group Psychotherapy*, Williams & Wilkins, Baltimore, 1971.

Malan, D. H., *Individual Psychotherapy and the Science of Psycho-dynamics*, Butterworths, London, 1979.

Mayer, B., and Chester, S., *Behavioural Therapy in Clinical Psychiatry*, Penguin Books, Harmondsworth, 1970.

Sperling, A. P., *Psychology Made Simple*, Heinemann, London, 1982.

Questions

1. How does psychotherapy differ from other methods of treatment?
2. What distinguishes behaviour therapy from dynamic psychotherapy?
3. What type of patients may most effectively benefit from psychotherapy?
4. What criteria do we need when evaluating the effectiveness of such a treatment?
5. To what extent is psychotherapy available at your local hospital? Is there a specialist psychotherapist on the staff of your psychiatric unit?
6. What is the value of (*a*) group therapy and (*b*) family therapy over individual therapy, and what is the disadvantage?

8
Electroplexy

Much ill-informed criticism has been directed against so-called shock treatment in recent years by various socio-political pressure groups both in the United States and in Britain. It is difficult to understand precisely why this particular therapy has been singled out. Much of the criticism could be applied equally well to many other medical and surgical techniques. The fact that the early treatments produced a convulsion, and the use of the term 'shock', have no doubt been largely to blame in making the public fearful, and the fact that the treatment was for the brain, as opposed to some less important area of the body, such as the kidney, added to the concern.

At the same time, to strap somebody to an operating table, to take a sharp knife and partially to disembowel them might also be seen as rather primitive! Yet this is the standard treatment for appendicitis. In both cases, of course, the patient has received an anaesthetic, and is not, therefore, consciously aware of what is going on; and the important point to remember is that in both cases the treatment is of value to the sufferer, while to withhold it can have considerable dangers.

Unfortunately for those in urgent need of electroplexy, a vociferous lobby has created a situation in some parts of the United States where so many restrictions are placed upon its use that it may be deemed wiser by the practitioner to withhold it altogether, or at any rate to prolong unnecessarily the patient's suffering by inordinate delays. Fortunately, this situation has not as yet come to pass in Britain, but it seems to the author that the public and the profession must guard against the imposition of minority views when they are against the best interests of individuals who are ill-placed at the time to speak for themselves.

ECT stands for **electro-convulsive therapy**, 'shock therapy' being another popular synonym. Both these terms should be discarded in favour of electroplexy, however, since their implications are frightening to those unfamiliar with the procedures.

The Nature of Electroplexy

The essence of this therapy lies in the production of a generalised seizure discharge within the central nervous system. The biochemical changes which take place in that system as a result of such a seizure discharge bear no direct relationship to the particular method used to induce it.

When the treatment was first developed, methods other than electrical induction were used. The development of a seizure discharge through electrical means has been desirable, making the treatment safer and freer from side-effects, since it gives the doctor a much more careful degree of control over the length and extent of seizure discharge than previous methods. Combined with the use of quick-acting anaesthetics, this procedure has been, therefore, a considerable advance, though it is merely a method of triggering off a generalised activity in the central nervous system.

The history of the development of electroplexy makes a fascinating study. Like so many advances in medicine, the beneficial effect was discovered almost accidentally, though it is fair to say that various research workers had for some time been piecing together bits of apparently unrelated information until the jigsaw became clearer.

It had been noted that sufferers from psychotic illnesses, if they were unfortunate enough in one sense to suffer an epileptic fit, sometimes appeared to have a temporary clearing, after the fit occurred, of the disorder of mood or thinking from which they were suffering. Moreover, it had been postulated by other workers that there was some mutual antagonism between epilepsy and schizophrenia on the basis—which subsequently proved erroneous, but the theory was originally propounded on this—that epileptics develop schizophrenia less frequently than would be expected in the general population, and that, as a corollary to this, epilepsy was less frequent in schizophrenics. It was postulated that **the artificial induction of a seizure discharge comparable to that found during an epileptic fit might, therefore, be used as a method of treatment**, in particular against the schizophrenic process, and could bring relief from the thought disorder which characterises that condition.

It must be remembered that at this time, some 40 years ago, psychotic illness was not the relatively mild condition we see today. Untreated, schizophrenia resulted in a gradual decline in personality and a total breakdown of the individual's ability to think and to relate socially. Behaviour was bizarre and disturbed. The patient withdrew into an autistic mutism, and bizarre delusions and auditory hallucinations were found. Such individuals finished up as long-term patients in psychiatric hospitals, cabbage-like husks of their former selves. The disease was and is found in 1 per cent of the population, and was dreaded as is cancer on the surgical wards.

Psychotic depression was equally severe, though fortunately the patients, if they survived, generally returned to a normal level of functioning when the disease process eventually burned itself out. Nevertheless, suicide was and is common. The depth of depression which obtained in pre-treatment days was such that severe cachexia, and wasting diseases such as tuberculosis or pneumonia (which could take over when such degrees of ill-health obtained, often for months at a time) were killers. Aspiring young psychologists and sociologists have no concept of what these diseases were like 30 years ago, and probably have never seen a case of this severity.

The advent of convulsive therapy revolutionised the treatment of psychoses. Suddenly and dramatically, patients who had been severely disabled by these diseases were restored to normal functioning, and many chronic patients discharged and sent home.

The initial attempts to induce seizure discharges were, not surprisingly, somewhat crude. Some workers attempted to use cerebral stimulants which were known to induce fits. Camphor was used by injection. This certainly induced a seizure discharge, but the epileptic fit which resulted was uncontrolled and might be severe and difficult to terminate. Thus, although the patient often showed remarkable improvement, there was, nevertheless, a sizeable morbidity and some mortality from the technique which prevented its wide acceptance and made it important to develop more reliable and safe methods.

Insulin Coma Therapy

Around the same time Sakel had been experimenting with the use of insulin, at that time a newly developed compound for the treatment of diabetes. It was found that if hypoglycaemia could be induced by means of injections of insulin, the hypoglycaemic coma so produced caused generalised seizure discharges to take place in the central nervous system, producing the same effect. The treatment on any particular occasion could be terminated by relieving the hypoglycaemic state with sugar. A course of treatment would consist of a number of such sessions spread out over three or four weeks. Depressive illness was found to respond dramatically to a course of as little as half a dozen sessions, but schizophrenic illness, which had initially been predicted as the condition likely to respond best to the seizure discharge, proved more difficult to treat. In some cases it proved of little benefit but in some 50 per cent the patients did show marked improvement if the course were prolonged to the extent of a dozen to twenty procedures. This was in contrast to what had been expected, since depression responded much more effectively.

Insulin coma therapy was, however, still not without its hazards. The onset of hypoglycaemia was not easily predictable, and it sometimes proved difficult to bring the patient out of coma, multiple seizure discharges being induced. The treatment period lasted a whole morning, and a high level of observation, nursing and medical skill was necessary. Side-effects from the fits might include injury to limbs from the tonic and clonic phases of the fit, or injury to the tongue. Occasional deaths still took place if the hypoglycaemia could not be terminated, and sometimes brain damage resulted.

It is important, however, to balance these serious side-effects with the fate of sufferers from the two illnesses before the advent of such treatment. There is a morbidity and mortality attached to many treatments in medicine and surgery, and indeed even to the simple process of having a baby. But the hazards of not giving treatment in terms of chronic hospitalisation, the risk of suicide, and the other well-recognised problems associated with psychotic illness, were in the view of most people—patients, relatives and therapists— more to be feared than the relatively slight risk attached to treatment.

Nevertheless, it was vitally important to develop ways of modifying the treatment so that, while remaining as effective, it became safer. To this end the induction of a seizure discharge through electrical stimulation was considered, and work by Meduna, Cerletti and Bini led to a highly significant breakthrough in the treatment of psychoses with the development of what has now come to be known as electroplexy or ECT.

Effects of Electroplexy

It should be made clear that the **use of electricity to trigger off a seizure discharge is purely a matter of safety and convenience.** The effectiveness of the therapy appears to lie in the biochemical and neuro-hormonal changes induced by the seizure discharge and not in the method by which it is provoked.

The advantage of electrical induction lies in the ability of the therapist to control the timing and onset of the seizure and its duration, through modification of the length of time the electrical stimulus is applied and by the strength of the current employed. Since the onset of the seizure can be accurately timed, precautions can be taken to prevent patients injuring themselves by, for example, biting their tongues, which is a not uncommon side-effect from the uncontrolled convulsion that a sufferer from epilepsy might experience.

Initially, an electrical stimulus passed across the forehead was found to be the most satisfactory method. The onset of a generalised cortical neuronal discharge rendered the patient only briefly unconscious but could still be somewhat frightening for the nervous patient. Further improvements to the acceptability of the treatment came with the development of anaesthetic skills, whereby a quick-acting intravenous anaesthetic such as thiopentone could be administered before the treatment, which allowed the patient to sleep through the procedure without any reduction in the effectiveness of the seizure discharge. Another improvement came with the development of muscle relaxants in anaesthetics, which meant that the unwanted side-effect of electroplexy—namely, the development of generalised muscle contractions, which always accompany an unmodified seizure—could be prevented by the use of scoline. Thus the patient could be given an injection in a vein in the hand, which would put him to sleep, followed by the rapid induction of muscle relaxation, followed by the electrically induced cortical seizure discharge; and when he was allowed to wake some ten minutes after, the effect of the muscle relaxant had worn off.

The therapeutic effect is in no way disturbed by the use of an anaesthetic or by scoline, which counters the common criticism of electroplexy that it has some kind of punishment value to a patient with delusions of unworthiness. The use of electroplexy in such circumstances is no more a ritual punishment that a course of attendances at the dentist. The prime object of the latter is to mend holes in the teeth, and the pain and discomfort are unnecessary concomitants which sensible therapists work to avoid.

The immediate after-effect of a generalised seizure discharge is a temporary confusion. This is a simple and expected consequence of a seizure. The same is found after an epileptic fit or a kick on the head at a game of rugby football. This feeling of confusion is of no value in the therapy, more of a nuisance. The aim of therapy is not to wipe out memory traces or in any way to 'brainwash'. The purpose of electroplexy is not to make people forget. It is to relieve the psychotic manifestations of a disease process. The vast majority of patients find little inconvenience from this side-effect as long as they have been warned in advance, and in most cases it wears off within an hour or so, though in some, particularly if a longer course of treatment has been necessary, it may continue for some days after the completion of the course.

In order to reduce this side-effect to a minimum the technique has been modified in recent years so that the electrical stimulus which triggers off the seizure discharge is applied across the non-dominant frontal cortex only, with the electrodes placed one on the centre of the forehead and the other on the temple of the non-dominant side. There is some evidence that this technique decreases the amount of post-treatment confusion but it also seems to be less effective in treating the severer psychotic breakdowns than is the application of electrodes to the temples. A seizure discharge that is induced in one hemisphere will, of course, generalise and spread across to the other side and down to subcortical levels, just as an epileptogenic focus will trigger off a generalised seizure discharge.

Reiterating what has been said in the historical introduction, it soon became apparent to researchers in the field that **depressive psychosis** had the most successful outcome. This has remained the prime indication for electroplexy, though it has continued to have a place in certain other fields, in particular in those cases of **schizophrenia** where there is a marked affective disturbance or where the patient's behaviour is disrupted by the delusional and hallucinatory thought content, when a considerable improvement may be expected in the acute stage of the illness, though long-term therapy with medication is still required and the outcome is still by no means always successful. **Acute manic psychoses** will show a much more rapid improvement if a short course of electroplexy is given initially while medication is given time to work.

Finally, and somewhat paradoxically, the confusion associated with **sub-acute delirious states**, which can sometimes linger on after the causative disease process has been removed, may respond very effectively, with a lifting of the clouding of consciousness, after one or two sessions of electroplexy. The same applies to the disturbed behaviour and altered consciousness that can sometimes be seen in **epilepsy** itself when a patient may be building up to a fit. A controlled administration of electroplexy in such a case may remove these symptoms and prevent the development of a more acute and uncontrolled grand-mal fit.

Evidence of Effectiveness

It has often been said, principally by those who appear to have little knowledge of the literature and argue from sociological premises, that the effectiveness of electroplexy has not been proven. What evidence is there that can counter this argument?

Four types of study of electroplexy have been carried out. First, there have been **comparative studies**, where the morbidity and progress of psychotic illness before the advent of electroplexy or convulsive therapy in general have been compared with matched groups of patients who had developed similar conditions following the advent of such treatment. This has been further extended in more recent years, to compare morbidity and outcome during the period when convulsive therapy alone was available and the period since the development of psychotropic drugs, when both types of treatment have been available.

Secondly, comparative trials have been undertaken whereby matched groups of patients have been given either electroplexy or such alternative forms of therapy as anti-depressant medication. Again, the morbidity and outcome between the two groups can be compared by means of a double-blind procedure. Trials have also been carried out to compare electroplexy with dummy therapy—that is to say, the use of an identical procedure, including anaesthetic, but where the seizure itself has not been induced. Thus, this acts as a **control group** and the active treatment is being compared with it.

Comparative trials have not been done very often for two very good reasons. First, it is ethically dubious to give a group of severely ill people a dummy treatment. Those who criticise research into electroplexy by saying that adequate double-blind control trials have been few and far between must remember that untreated psychotic illness can have a considerable mortality and morbidity. To give an example, it might be suggested that the use of appendicectomy as a treatment for appendicitis is not without risk and may sometimes be performed unnecessarily when the appendix at operation turns out to be normal. It might be justifiable, therefore, to do a trial, treating appendicitis by appendicectomy for one half of the group and using, say, penicillin for the other half. This would establish whether penicillin was as effective, or more or less effective, than appendicectomy in the condition. The fact that a number of people might die of appendicitis spreading to peritonitis in the process would have to be a so-called justifiable risk. To take a further group who had appendicitis and administer a placebo treatment as a control, i.e. in effect giving no treatment, would probably be even more hazardous. Patients would have to be asked if they were prepared to join in this kind of experiment, and the risks explained.

Exactly the same argument applies to psychotic depression or severe schizophrenic breakdown. The consequences of not doing one's best to treat such individuals can be dangerous and lethal. The comparison with appendicitis, therefore, while not being entirely valid, has similarities in this respect.

The second reason, however, that there is rather a dearth of such controlled trials is that the treatment has been proven effective to the satisfaction of the majority who have worked with such diseases over a span of a quarter of a century—in both private and Health Service practice—and in virtually all parts of the world, regardless of social structure or political leanings. Thus, to most workers in the field the need to prove the point further at this stage is superfluous.

The third type of trial that has been conducted with regard to electroplexy has been to compare not the effectiveness of the treatment but the **potential side-effects** or harmful effects with those of other forms of treatment used for psychotic illness. Thus, the morbidity associated with electroplexy can be compared with the morbidity associated with anti-depressant medication under various circumstances, and with different age groups and types of disease. It is fair to say that virtually all trials of this type that have been done have shown electroplexy to be extremely safe, and the morbidity to be less than that found with other forms of treatment. No long-term deleterious results have been identified despite considerable world-wide research into the subject. There is, indeed, little reason to think that there would be long-term effects from a course of artificially induced seizure discharges. The bulk of epileptics will have had hundreds more such seizure discharges in their lives than ever a patient with depression or schizophrenia will receive. These are uncontrolled fits and likely to have far more hazards than a medical treatment, yet even in epileptics the vast majority suffer no long-term consequences from such fits as long as they do not injure themselves by falling or suffering a period of anoxia.

The fourth and final type of trial has been to **compare the effectiveness of different types of induction** to produce seizure discharge—for instance, to compare unilateral with standard application of the electrodes, or to compare electroplexy in the induction of a seizure discharge with some other method, such as indoklon or insulin coma techniques.

The double-blind control trial, using modern statistical methods, is a relative newcomer to the medical scene. Thus such trial work is not available for work done 20–25 years ago. Most research into the efficacy of electroplexy has devoted itself to depressive psychosis, since this is undoubtedly where it has been most effective.

Those who worked in the field of mental illness before the introduction of electroplexy have been impressed by the dramatic changes in terms of length of stay, morbidity and prognosis when the two eras are contrasted. The improvement was as dramatic as that which had occurred some decades before when *dementia paralytica* or GPI had first been shown to respond to hyperthermia or hyperpyrexia.

A study of depressive psychosis occurring in the puerperium, i.e. after childbirth, investigated all the admissions to hospitals in Newcastle-upon-Tyne with this diagnosis in the decades before electroplexy was introduced, during the time when electroplexy alone was available, and the first decade in which both tricyclic anti-depressants and electroplexy were equally available. This showed a dramatic improvement between the pre-electroplexy and the electroplexy decades. The mortality dropped, and the chronicity of the condition, whereby in earlier days many patients had remained as long-stay hospital cases, improved so much that after electroplexy was introduced this situation occurred very rarely. The principal difference since the introduction of anti-depressant drugs has been a shortening of the length of stay needed in hospital. Recurrence rates do not seem to have been appreciably affected by the introduction of drugs.

Another criticism that is voiced concerning electroplexy is that it does not 'cure' depression. The use of the word 'cure' is a curious one. There are relatively few treatments in medicine which, strictly speaking, cure rather than relieve. Antibiotics are perhaps one exception to this. Insulin does not cure diabetics. The removal of the appendix hardly cures appendicitis, in the sense that the patient is not left with a normal healed appendix at the end of the treatment. Filling a hole in a tooth with amalgam does not 'cure' dental caries. Yet people do not criticise these treatments because they do not cure.

Similarly, the effect of electroplexy on an acute depressive psychosis is to clear it up more quickly. This is humane and sensible. Not to do so would increase the risk of incidence of suicide, increase the patient's length of stay in hospital, increase the length of total suffering, and cause a minority of the patients to become chronically hospitalised. In the majority, however, given time—and here we are talking about six months to a year in most cases—a natural remission would occur. All electroplexy is doing is restoring the patient to health from that particular attack more rapidly. But depressive psychosis in a sizeable proportion of patients is an illness which can recur at some later stage in their lives, and there is no evidence that electroplexy will reduce the possibility of a subsequent recurrence in two, five or ten years' time: no more than giving penicillin to a case of pneumonia can ensure that such a patient will never get pneumonia again.

Research and Efficacy

Let us now turn to some key research papers which have been devoted to the effectiveness of electroplexy.

Bratfos and Hauge from Oslo reported (in the *Acta Psychiatrica Scandinavica* in 1965) on the effectiveness of electroplexy and compared it with drug therapy. In their study they showed that the effect of electroplexy was considerably better than that of anti-depressant drugs in manic-depressive disease. A significantly greater number of patients were discharged recovered, and the shorter duration of hospital stay in the electroplexy group justified the conclusion that electroplexy should be the treatment of choice in manic-depressive disease.

Bruce in 1960 and Kristiansen in 1961 found that electroplexy and imipramine were approximately equally effective. Kiloh in 1962 found that electroplexy gave better initial results. Hutchinson and Smedberg in 1963 compared electroplexy with six different anti-depressants in a total of 200 patients, and showed that electroplexy gave significantly better results than drug therapy. Greenblatt in 1964 published a similar study of 281 severely depressed patients in whom electroplexy was found more effective than tricyclic anti-depressants and MAOI drugs.

In 1965 the Medical Research Council in Britain compared the efficacy of electroplexy, anti-depressant drugs and a placebo, 250 patients with a diagnosis of affective psychosis being randomly allotted to the different types of treatment. It was shown that both on a short-term basis (after four weeks' treatment in hospital) and on a long-term basis (six months later) electroplexy markedly increased the frequency of recovery over the spontaneous rate shown by patients on the placebo. An anti-depressant drug showed a slower action that electroplexy but also increased the frequency of recovery over a placebo.

With regard to the effectiveness of electroplexy in the treatment of acute schizophrenia, it has been shown by comparing electroplexy and drug therapy alone, with drugs plus psychotherapy, and with standard ward care only, that electroplexy is more effective than standard ward care or psychotherapy alone but less effective than phenothiazines in the long term. Smith, however, in 1967 showed, when comparing phenothiazines alone with phenothiazines plus electroplexy, that the group receiving the latter treatment responded more rapidly in some symptom areas and were discharged more quickly from hospital.

Mode of Action

A criticism often made is that the treatment is given without any clear idea of the way it works. This is to some extent justified but has been equally true of many discoveries in medicine, where the effectiveness of the treatment has pre-dated the discovery of the reasons. It applied to quinine in the treatment of malaria, the first use of penicillin, and early methods of treating syphilis, to name but a few.

It should be clear from what has been said earlier that the effectiveness of electroplexy lies in the production of a generalised seizure discharge. A number of investigators have compared electroplexy with a pseudo-electroplexy (i.e. anaesthesia without the shock). Ottosson, however, in 1970 showed that shortening the seizure discharge decreased the therapeutic efficacy of electroplexy. He established that the depression-relieving effect of electroplexy was bound to seizure activity. His article quotes a large number of other relevant trials.

The mechanism of the depression-relieving action has been the subject of a number of hypotheses, and there are conflicting opinions on the fundamental question of whether the therapeutic effect is the result of bio-chemical or neuronal changes induced by the seizure. However, Modigh showed in 1977 that the main effect was via seizure activity in the brain stem, where there is a high concentration of mono-amines. A consequence of the seizure discharge is an increased release of noradrenalin, dopamine and 5–hydroxytryptamine. An increase in turnover of noradrenalin is found 24 hours after the administration of treatment, and there appears to be a facilitation of neuro-transmission. The chain of action through tyrosine, dopa, dopamine and noradrenalin and through tryptophan to 5–hydroxytryptamine is facilitated especially in the corpus striatum and limbic lobe, where there is an increased sensitivity in dopamine receptors. Thus the action would appear to be an increase in noradrenalin synthesis, an increase in the sensitivity of the receptors and, therefore, a reversal of the type of changes that have been shown to be present in affective psychoses —namely, a diminution of availability of mono-amines at the synapse in certain parts of the central nervous system and an alteration in membrane permeability, with increase of intracellular sodium levels, associated with a decrease in electrical efficiency of the cell. These findings have been confirmed by many biochemical studies relating to the mode of action of tricyclic and mono-amine oxidase inhibitor anti-depressants and the prophy-lactic effect of lithium in manic-depressive disease.

One piece of 'evidence' which has often been adduced in attacks on electro-plexy appeared in *World Medicine* on 11 September 1974. An anonymous author stated he had worked as an anaesthetist in a hopsital where an ECT machine, in use over a long period of time, had not been noticed to be faulty, but had not seemingly caused any lessening of the effectiveness of treatment noted by the clinical staff in patients referred. It has never been possible to substantiate this report. Quite clearly there was no question of a controlled trial, and the report is at best anecdotal. No indication of how many patients were treated through the faulty machine is given, whether anti-depressant drugs were used concurrently, and whether in fact the length of stay of these patients in hospital was longer than would have been anticipated if electroplexy had been given successfully in addition to anti-depressant therapy. It is difficult to see how the staff could have failed to notice that the treatment was not inducing a seizure discharge, since anyone who has watched electroplexy being given will know that the seizure discharge, although modified by anti-convulsant drugs, is quite obvious when it occurs. Notwithstanding this, the lobby operating at present in the field of consent to treatment in mental illness has chosen to quote this unsubstantiated article widely, presumably for want of any better evidence. *World Medicine* on 16 November 1977, in an editorial, was constrained to state: 'People who use this story as evidence that ECT is an ineffective treatment must accept that it has the status only of an unconfirmed, uninvestigated anecdote'.

Hazards

Another way critics have attacked electroplexy is through ill-informed quotations about its dangers. Thus Michael Stern in an article entitled 'ECT Under Attack' in *On Call*, 10 November 1977, states: 'An increasing catalogue of alarming side-effects has over the years brought even the more conservative observers to quesion its widespread use'. It is curious, however, that those authors critical of ECT are anecdotal and that properly conducted trials are never quoted in their articles.

It must be remembered that one of the main symptoms of the psychoses is disturbance in concentration. The brain, because of the disease process, is not functioning fully effectively—hence the distortions of mood or thinking which can occur. Furthermore, these diseases can often be recurring, so that to quote an individual who happened to have a course of electroplexy some years before and who now states that he suffers impairment of concentration and blames this on the electroplexy is something that should not be accepted at face value nor naively. Indeed, trials comparing electroplexy with placebo (reported by Greenblatt in 1964) showed that, while post-treatment headaches were reported more frequently in those who had received the active treatment, headaches were also reported, although less frequently, in patients who were on the placebo, and some symptoms were actually reported more frequently in those on the placebo, presumably because they related to the disease process itself rather than being a side-effect of treatment.

It has, nevertheless, been recognised that there is some short-term impairment of memory following electroplexy, though, as Sternberg and Jarvik point out, memory functions are impaired in depression and improve with improvements in the mental state. Cronholm and Ottosson comment that patients who showed the most improvement following electroplexy experienced least subjective memory impairment. These authors suggest that electroplexy impairs retention temporarily, whereas depression itself is associated with deficiencies in the learning or acquisition process.

Squire and Miller found that the ability to learn new material was initially impaired but then recovered in the hours following each treatment, and that ability to retain material for 24 hours was more impaired following the fourth than the first treatment. However, using a wide battery of tests, they could find no objective impairment of memory disturbances at six months and nine months after a course of electroplexy.

Professor G. D'Elia from Sweden, reporting in 1977, stated his research had shown that the main side-effect of ECT was on retention. There was a retrograde effect, but within six hours of treatment 39 per cent of the original level of retention had returned. After a week 69 per cent had returned, and after a month patients were shown to be functioning at 101 per cent of their pre-treatment ability. The fact that they were functioning marginally better should be no surprise, since there would have been some diminution of function as a result of the disease process itself.

Further studies in Denmark have shown that **no memory disturbance at all could be detected in patients who were followed up for a three-month period.**

Anaesthetic Risks

Some side-effects to the cardiovascular system are the direct result of the anaesthetic rather than of electroplexy. There are, of course, the same risks attached to anaesthetics for electroplexy as to any other short-term anaesthetic administration, but the use of quick-acting intravenous anaesthesia is an extremely safe procedure and the mortality associated with it negligible. A brief rise in blood pressure has been shown during electroplexy, and it is, of course, prudent not to give such treatment to individuals with severe heart or lung disease or with evidence of a dementing state, which could be worsened.

D'Elia and Raotma (1977) studied the influence of age and the number of treatments on memory impairment. They showed that before treatment older age groups had decreased ability to learn but that their post treatment forgetting score was not significantly higher than in other age groups. Increasing the number of electroplexies in the treatment series did not alter the degree of memory impairment. **No apparent influence on memory could be shown after electroplexy.**

Dangers of Withholding Treatment

A highly important consideration in the application of any type of treatment in medicine or surgery must be the morbidity and mortality associated with withholding treatment. There are, for example, side-effects associated with the giving of insulin over a long period of time, but these are far outweighed by the seriousness of leaving diabetes untreated. It must be emphasised that **electroplexy is safer than using aspirin, safer than the contraceptive pill, and safer than the dentist's chair! It is also safer, particularly in older people, than the use of tricyclic anti-depressants.** Furthermore, psychotic depression is a killer disease, and, untreated, can result in death from suicide. Indeed, it often does.

D. H. Blachly from Oregon, reporting in 1977, showed that there were less mortality and morbidity associated with electroplexy than with tricyclic anti-depressants. An important article by Avery and Winokur (in *Archives of General Psychiatry*, Volume 33, September 1976) showed in 519 patients suffering from depression and hospitalised in the decade 1959 to 1969, and subjected to a three-year follow-up study, that the group treated with electroplexy had a significantly lower mortality than the group not so treated. Non-suicidal deaths and myocardial infarction were significantly more frequent in the group not treated with electroplexy. This endorsed the importance of adequate treatment of psychotic depression, especially in the older men in the trial. This article is well worth further study.

Thus we have seen that there are numerous research projects which have considered the effectiveness and mode of action of electroplexy, compared it with other current methods of treatment for depressive and schizophrenic psychoses, and assessed morbidity, compared with these treatments. There has proved to be singularly little cause for the scaremongering which has been put about. No deleterious effect on the brain function has ever been established. On the contrary, the improvement effected by the relief of the psychotic state is of considerable benefit to sufferers.

The side-effects associated with the seizure and with the administration of anaesthetic have become minimal as a result of advances in the technique. The types of side-effect which occurred with earlier methods of inducing seizure discharge are no longer relevant or valid. No more effective method of treating affective psychosis has yet been devised, and until convincing evidence can be shown that the new anti-depressants are as safe and as rapidly effective, there seems no justification for discarding ECT, bearing in mind the seriousness of the disease process.

It seems to the author a strong argument that seizure therapy for psychoses has stood the test of a quarter of a century, since it revolutionised the treatment of affective psychosis in psychiatric hospital wards in the 1950s. Furthermore, it has been found acceptable and useful among practitioners working within widely differing social structures and political systems. Psychotic illness has a worldwide distribution which seems little affected by race or creed, and the use of electroplexy has been equally worldwide.

Further Reading

Fink, M., *Convulsive Therapy: theory and practice*, Raven, New York, 1979.
Medical Research Council Report, *Clinical trial of the treatment of depressive illness*, 1 (881), 1968.
Miller, F., 'Psychological Theories of ECT. A review', *British Journal of Psychiatry*, 113 (1967) 301.
Pippard, J., and Ellam, L., *Electroconvulsive Treatment in Great Britain, 1980*, a report to the College of Psychiatrists, Gaskell, London, 1981.
'Royal College of Psychiatrists' memorandum on the use of ECT', *British Journal of Psychiatry*, 131 (261) 1977.

Questions

1. What are the indications for the use of electroplexy?
2. How does it appear that electroplexy exerts its mode of action?
3. What types of trial can be used to assess the effectiveness of a treatment?

9
Relationship of Psychiatry with other Disciplines ('Liaison Psychiatry')

Psychiatry is a branch of medicine and cannot therefore be seen nor can it operate in isolation from other disciplines. In order to understand the interaction between mental processes and disturbances of bodily function or disease, the psychiatrist must have a medical training and all other doctors should now have at least a ground-work of training in psychiatry.

Certain areas, however, will have closer affinities with the speciality than others. Perhaps the most important contact is with the primary care team headed by the general practitioner. The majority of referrals to the psychiatrist will come through him and in due course those who leave hospital will be referred back to him.

The psychiatrist, however, more so than in many other specialities, must develop close contacts with non-medical specialities and colleagues, particularly in such areas as social work, occupational therapists and clinical psychologists.

Many diseases may manifest themselves in different ways and because of their presentation arrive on the doorstep of one speciality or another. This is perhaps particularly so in neurology and neurosurgery, though is also true in endocrinology, dermatology and other medical specialities.

Indeed, in many countries neurology and psychiatry are combined, the specialist acting in both areas and combining both roles. This is not the case in Britain but in recent years there has been the development in some regions of neuropsychiatric units where there are staff trained in both disciplines, neurology and psychiatry, and where the problems associated with epilepsy, brain tumours or cerebral infections may be studied. Here those patients who present with psychiatric disturbance but in whom there is an underlying neurological disorder may be assessed and treated.

We shall now look at some of these areas of overlap in a little more depth.

General Practice

The majority of the milder psychiatric disorders, in which we include many of the neuroses and depressive states, never reach the psychiatrist at all but are dealt with entirely by the family doctor. Furthermore, the majority of cases that are referred for a second opinion to a psychiatrist will be followed up and treated subsequently by the family doctor. Probably some 25 per cent of the general practitioner's work is concerned with psychiatric problems, and he or she, as the primary care team, will be the first to be consulted, even in those cases that require hospital admission.

With the development of community care and the expansion of community psychiatric nurses working with the primary care team and the health visitor, the community is increasingly taking over the day-to-day treatment of all but those needing acute hospital care. The average length of stay within hospital is now less than six weeks. Thus the majority of patients, even those with psychotic conditions such as schizophrenia, will be well enough to return to the community and again come under the primary care team at an early stage.

Neurology

In Great Britain neurology and psychiatry have traditionally developed as separate specialities. In many countries, however, one single speciality of neuro-psychiatry has been felt to suffice. There is logic in both traditions. There is obviously considerable overlap between neurology, which has studied diseases affecting the brain and the peripheral nerve supply, and psychiatry, which has studied diseases affecting thinking and emotion. Many of the conditions are common to both, and as the organic aspects of psychiatry develop, more diseases are recognised as having an organic basis to them.

Nevertheless, there is logic in separating the two specialities, particularly with regard to in-patient hospital care, since the needs of the sufferer from a neurological complaint are basically the same as those of general medicine, and the mental processes are not in general affected. In psychiatry, the nursing of patients with mood changes, thought disorder or memory disturbance requires special skills and a different type of daily routine and ward organisation. Much of the investigative procedure will, however, be the same, though in neurology the emphasis will be on discovering specific organic dysfunctions affecting brain or nerve cell activity, and this will reflect itself more in abnormalities of movement, sensation, posture and speech.

Conditions more specifically the province of the neurologist, therefore, would be such diseases as multiple sclerosis, nerve injuries, and tumours or other physical diseases of the brain. We are more interested in the areas of overlap, which we shall now consider.

Epilepsy

The majority of individuals who develop blackouts or fits will be referred to a neurologist for an assessment of their cause. Psychiatric consequences are unlikely. A number of degenerative conditions of the brain, however, may well present with disturbances of this kind, and some degree of confusion or memory disturbance may also be present. Disturbed patterns of behaviour may be associated with epilepsy affecting certain parts of the brain, and in particular the temporal lobe. Temporal lobe epilepsy may mimic some neurotic conditions.

A tendency to epilepsy may also be present in many of the conditions that cause mental retardation, and the proper management of such fits is, therefore, an important part of psychiatric knowledge. The various causes of dementias, which will be considered in Part 2, and in particular the main groups of senile and arteriosclerotic dementia, may well produce epileptic fits as part of their symptomatology.

Looked at in reverse, some cases of serious epilepsy, where fits are only poorly controlled and are frequent and long-standing, may produce damage to the central nervous system eventually through repeated minor episodes of oxygen deprivation during the fit, through the traumatic effects of falls and blows to the head, or from whatever the underlying cause of the fits themselves may be. Furthermore, psychotic conditions are occasionally seen associated with epilepsy, usually similar in character to the symptoms of paranoid schizophrenia. Not uncommonly, the epileptic patient may develop a personality disturbance as a result of the frustration associated with the condition. Epileptics may be feared and socially less acceptable in some societies; their activities are restricted through fear of injury and their career openings are reduced. Not being allowed in control of a vehicle, in the armed forces or police force, or in diving and scaffolding are obvious examples. All this may combine to make the more severe epileptics somewhat bitter and discontented with their lot.

Headache

This symptom is frequently found in states of anxiety and depression, but can also be associated with neurological disturbance within the brain, with high blood pressure or with other general diseases—for example, of the kidney or liver. Thus the proper investigation of headache needs to take into account both fields of expertise. Migraine is one such condition where the two areas overlap.

Syphilis

This condition, the great mimicker of other disease, has, as we have seen, a great historical importance in psychiatry. The long-term effects of the infection reaching the central nervous system can induce a dementia, and untreated may result in eventual long-term psychiatric hospital care. The earlier meningovascular effects, however, may very much be the province of the neurologist. The early infective phase will be the province of the venereologist, and even the skin specialist, who may be called upon to decide on the cause of the rash. Some manifestations of the disease, such as involvement of the heart valves, may be treated by the general physician or cardiologist, and the social implications and preventive aspects will lie with fields even outside medicine such as sociology. Thus some diseases may encompass many disciplines, owing to the great variety of the nature of their symptomatology.

Brain Tumour

The discovery of a new growth affecting the central nervous system would, when diagnosed, be the province of the neurologist and neurosurgeon, should operative intervention be necessary. Here psychiatry and neurosurgery may overlap, in that a significant proportion of brain tumours present with disturbances of emotions, thought or behaviour, and are initially seen by the psychiatric services. Furthermore, a number of cases of apparent generalised dementia that come to post-mortem may prove to have unsuspected brain tumours, which have not been diagnosable during life.

Tumours affecting the frontal lobe of the cortex in the brain are particularly liable to induce emotional or personality changes, and such a possibility must always be borne in mind when somewhat atypical neurotic or hysterical features are present in a previously stable personality and some level of intellectual deterioration is noted. Some 10 per cent of brain tumours are picked up during psychiatric assessment in hospital or out-patients' departments.

Neuropathy

Peripheral nerves in the limbs are particularly susceptible to damage from deficiency states or toxic processes acting on the nerve cell. Such changes, if they occur in the limbs, will present with disturbances of coordination, position sense or the ability to distinguish touch or pain. If the autonomic nervous system is involved, then disturbances of internal bodily function and, in particular, sexual dysfunction may be present. Bladder or bowel function may also be disturbed. If the condition affects the central nervous system, then the usual disturbances of memory, emotion or thought may appear. In such a case referral to a psychiatrist may be most appropriate.

Common causes of peripheral neuropathy are some anaemias, particularly pernicious anaemia due to deficient absorption of vitamin B12, diabetes and thyroid disease. Hypertension, nicotine poisoning, and many other toxic products, including heavy metals such as lead, can produce similar symptoms. Some other neurological diseases, such as multiple sclerosis and some collagen diseases, can produce similar effects, and all must be distinguished from the glove and stocking anaesthesia, which is occasionally seen as part of an hysterical neurosis.

A wide variety of rarer conditions sometimes also needs to be excluded when making a neurological investigation of a psychiatric problem. Various specialised tests, including electro-encephalogram, brain scan and X-rays will need to be employed. The central effects of worm infestations such as cisticercosis, slow infective processes such as tuberculosis and leprosy, tropical diseases such as sleeping sickness, and the rare case of deliberate poisoning by another individual with such substances as cadmium or beryllium, should always be at the back of one's mind.

Psychology

A study of psychology must naturally form a major element in the training of any psychiatrist.

Psychology can be defined as the study of the **normal functioning of the mental processes or mind**. It is as anatomy is to the surgeon. Pathology, on the other hand, is a study of what goes wrong in the anatomy of an individual, and psychopathology is the study of abnormal psychological mechanisms. An understanding of mental mechanisms and the theories underlying such processes as learning, personality development and perception form a basis on which much psychiatric disturbance can be understood.

The examination for the Diploma in Psychological Medicine required a year's study of psychology, and written and oral examinations at the end of the course.

The psychiatrist should also learn how to make the best use of the expertise of the clinical psychologist on the staff of most psychiatric units, in order to collaborate effectively. He will need an understanding of the uses and limitations of psychological testing—particularly in the fields of intelligence, personality and emotion—and the contributions made by behavioural treatments deriving from the early work of Pavlov and his studies of learning; and also the psychodynamic theories deriving from Freud and later workers, which form the basis of psychoanalytical and, indeed, most psychotherapeutic treatment models, both individual and group.

The reader is recommended to study a companion volume, *Psychology Made Simple*, in order to obtain a wider knowledge of this area than is appropriate in this volume.

The Clinical Psychologist

The clinical psychologist has played an increasing role within the psychiatric hospital and, indeed, in other branches of medicine in recent years. We might compare him to the biochemist in the general hospital or the pathologist associated with a surgical team.

The earlier and traditional role of the psychologist working in the clinical field was to provide assessment and evaluation through psychological testing of such factors as intelligence quotients, memory impairment or personality distortion. These tests would provide an objective and quantified measure which might be helpful in forming a proper diagnostic appraisal or used for serial comparisons of progress.

The usefulness of some of these tests is limited, however, and, increasingly, clinical psychologists have worked in therapy, especially as it relates to behavioural treatment for such conditions as agoraphobia or obsessional neuroses, and the removal of deviant behaviour, such as is found in some sexual problems. At a ward level they have also taken part in monitoring progress of rehabilitation programmes, group work, programmes of further training for staff, and research.

Thus, on the one hand, an active clinical psychology department within the hospital can provide a very useful service to patients and to the psychiatrists responsible for such patients; and, on the other hand, the psychiatrist or doctor-in-training working in the hospital must obtain a working knowledge of the skills available through the clinical application of psychological principles in order to utilise these services to the full. The working knowledge acquired will also give increased depth to his own understanding of mental illness.

Sociology

The study of the social mechanisms which operate in society has in recent years increased its scientific status. Departments of Sociology and of Social Studies, with their own academic staff, have been set up in most universities. The sociologist studies the way in which society orders itself and the factors which operate within social groups, including the pressures affecting such groups and the individual.

Thus sociology, like psychology or anatomy, is a study of normal structure, but abnormal sociology may also be a legitimate area of study. Its purpose is to investigate those factors which cause societies to disintegrate and which produce disruption and stresses on the individual when the society is not a healthy one, or the individual is unable to adapt to the society in which he finds himself.

Sociological theories relating some types of psychiatric illness to social stress have been developed and it is in this area that the work of the psychiatrist and sociologist can overlap. The psychiatrist, furthermore, needs to keep abreast of research in this field if he is to pay proper regard to the significance of the environment in which the patient must live.

The Social Worker

Before the passing of the 1959 Mental Health Act, the arrangements for admission to hospital under compulsory orders rested with the duly authorised officer, who had certain statutory duties conferred through the courts. Mental welfare officers, subsequently introduced, developed considerable expertise in dealing with community psychiatric problems, and had statutory powers under the Mental Health Act to detain and convey patients and make applications to the hospital if compulsory admission was necessary. They also played a considerable role, however, in following up patients who had been discharged back into the community, and liaising with the psychiatric social worker in the hospital.

This arrangement was changed with the reorganisation of the social services in the early 1970s. Mental welfare officers and other care workers who had specialised in the care of the elderly, of children and such special services as care of the deaf, were combined into a generic social service department, so that in theory all social workers should have skills in handling the problems of mental illness and should be able to provide case work for families, but in addition continue to act in the capacity of mental welfare officer as designated under the Mental Health Act.

Such social workers have gradually devolved special interests. Most will have received training through the Department of Social Administration at a university, and they are employed within the Department of Health and Social Services to deal with the social problems that occur in the community. Thus they have a very wide range of interests and must deal with a very wide range of problems. They have certain statutory powers concerning children in care, and many other commitments apart from those under the Mental Health Act. Most psychiatric hospitals have social workers attached or working from the hospital as a base, who, therefore, work closely with the psychiatrist, dealing with a range of problems extending from the old almoner duties of helping patients and relatives with practical matters such as housing and bedding and accommodation, through to the more skilled use of case work, particularly with the families of those with psychiatric problems.

Therefore, as with clinical psychology, the trainee psychiatrist should establish a sound knowledge of the role and function of social workers and have some understanding of the way in which such provision can be best utilised for the patient's benefit. In many types of psychiatric problem there is a considerable overlap between social problems and mental disorder, and the concept of the multidisciplinary team, with a psychiatrist, community psychiatric nurse, social worker and family doctor all working together so that the family unit can be helped to cope with the problems that a psychiatrically ill member may produce, has promoted a level of cooperation which has enabled much more effective work to be done within the community itself, frequently to the extent of hospital admission or relapse being prevented.

Biochemistry

Major advances in the knowledge of the chemical processes within the central nervous system and the role these play, certainly in the development of psychotic illness and in the dementias, is making a knowledge of biochemistry increasingly important to the psychiatrist. While this subject is an integral part of the basic training of all doctors, the particular application of neurobiochemistry must be studied in more depth if a proper understanding of such matters as the mono-amine metabolism mentioned in earlier chapters is to be understood.

Pharmacology

What has just been said of biochemistry is equally true of the study of the chemical action of drugs and medicines, and the effects which such products have on the body and, particularly, on the central nervous system. Again, pharmacology is an integral part of the basic medical training, but in psychiatry a particular knowledge of neuropharmacology is required so that the application of biochemical advances in the understanding of brain function can be translated into an understanding of how such drugs as the anti-depressants, phenothiazines and tranquillisers work. Not only the mode of action but the side-effects, both short- and long-term, which these products may have is essential before anyone should presume to prescribe them.

Statistics

Finally, in psychiatric research a knowledge of statistics is becoming increasingly important. Research in psychiatry must rely to a large extent on the controlled clinical trial, where double-blind procedures are utilised to compare one group of people with another in, for example, assessing the effectiveness of a new method of treatment.

In the double-blind cross-over trial a product whose effect is already well tried may need to be compared with a new product recently on the market. A group of patients suffering from the appropriate disorder are placed randomly on either of the two active drugs or, conceivably, with the patient's permission, on either an active drug or a placebo—that is to say, a non-active preparation—for comparison. The two preparations to be administered are made up identically and the prescriber does not know which of the two products is being given. He rates improvement, the presence of any side-effects that develop and so on at regular intervals, and at the end of the trial the key is broken and the results of the two preparations can be compared. This blind procedure eliminates observer bias and prevents the patient and the ward doctor from making value judgements about a product, which might interfere with the proper assessment of its effectiveness.

In order to assess critically the value of results from such therapeutic trials, which are frequently written up in the medical journals, a knowledge of statistical method, in particular as it relates to correlation matrices and techniques such as standard deviation, chi², T tests and distribution curves, is highly desirable.

Neurosurgery (Leucotomy)

Operations on nerve tracts within the central nervous system, i.e. within the substance of the brain, have been practised at a primitive level for a long time, certainly as far back as Egyptian ancient history. The substance of the brain being very complex, however, and its workings associated with personality and mood, much mystique has surrounded the problems of surgical interference, and emotion at a somewhat primitive level has been allowed to colour the thinking of some who should have been able to apply a more rational judgement.

Early operations on the brain were principally to relieve depressed fractures, to remove foreign bodies or attempt to drain blood clots. It became apparent over the years, however, that damage to certain areas of the brain produced specific types of defect. Thus, mapping of the motor and sensory areas of the brain was able to take place. It also became apparent that certain areas of the brain, particularly the frontal cortex, were concerned with the control of personality function. More recent research into deeper structures has shown areas relevant to emotional states. Traumatic injuries during the World Wars added to our knowledge, as has experimental work on animals.

Some 50 years ago it had been established that the division of certain nerve tracts travelling between the emotional centres of the brain in the limbic lobe and the frontal cortex were particularly relevant in the control of mood states. The division of these tracts was found to create a state of euphoria and relief of tension. The more careful application of research into the function of these areas showed more specifically which nerve centres were significant.

Since nerve cells, once severed, do not regenerate in the nervous system, the division of such tracts should not, of course, be undertaken lightly. It is a final attempt, comparable with the removal of a limb when gangrene in the periphery would otherwise threaten life. It is a poor way to solve the problem but it is better than the alternative.

Egas Moniz first developed the operation that has come to be known as leucotomy in 1936 in Portugal. The operation was found to be effective in chronic unremitting depressive states, severe obsessional states, and in some cases of schizophrenia. As has been described in our historical section, the early operation, while allowing many seriously and chronically ill mental hospital patients to lead more normal lives and in some cases return to the community, which was a considerable step forward compared with their prospect of life-long hospital institutionalisation, was too radical a procedure to be used in less serious cases. Personality disturbance was excessive, causing a somewhat fatuous and sociable mood which, while better than the previous state, still made such individuals a problem to themselves and their relatives.

Moreover, the operation itself had serious hazards to it. The procedure was done blind through two burr holes drilled into the frontal part of the skull and a knife known as a 'leucotome' was used to divide the particular tracts in the central nervous system which seemed associated with this excessive level of tension and stress. There was some danger of bleeding, and subsequent scar formation led in some 10 per cent of cases to the development of epilepsy. Nevertheless, this was perhaps a relatively small price to pay compared with the prospect, as there was in those days, of permanent need to be in a mental hospital.

Subsequent workers, however, have striven to make the operation safer and to clarify the indications. In the early days the procedure was un-doubtedly used over-enthusiastically, and it has subsequently become clear that in schizophrenic illness the operation has not achieved dramatic results, though certainly good results were obtained in some severer cases at a time when other procedures were not developed. The standard operation has become modified and new techniques of brain surgery, whereby the opera-tion can be done by means of stereotactic techniques under X-ray control, have made the operation much more accurate. Techniques of electro-coagulation have reduced the danger of bleeding and allowed extirpation of the tissue to be carried out in a clear field. Finally, the use of radioactive implants, which can be accurately localised, has reduced further the dangers of long-term side-effects from scarring.

The function of the fibre tracts have also become much more clearly under-stood, and particular areas can now be cut for particular types of problem. The present indications are in chronic recurrent depressive states which have not responded effectively to drugs or electroplexy, in severe obsessional states, and states of chronic high levels of tension. Fortunately, new methods of treatment have allowed this procedure to be used only rarely and as a last resort. Obviously, no one wants to damage or remove any part of the body if its normal function can be restored without recourse to operation. It must be recognised, however, that in occasional cases normal function cannot be restored without recourse to operation, and the end result justifies the procedure in such individuals.

A survey of leucotomy practice in Britain was published in the *British Medical Journal* of December 9, 1978, by Barraclough and Mitchell-Heggs. All forty-four neurosurgical units in the British Isles were surveyed during the period 1974 to 1976, when 431 operations had been carried out, represent-ing a yearly rate of 3.4 operations per million of the adult population. During this period the number of operations had declined from 158 in 1974 to 119 in 1976. This reflected the increased effectiveness of alternative methods of treatment, principally with drugs or behaviour therapy, which have been developing in this last decade.

In some 300 of the operations, stereotactic methods had been used to locate the site for the lesion. The principal psychiatric conditions treated by neurosurgery were severe mood disorders, chronic states of anxiety and tension, and obsessive compulsive neurosis. Other conditions treated were Parkinson's disease and epilepsy.

Two-thirds of the operations were performed in four national centres where specialised expertise was available. A variety of procedures was used, depending on the particular symptoms or desired result. The diagnostic categories in one survey quoted were broken down as follows: depression 24, anxiety 20, obsessional compulsive states 19, violent behaviour 6, anorexia nervosa 5, intractable pain 4, schizophrenia 4 and self-destructive behaviour 3.

It must be recognised that adverse publicity has also been a factor in reducing the number of operations performed. As the article in the *British Medical Journal* points out, if this reduction is based on an improved outcome through alternative methods of treatment and a reduced necessity for operative interference, then that is fine. However, if the reduction is the result of pressure from ill-informed bodies creating an atmosphere of scepticism and loss of confidence among the public, this may have caused a number of sufferers from mental illness who might otherwise have benefitted from such procedures to be deprived of the most effective method of treatment at present open to them.

Minority groups are given the opportunity to be vociferous through the media of television and the press, and there is no doubt that in the United States doctors may be intimidated into carrying out only the most conservative and uncontroversial therapies by the fear of disproportionate claims when things do not go exactly according to plan. Unfortunately, this stifles progress and makes people chary of applying new advances in treatment. One must hope that a similar development does not occur in Britain. To quote Barraclough and Mitchell-Heggs, referring to the decrease in the numbers referred for operation in the last few years: 'Opponents of the operation may approve of the change, but if it successfully relieves mental illness resistant to other treatments ill people may have been deprived of effective treatment. The public's best protection when there is doubt about a controversial treatment is a controlled evaluation'.

Further Reading

Barraclough and Mitchell-Heggs, 'Bifrontal stereotactic tractotomy', *British Medical Journal*, December 9, 1978.

Birley, J. L. T., 'Modified frontal leucotomy', *British Journal of Psychiatry*, 110, 1964.

Laitinen, L., and Livingston, K., *Surgical Approaches in Psychiatry*, MTP Press, Lancaster, England, 1973.

Meyer Gross, Slater and Roth, *Textbook of Psychiatry* (3rd edn).

Sperling, A., and Marlin, K., *Psychology Made Simple*, Heinemann, London, 1982.

Ström Olsen, R., and Carlisle, S., *British Journal of Psychiatry*, 118, 1971.

Questions

1. What is temporal lobe epilepsy?
2. Is it a good idea to have two specialities (neurology and psychiatry) as in Britain?
3. What neurological disorders may present to a psychiatrist?
4. What is a leucotomy operation?
5. What are the modern indications for such an operation?
6. Are these operations performed at your local neurosurgical unit?
7. How many are performed per annum?

Part 2: Psychiatric Syndromes

In the second part of this book we shall be considering individually those conditions normally treated by specialists in psychological medicine, finishing the book with chapters on sub-specialities which have problems unique to themselves, such as child psychiatry and the treatment of psychosexual disorders. Before embarking, however, some further thought should be given to the question of classification of psychiatric problems.

In the absence of clear confirmation of the underlying causes of many psychiatric disorders, it has been customary to describe syndromes where a characteristic pattern of symptoms presented with sufficient regularity and consistency to be identifiable as an entity in themselves. It has further been customary to divide what have been known as functional illnesses—that is to say, where no organic cause had as yet been discovered at the time that the syndrome was identified—into two types, known as psychotic and neurotic, the former being those where insight in severer cases was lost.

Another logical way to classify disorders might be on the basis of response to treatment. This at present may be particularly appropriate in psychiatry, since it is symptom clusters that are being treated, in terms of physical methods of treatment, and thus the predominant symptom might be used as a method of grouping. This procedure has been adopted in the second part of this book. It will be recalled that psychiatry was defined as being **that branch of medicine which dealt with conditions that presented with disturbance of thinking, emotion and, arising out of these, behaviour.** To this might be added a separate group of disturbances of memory and intellectual function. As many of the so-called functional disorders are likely to have an organic basis and thus be just as physical in the long-term as, say, diabetes, a subdivision into functional and organic is likely to prove increasingly artificial.

The first conditions to be considered will be those where a **disorder of thought is the predominant and primary condition.** We must qualify this by stating that it is those conditions of disordered thinking which arise in a clear consciousness, removing from the group such conditions as acute delirium following, for example, a febrile illness. The conditions to be included will contain the schizophrenias, paranoid states and paraphrenia.

The second major group to be considered will be those where **a disorder of affect** is found. Affect may be disturbed in four primary ways, namely, depression, elation, anxiety or fear, and aggression. We shall include under those conditions where the mood change is one of depression or elation the psychotic manic-depressive illnesses, and also depressive reactions which may be found in company with anxiety states.

Anxiety is the predominant symptom in most psychoneurotic illnesses. It will thus include pathological anxiety, felt as a continuous or pervasive process by the individual and probably endogenous in character, and also those states of anxiety reactive to elements in the environment, particularly phobic states, in which the anxiety relates to a particular situation or object. Some phobic states may be monosymptomatic, referring, for example, to such things as fear of heights or the dark; or they may form a symptom pattern usually known as **agoraphobia**, which in its original translation means 'fear of the market place', where the fears are congregated on a group of situations dependent upon leaving the home and entering crowded places, shops, travelling on buses and so on.

In addition to the anxiety states and depressive reactions found in psychoneurotic conditions, there are certain other specific kinds of symptom. **Obsessional compulsive states** occur where the individual feels compelled to reiterate a thought or a phase or carry out some ritual action often associated with tidiness or cleanliness; or patients may have a recurrent thought, sometimes of a phobic quality, where, for example, they may fear they will utter a swear word out loud in church or perhaps fear that they will commit some crime or harm their child. Often the performance of some ritual comes to be associated with relieving such fears, and because it temporarily relieves anxiety, becomes a fixed pattern of response. Such rituals may get out of hand and completely disrupt the individual's life.

Another pattern of condition found in psychoneuroses is that of **hysteria**. This word has come to be used almost as a term of abuse in general conversation, but technically we are referring here to a condition of disturbed function which can affect any part, and which is not a symptom of any underlying physical disease. Often an hysterical symptom can be recognised by the fact that the disability does not follow the characteristics that would be expected of an organic loss of function in such a part. The disturbance may be a loss of sensation, a loss of movement or loss of awareness for pain. There may be a loss of memory (hysterical amnesia) or a loss of vision or hearing. Indeed, any function of the body can be affected in this way. The condition is an interesting one, and perhaps has some sort of switching-off function in a brain which is faced with an intolerable anxiety-provoking situation. Commonly, secondary gain develops as a result of the disturbance of function, and tends to perpetuate it. Such disturbances of function can be induced under hypnosis and often the hysterical symptom itself can be removed by hypnosis or suitable drugs, and the element of hyper-suggestibility is, therefore, apparent. Commonly, the patient shows a lack of concern for the disability which is surprising to the observer, and this was referred to by Janet as *la bel indifférence*.

A further symptom complex found in psychoneuroses is that of **deperson-alisation**, which is perhaps somewhat allied to hysterical symptoms, since again a switching-off mechanism seems to be brought into play. Basically, there are three types of symptom quite commonly found in association with anxiety states but sometimes also seen in normal individuals under stress and sensory deprivation, in hypnogogic states before sleep or just on awakening, and in certain types of epilepsy. In the first type there is an altered awareness of one's self-image. Thus, on looking in a mirror the individual fails to recognise the image as being that of himself. Something seems to be changed, or, in awareness of body size, parts of the body seem to be bigger or smaller than they really are.

A second type, often known as **derealisation**, is the same thing applied to the external environment. Here, the individual on looking out perhaps at a familiar view, lacks a sense of recognition, although knowing full well that the view is familiar. The same recognition problem may arise with regard to other people.

Finally, there may be a switching-off of emotional feeling whereby the patient, for example, although in a situation of sadness and apparently displaying the signs of grief, denies being able to feel the inner experience which would normally accompany it. This is sometimes found in psychosexual problems also, where the patient, while showing evidence of sexual arousal, denies any feeling for the same.

The final group of conditions where a change of affect predominates is that of **aggression**. This as an entity in itself has received little attention in orthodox psychiatric textbooks. Nevertheless, it is a predominant part of many of the personality disorders and is widespread as a symptom of many conditions. It seems probable that there is a condition of endogenous aggression where the mechanisms in the brain concerned with levels of arousal are overactive. The opposite pole of this is **apathy**, which can again be seen as an entity in itself. This theme will be taken further in the relevant chapter.

This leads us to the third major category in our general classification, that of **disorders of behaviour**. Under this category would be included the personality disorders, in which character traits in terms of mood, obsessionality, aggression, inadequacy or immaturity reach extremes that bring them to medical attention. The severest form of this is seen in the diagnosis of psychopathy—a condition which has a special place in the Mental Health Act—where social awareness and the ability to empathise are minimal. In this group we also include deviant personalities, where addiction to drugs or alcohol is a main feature, and those where sexual deviation is the presenting complaint. It will be realised that this group encompasses a heterogeneous mixture, often with differing aetiologies.

The fourth main group of conditions are those where **intellectual function, memory and orientation** are impaired. Such conditions usually arise as a result of temporary or permanent damage to the brain function, either from the toxic effect of substances in the circulation or from degeneration of the brain cells themselves. A very wide variety of physical organic illnesses can produce states of confusion. In general they can be divided into the acute problems of **delirium** and the longer-term problems encountered in **dementia**. Certain conditions in the latter category have been of historical interest in psychiatry, particularly the dementia resulting from general paralysis of the insane, the old term for the late effects of syphilis affecting the nervous system. A further heading under this group of conditions is that of **epilepsy**, which can commonly manifest itself with psychiatric problems.

Finally, there are disturbances of brain function occurring from birth, where **amentia** or **subnormality of intelligence** is the major problem.

Three other subgroups that do not fit readily into the categories described above will be considered. First, there are **psychosexual disorders**, where psychological factors often predominate in conditions such as impotency and frigidity. Secondly, there are conditions found exclusively in **childhood**, and it is convenient to group these under a separate heading. Autism is perhaps the most significant of the psychotic problems, but many behaviour disorders in children and adolescents require special consideration.

Finally, a special chapter has been devoted to **forensic psychiatry**—that is to say, those aspects of psychiatry which have medico-legal implications.

Much learned thought has gone into providing satisfactory classifications for disease and in particular in this book for psychiatry. The exercise need not bother us over much, except to be aware that systems of classifications have been developed and are under review. The system that operates within Britain is known as the international classification of disease (ICD) and has now reached its tenth revision. Such classifications are useful in terms of statistical research since they provide a standardised form of classifying and describing conditions and these can be converted into computerised records in terms of defining the incidents and prevalence within a community and trends in diagnosis.

In the United States of America another system is found and this has now reached its third revision (DCM 3). Both systems have their advantages and are a little different in the way they approach the problem. The major criticism of such systems in psychiatry is that at the present time it is not really possible to classify conditions other than as symptom clusters when we do not have much knowledge of the underlying pathologies or these conditions.

10
Conditions Where Disorder of Thought Predominates

Summary

Thought disorder is the dominating symptom in a group of conditions that come under the heading of schizophrenia, and in conditions originally referred to by Kraepelin as paranoia. Schizophrenia is here defined as a number of syndromes, possibly with differing aetiological factors, characterised by a disorder of the thought processes, of emotional response and of behaviour. Delusional ideas and hallucinatory experiences are common. Untreated, the majority of cases progress to a residual schizophrenic defect state. The cause remains unknown, though research points towards a genetic factor being implicated, biochemical disturbances in brain mono-amine metabolism causing a generalised distortion and fragmentation of the thought process, and environmental factors probably acting as triggers in the presence of such predisposition.

Subdivisions

Certain sub-types of schizophrenia where particular symptom clusters predominate can be identified:

1. **Hebephrenia.** Disorder of thinking is the most marked feature, with delusions and hallucinations. Common age of onset, late adolescence.

2. **Catatonia.** A type of schizophrenia where motor activity and behaviour are predominantly disturbed.

3. **Paranoid schizophrenia.** Delusional systems are usually the presenting symptom, principally of a persecutory nature. The onset tends to be in middle age, and the personality remains more intact.

4. **Simple.** An additional category introduced by Bleuler, where loss of drive and emotional flattening are the principal features.

5. **Residual schizophrenia.** The late effects of schizophrenia common to all groups, where emotional flattening and lack of drive, with some general deterioration of personality, are seen.

6. **Paraphrenia.** A type of schizophrenia seen in the elderly, and characterised by a fixed delusional system without the deterioration of personality seen in younger cases.

7. **Paranoia.** This term has now come to refer to a group of rarer conditions, characterised by monosymptomatic delusional systems, which are held with obsessional intensity, but without evidence of other psychotic thought process developing, as usually occurs in schizophrenia.

General Incidence

Worldwide research has found an incidence of a little under 1 per cent of the population, with only minor variations.

Main Symptoms of Schizophrenia

1. A disorder of thinking.
2. A disorder of emotion, characterised by flattening or incongruity.
3. A disorder of motor behaviour, often manneristic behaviour.
4. Delusional ideas.
5. Hallucinations, predominantly but not always auditory.
6. A general fragmentation and deterioration of the personality.
7. An absence of any disturbance in the level of consciousness.

Differential Diagnosis

Other conditions that can mimic and may be confused with schizophrenia, particularly in the mild or early stage, are other types of psychosis, such as manic-depressive illness, hysterical phenomena, temporal lobe epilepsy, and organic disturbance of brain function from a wide variety of causes.

Treatment

The mainstay of the control of schizophrenia now lies in anti-psychotic drugs. Electroplexy may still play a part in the acute stages. In the long term, re-habilitation and careful follow-up to monitor the patient's environment and progress are essential.

Prognosis

The outcome for recovery from an individual attack is now good, but the necessity for long-term maintenance therapy remains in the majority of cases. The outcome becomes more guarded in those cases where recurrence becomes frequent and present therapy is unable to maintain control.

Description

In this chapter **we shall be considering those syndromes found in the group of schizophrenias and paranoid states.** Some confusion arises over the term 'schizophrenia'. The word is often used incorrectly by the mass media, and the general public will immediately respond to schizophrenia by saying: 'Oh yes, split personality: Jeckyll and Hyde'. In fact, this sort of picture is usually more characteristic of the hysterical personality, and bears no relationship to the type of fragmentation of the thought processes which occurs as part of a schizophrenic breakdown. What may show as an incongruity of thinking in some kinds of schizophrenic breakdown is the ability of the patient to hold two conflicting beliefs while apparently being uninfluenced by the incongruity of this fact. For example, an individual with a grandiose delusion that he or she is a person of some importance in world affairs may, at the same time, be quite contented to be on a hospital ward assisting a nurse with some menial task which would be quite inappropriate to his or her delusional beliefs.

What does seem to happen is that the individual is unable to sort incoming sensory data and to perceive these in a logical way. This inability on the part of the patient to make clear judgements, and the false beliefs that may arise therefrom, explain much of the bizarre ideas and the apparently incongruous emotional behaviour which may follow.

A number of theories have been put forward in an attempt to explain what happens to the thinking processes, and these theories often reflect the particular interest or bias of the research worker putting them forward. Some workers have suggested that there is an **over-inclusive thinking**, i.e. the individual is unable to filter incoming data and decide which should be retained at a conscious level and which discarded as background. Patients may complain that their **thinking becomes fragmented**, in that they cannot hold a visual image in their mind, or that it becomes distorted. When reading, they may find that a sentence becomes fragmented, and they cannot make sense of the whole by the time they have completed reading it.

There appear to be **certain discrete patterns of presentation** of such illnesses. These are characteristic, regardless of the populations considered, and there are probably discrete underlying chemical disturbances in brain function which explain this. It may well be that the symptoms of thought disorder are the outward expression of these inner disturbances but are quite non-specific in the same sense that a cough may be an expression of a variety of diseases in the chest, and the subtle differences between one cough and another are the only way of distinguishing the differences in the underlying problems.

Kraepelin in the nineteenth century first distinguished three characteristic types of presentation of such illnesses, which were then known as *dementia praecox*, since, untreated, the disease often progressed to an apparent dementia, and often began in adolescence. Bleuler in 1911 added a fourth group. It seems probable that there is some interchange of these groupings, but their descriptive value has nevertheless remained valid.

Incidence and Causation

The incidence of schizophrenia is in the region of 1 per cent of the population. This holds true, with small regional variations, whether the survey is carried out in Britain, the United States, Russia or China, in primitive areas in Africa and South East Asia, under capitalism or communism, Catholicism or Confucionism. It thus follows the pattern of other diseases which appear to have an inbuilt and often genetic cause. Under these conditions the prime problem seems most unlikely to be of a sociological nature or to arise from cultural determinants in the shape of parent–child relationships. Epilepsy is a similarly common condition, but no one has suggested that it might be caused by peculiar mothers!

The incidence is higher in those families with an already affected close member. It is higher still among brothers and sisters, even higher than that among twins, and highest of all among identical twins. This is so whether the identical twins have been reared together or apart, which is another strong argument that inheritance plays a large part in causation. However, the genetic mechanism is not a clear-cut one, as it is with such things as eye colour or the inheritance of a disease such as haemophilia. It seems probable that a number of genetic mechanisms come into play, and that this may predispose the individual in some way (presumably through a biochemical disturbance of mono-amine function in the brain, since these are the chemicals which make nerve cells work) to the development of the disease in certain cases. Some sort of environmental or emotional trigger may be required to set off the disease process. This is not unknown in other conditions where emotional factors can be important.

Biochemical Disturbance

Attempts have been made to isolate the biochemical disturbances in this group of conditions, with some success but at times with conflicting results. One snag in investigating diseases of the central nervous system is that it is not in general possible to make direct observations in the living person, and biochemical changes are usually impossible to trace at post-mortem, since the enzymes concerned will deteriorate very rapidly once death has occurred. Observations must, therefore, be made of parts indirectly affected, such as cerebrospinal fluid, the blood and breakdown products which may be found in the urine.

An abnormal breakdown product of mono-amine metabolism has been found in the urine of some patients with schizophrenic breakdown. This is known as DMPE for short, or dimethyl phenyl ethylamine. Animal studies have shown that if a purified extract of the urine or cerebrospinal fluid from such a patient is injected into an experimental animal, disturbances in behaviour occur, though they are not shown with a control group. Furthermore, a metabolic disease known as **homocystinuria**, which, as one of its effects, produces abnormal mono-amines in the circulation, often produces in such patients psychological changes very similar to those of a schizophrenic breakdown.

Other research has shown an abnormal pigmentation in some patients suffering from schizophrenia. This pigment is melanin and is probably produced in response to a hormone within the pineal gland in the brain. Again, melanin and its breakdown products are related to the mono-amines that are important in central nervous system function.

Finally, the **effect of hallucinogenic drugs** and stimulants such as **amphetamine** (which is again a mono-amine related to those used in brain function) is sometimes to produce a syndrome in many ways indistinguishable from schizophrenic illness. Hallucinogens such as lysergic acid and mescaline are also related to mono-amines. Some fascinating botanical and pharmacological studies have been made on the use of plants from which the substances have been derived. Many are found in Central America, in particular in extracts of certain cactuses and toadstools. These have been used by the native people for centuries, and it is interesting to note that different varieties of the plants produce slightly different hallucinogenic experiences, though the underlying chemical reason for this has yet to be ascertained.

Epidemiology

Much **epidemiological work** has been carried out on schizophrenic syndromes, showing, for example, that schizophrenia is commoner in immigrant populations and in the lowest two socio-economic groups (4 and 5). If, however, the socio-economic group of the parents is considered, the scatter of the disease shows itself equally spread over all groups in the community. This suggests that the higher incidence in groups 4 and 5 is due to the effects of the illness rather than the reverse. In other words, people who have suffered a schizophrenic breakdown tend by and large to drop in the social scale as a result of the after-effects of the illness.

Some workers have suggested that there may be carriers of the disease who show a muted form in terms simply of some personality disturbance. They have found that, through the use of hallucinogenic drugs, such carriers can be spotted, and a pedigree plotted as a result of the temporary induction of psychotic symptoms.

The theory of the schizophrenogenic mother, as put forward by Lidz, would seem to have little to commend it. In the present state of our knowledge it seems regrettable to suggest that parents may have any influence over the creation of a state such as schizophrenia in their offspring, though it is possible that parents may show a carrier state themselves and, therefore, have some difficulty themselves in making relationships More likely the parent is affected secondarily by the poor ability to empathise of a schizoid child. There is no properly tested research showing that parental behaviour can in any way cause schizophrenia in someone who would not otherwise develop it.

Symptom Patterns

It is possible to identify a number of typical patterns in the symptoms and course of schizophrenia, which could imply slightly differing underlying chemical disturbance. This seems particularly to separate the **paranoid schizophrenia** group from the others; some of the biochemical changes and abnormal breakdown products found in the urine seem to be found in the non-paranoid groups and not in paranoid schizophrenia.

Hebephrenia

The first pattern we shall describe corresponds broadly to the type which Kraepelin referred to as hebephrenia. The onset of the disease can usually be identified as occurring in adolescence or early adulthood—hence the old term of *dementia praecox*, describing an illness which came on in the post-pubertal years. With hindsight, abnormalities of personality can often be identified even earlier, the individual being solitary, introverted and schizoid, with slightly bizarre and isolated interests, an aesthenic build, and, showing in the year or so before obvious symptoms appear, a deterioration in work record, in personal social graces, and in generally withdrawing from contact with his fellows.

There follows a breakdown in individuals' ability to handle rational arguments and to absorb abstract concepts. Their thinking and conversation become obscure. People talking to them may fail to make much sense of their answers. In the less intelligent adolescent who vocalises less well this may not be immediately apparent, and in the highly intelligent individual, who perhaps decides to study philosophy at university, it may be difficult at first to distinguish immature ideas from thought-disordered ones.

After these early symptoms, evidence of a more marked disturbance of thinking usually becomes apparent, along with **delusional ideas**. This may be gradual but can in some cases occur quite suddenly, with the development of a primary delusion in the shape of what is known as an autochthonous idea. The individual may suddenly come to the realisation that something has changed: that he or she has an important role to play or that some inspiration has been given to them in some vision-like way. This may be associated with an **hallucinatory experience**, and, out of this, secondary delusional ideas develop to explain to the individual's satisfaction the presence of the hallucination. The content of these delusional ideas and the explanation for hallucinatory experiences will vary with the individual's culture and beliefs. Thus his or her interpretation may be given a religious flavour or be thought of in electronic terms or telepathy. The experience may leave the sufferers frightened or exhilarated. People have described feelings of ecstasy associated with some of these manifestations of disordered thinking.

Hallucinations

The hallucinatory experiences in schizophrenia are most commonly auditory. There are certain typical patterns. First, **the individuals may feel that their own thoughts are being spoken aloud or echoed**. The thought is their own but is externalised—it appears to come from outside. Probably the simplest way to understand this is to imagine that the impulses that are tracking through the central nervous system track in on the wrong line. If something which is actually a thought tracks in on nerve routes which are appropriate to hearing, since they come from nerves derived in the inner ear, then the brain will interpret these consciously as hearing impulses even though their origin may have been in another part of the central nervous system itself. This apparent externalising of impulses which derive from the cortex is very characteristic of schizophrenic thinking.

Secondly, the **auditory hallucinations may appear as if overhearing a conversation**, a group of people talking, or other sounds such as music. As these become stronger and impinge on consciousness, the sufferer is aware of their content and may feel that the voices are recognisable, sounding like people that he or she knows. What they are saying may also be recognisable, and is often derogatory to the individual. These thoughts are again, of course, originating in the brain of the sufferer but are interpreted as coming from outside. The loss of insight associated with this illness may make the sufferer genuinely believe that these people are indeed saying things about him, and he may then act on this, to everybody's discomfort. This sort of projection may lead to ideas of persecution, but this is more typical of the paranoid schizophrenia described later.

The third kind of hallucinatory experience is that where the voice appears to be directed at the patient, telling him to do things or in various way directing his life-style. Again this may be thought of as an externalised thought, and it often has a compulsive quality whereby the sufferer feels that he must obey the voice even though a part of him may recognise that this is foolish. It was with these cases in the past, where the illness had become more severe, that some danger of aggressive outbursts was present.

Hallucinatory experiences may not only be auditory but can be experienced through any of the senses, though those experienced through hearing are the commonest in this disease. Visual hallucinations are unusual, but may consist of seeing figures of a threatening type or distortions of shapes. Often these are frightening to the patient. Occasionally, hallucinations of smell or taste are found, leading to the belief that, for example, food is being poisoned. Finally, tactile hallucinations may occur, the sufferer believing that he or she is being touched or that things are crawling over the skin. These hallucinations may be experienced as electrical-like shocks which the individual believes are being applied deliberately by outside people, perhaps neighbours, and, particularly in the elderly, these often seem to have a connotation of sexual assault.

Other Symptoms

We have covered in some detail the type of thought disorder found with delusional and hallucinatory experiences. Three other symptoms are common. There is usually **a change in emotional state** or feeling, commonly described as a **flattening of affect** or an **incongruity of affect**. Here the emotion appears inappropriate to the situation and is often shallow, the patients recognising that they do not feel things as strongly as they used to do.

In addition, there is commonly a **loss of drive** or energy level, the patient becoming rather lethargic and lazy and unable to concentrate on his normal activities. He may get up late in the morning and lose jobs as a result of this inability to get going. The housewife may become sluttish through lack of attention to her work. This is one of the most difficult aspects of the disease to treat, and one which often carries over into the residual after-effects of the acute illness.

Finally, there may be **motor symptoms**. The patient may develop **mannerisms** or may seem to have a rather stilted wooden gait. Movements do not seem to come quite as naturally and automatically as in the well person.

H.Y., a girl of 19, had been quite successful at school, taking O levels and two A levels. A bit of a loner, she had nevertheless got into teacher training college. For the first two terms things went well enough but in her third term she began to be reported for non-attendance, found great difficulty in getting up in the morning and began to neglect her personal appearance and hygiene. By the beginning of her second year she had become more strange in her habits and would spend long periods of time alone writing material of a vaguely philosophical nature which had little purpose or content to it. Her admission to hospital was arranged at a point where her parents became aware that she was leaving used sanitary towels around the house inappropriately and with no reasonable explanation.

At this first admission there was little to identify except some mild degree of thought disorder and it was difficult to be certain if this was the diagnosis. After a period of observation she was discharged and went back to college on medication, which she apparently did not continue. Tragically her next admission came when she was pregnant some six months later and could only give a short list of possible fathers. Her habits had deteriorated further and she now admitted to thoughts being repeated in her head and seeming to come from somewhere outside and which influenced her behaviour. Clear-cut first-rank symptoms had therefore taken somewhat more than a year to become fully developed. Untreated these would likely progress to the more florid stage of schizophrenia seen 40 or 50 years ago with unpredictable and impulsive bizarre behaviour, retreating into a little twilight world of their own and unable effectively to communicate with others. This girl fortunately responded well to delayed release injections after an initial course of phenothiazines and was able eventually to take up and complete a librarianship course.

Simple Schizophrenia

The second pattern of illness is that which was in 1911 described by Bleuler as simple schizophrenia. Here again the problem usually starts **in late adolescence**. The more florid symptoms such as delusional thinking and hallucinatory experiences are not found, and the characteristic problem is the development in a previously stable and hard-working individual of a progressive withdrawal from social contact, a **loss of drive** and a **loss of interest** in the person's previous pursuits. Thus a bright adolescent perhaps working at school for GCE examinations may begin to show a deterioration in school reports and in output of work. At first this may be put down to the development of some adolescent crisis, but over a period of time the true nature of the situation becomes apparent. At a later state hallucinatory experiences may appear, but the autistic withdrawal remains the dominant feature though the end result of a schizophrenic residual defect state is very much the same in both syndromes described. Many such patients become vagrants and itinerant wanderers, and fail subsequently to keep a job, though this may be less so with modern methods of treatment.

B.T. was a young man of 24. Interested in somewhat esoteric hobbies from his teens, he had nevertheless qualified in a trade and had been working for two or three years as an electrician. He had always been considered reliable and trustworthy. Over the course of some six months, however, his work record steadily deteriorated. He became lacking in drive and enthusiasm and when asked just said he didn't feel well. Some emotional blunting was evident and his personal relationships with a girlfriend and with his friends in general tended to wither. Then he threw up his job altogether and stayed at home, living with his parents, spending most of the time in his own room listening to records, becoming virtually a recluse in his own house. Later he decided to eat in his own room and sometimes for days would not speak to other members of the family. At one stage his parents wondered whether he was taking drugs but this was never the case and full investigation failed to reveal any physical abnormality.

The youth resisted attempts to get him into hospital for rehabilitation and his parents were in a great dilemma as to what to do with him. Eventually it did come to hospital admission and once there the youth showed very little drive or desire to do anything or even to leave. Sometimes more obvious signs of thought disorder develop. Usually the residual defect state is resistive to therapy and in this young man's case it was not until the advent of pimozide after he had already been in and out of hospital over a five-year period that real improvement was noted and he was eventually able to get back to a more useful life-style.

Catatonia

A third type of presentation is that known as catatonia. Here the dominant feature is a **disturbance of behaviour**, though an underlying thought disorder is also present. Individuals may become **mute or stuporose**, not making any movement and ignoring all attempts to rouse them. This may be interspersed with **sudden outbursts of bizarre over-activity** which are unpredictable and may be self-destructive. The patient retains a clear consciousness and is often able to recall such episodes quite lucidly when in due course he recovers. **Negativistic behaviour** may appear, with the patient doing the opposite of what is requested in an apparently compulsive manner. A condition known as **flexibilitas cerea** may also be seen: translated this means 'waxy flexibility' and refers to the situation where an individual may posture and remain in a position, say, with hand raised if the doctor has put it there while doing an examination, instead of bringing it down again, or may sit in the bed in this position, if allowed to, for many hours. The normal individual would find such a posture extremely tiring on the muscles. It will be appreciated that in the acute phases of such an illness the nursing care must be very attentive if problems are to be avoided.

A woman of 32, when seen in the hospital bed, sat bolt upright with one arm outstretched. Seemingly she had held it like this for some time when, in any normal individual, the arm would have rapidly become tired. It was a hot summer day and the windows were open but she did not move even when an insect flew in and settled on her face and made no attempts to brush it off. She did not speak and made no sign of acknowledgement when spoken to. She remained in this state for some hours before suddenly and unpredictably leaping out of bed and rushing to a window which she smashed with her bare arm, cutting herself in the process. When questioned some weeks later, when recovered, as to whether she recalled the episode she had a clear memory of the events. She recalled that at the moment that her arm was cut by the glass she had a feeling of ecstasy rather than pain akin to a religious experience.

Sometimes the main presentation is that where **mood change** is the striking feature. This may be a mood of elation, with a fatuous shallow jocularity, or a depressive picture, with morbid delusional ideas. Sometimes the picture may be one more of psychopathic behaviour, with the individual developing an apparently amoral attitude, lacking in conscience, and not uncommonly promiscuous. This picture can be confused with manic-depressive illness or with psychopathy.

The key to the diagnosis in these syndromes lies in the change in personality from a previously stable-functioning individual. This contrasts with the pattern seen in disturbed personalities from emotionally deprived backgrounds who have shown a pattern of disturbed behaviour, though admittedly without the bizarre thought disorder that may occur in schizophrenia, right from childhood. More careful psychological testing will often show a deterioration in abstract thinking and an inability to cope with cognitive tests. Thus the ability to give the meaning of a proverb and the tendency to answer in concrete terms is commonly found. When schizophrenic thought disorder is described as showing over-inclusive thinking, this means that the individual is unable to filter out the important salient features of a problem or a sentence spoken to them, and is continually confused by the simultaneous presentation in consciousness of things which the normal individual would exclude as being irrelevant.

Schneider has considered the problems of diagnosis in conditions where confirmatory laboratory tests are not as yet available. He proposes in schizophrenia that a set of first rank symptoms are *pathagnomonic*. These include particular types of hallucinatory experience of voices commenting on one's actions, thought echo, and the development of the primary delusion.

Furthermore, the presence of any degree of confusion or intellectual deterioration should put one on one's guard for an organic cause of some other sort affecting the central nervous system, since in schizophrenia this should not occur. Further diagnostic tests to eliminate these, including blood tests, EEG, X-rays, etc., may need to be performed.

Paranoid Schizophrenia

The group of schizophrenias where **paranoid delusional ideation** is the predominant feature seem to form a slightly different population. There is some evidence that the underlying biochemical changes may be different, since in the paranoid group the presence of abnormal metabolites in the urine has not been so consistently found. Furthermore, the onset of the condition is usually **in middle age** or even later, and the personality structure seems to be better maintained. Thus the loss of drive is not so apparent, and if in conversation the presence of the fixed delusional system is avoided, then the individual may present a relatively normal picture to the untrained observer.

Paranoid schizophrenia usually presents as **an abnormally suspicious individual believing himself to be badly done to** and showing **persecutory ideas** which may develop grandiose elements, the patient feeling that the very fact of persecution provides evidence for his or her importance in some special way. For example, the belief that the police are watching may develop, or there may be an occurrence of **ideas of reference**, where particular significance is attached to cars passing in the street, or items in the newspaper or on the television which seem to the patients to be directed personally towards them. They may believe that this is because they have some personal knowledge of great importance or have been chosen perhaps by some power to lead people. This may turn into a **messianic complex**, and, indeed, such individuals have been known to acquire quite a following before the more bizarre elements of their illness make it plain to even their devotees that something is wrong. The type of delusion may follow a current fashion and relate to German, Russian or Chinese spies or some religious group, depending on the individual's previous interests, age and experience.

An accountant aged 47, shortly after the first Telstar satellite had been put in orbit, began to hear things in his head which seemed to come from outside. Although these voices seemed to be saying that he should go to Germany because he was a reincarnation of Hitler he illogically decided that he must be hearing radio waves from the satellite. This is a good example of the fragmentation of thinking which can occur in schizophrenia whereby two mutually incompatible beliefs can be seemingly held at the same time.

Secondary elaboration of this primary delusional system was for the man to assume that in order to pick up this transmission someone must have implanted a receiver in his ear when asleep. Acting on these ideas he did indeed go to Germany for a few days but returned to this country where his increasingly irrational behaviour led his wife to consult the doctor.

A woman of 48 became convinced, perhaps because of some gustatory hallucination, that somebody was poisoning her food. Before her illness she had been a keen Conservative party worker in a local town and became convinced that members of the Socialist party were trying to do away with her because of the keen work she had done. Later she became convinced that Mr Heath, the then Prime Minister, was in love with her and wrote him frequent and amorous letters. When pressed she showed evidence of his returning her love by a letter which had the House of Commons stamp upon it. When persuaded to show the contents of this letter it proved to be a routine letter to all party workers issued after the election thanking them for their work in a successful campaign.

Paraphrenia

This condition is best described as a schizophrenia that occurs in the elderly. Again, as in paranoid schizophrenia, the personality remains intact, and the more generalised symptoms of disturbance, such as are seen in the younger hebephrenic, are rarely found.

A fixed delusional system often of persecutory type generally develops, often associated with hallucinations, which may affect any of the senses, including touch and smell. Not uncommonly such individuals are found to be rather deaf.

The typical presentation is an elderly person who believes that neighbours are stealing her possessions or breaking into her house, or that the upstairs lodger or burglars in the attic are interfering with her, perhaps in a sexual manner, by means of electric shocks through the floorboards or some such delusion. Sometimes these delusions are misinterpretations of real feelings in the body due perhaps to rheumatism. If taste is distorted, then the old person may believe her food is being poisoned and refuse to eat. If smell is distorted, then such persons may believe they are being gassed by a leak or by some deliberate act of neighbours piping poisonous fumes into their house through the wall.

Such elderly people may become a nuisance to the police or to neighbours by their persistent accusations, or by aggressive behaviour in response to these delusional ideas. They may make frequent unwarranted complaints, and may even act on their suspicions by becoming aggressive towards those whom they see to be persecuting them. As paraphrenia is a psychotic illness, insight is lost and simple reassurance has no beneficial effect. It is always important to recognise in the elderly person that these symptoms may be a manifestation of a pure paraphrenia or may herald the development of a dementing process, with impairment of memory and intellect, as will be described in a later chapter.

An elderly lady lived in a block of old people's flats. She became convinced that the equally elderly lady in the flat below her was entering her flat through a forged key and doing mischief while she was out. She attributed tiny scratches on her furniture and articles she believed had been moved to the attentions of this other lady.

Her problem continued despite changing the lock on the door and she branded the lady below as a demon. Matters came to a head when she marched downstairs and hit her neighbour over the head with a frying pan.

Until recently paraphrenia was difficult to treat. Fortunately, some of the newer drugs that have come along in the last few years, in particular haloperidol and pimozide, have led to considerably better control. Persuading such elderly people after they leave hospital to continue taking their medication, particularly as many of them live alone, is, however, often a difficult matter.

Paranoia

The term paranoia, an ancient one, was used in Kraepelin's classification. It is the word from which the term paranoid derives. It is customary now, however, to use the term to describe a fascinating group of rarish syndromes having in common that they are monosymptomatic psychoses, i.e. there develops a fixed idea, often with a persecutory element to it, which the patient then holds as a unshakeable belief irrationally and despite evidence to the contrary. The difference between these conditions and those of paranoid schizophrenia or paraphrenia is that in the pure state there seems to be no progression to a schizophrenic type of illness, with generalised thought disorder, hallucinations or personality disintegration.

Many of these fixed delusional ideas have been given specific names, usually that of the person who described the syndrome. French psychiatrists seem to have been particularly interested in describing some of these rare forms, but it seems probable that although all are interrelated, and while in some cases external events may produce what could be called a reactive psychosis, in many cases some internal mono-amine malfunction is at the root of the development of some of these patterns of false recognition and distorted thinking.

Perhaps the commonest of the paranoias is that known as the **Othello syndrome**. This syndrome gets its name from the character of Othello in Shakespeare's play and refers to persons who develop a fixed idea that their partner is being unfaithful to them. While genuine infidelity is, of course, common enough, sufferers from the Othello syndrome develop a bizarre, fixed delusional syndrome relating to their partner's infidelity, usually on the flimsiest of evidence, without the partner in fact being engaged in an illicit affair. Often it seems to be associated with feelings of sexual and other inadequacy on the part of the sufferers, who may go to quite extraordinary lengths to provide proof of their partner's misdeeds. The way in which milk bottles are arranged on the back step is adduced as evidence of a message to a would-be lover. The sufferer may return from work during the day and insist on stripping beds and examining underwear for evidence of recent sexual activity. Physical assault may take place in efforts to extract a confession, and murders are not unknown. Evidence of the presence of psychosis as opposed to a genuine suspicion usually comes from the bizarre and increasingly absurd nature of the evidence which is being provided, and the patient's total lack of ability to see a reasoned argument on the subject.

A man of 45 suffered some degree of erective impotence and was an unsatisfactory lover to his wife. His self-image was poor, being unable to get reasonably paid employment, while his wife, somewhat larger than himself physically, worked as a successful secretary. Gradually the idea began to form in his mind that his wife was having an affair with a man who lived in a house abutting their back garden. There was, in fact, no real evidence for this at all but he deduced from bizarre evidence such as the order in which the empty milk bottles had been put out at the back door and other such trivial matters that she was indicating her readiness for some illicit liaison. Eventually this man killed his wife while trying to extract a confession from her by choking her with a stocking tied round her neck. The charge of murder was reduced to manslaughter on the grounds of his diminished responsibility due to mental illness and he was sent to Broadmoor Hospital.

Many more such syndromes are detailed in *Uncommon Psychiatric Syndromes*, by Enoch and Trethowen. The **Cap Gras** syndrome is another intriguing one. It is also known as the 'delusion of doubles', and in it patients become convinced that their partner has been replaced by an impostor. A schizophrenic element to such thinking shows in the fact that such patients go to tremendous lengths to convince people that the person they are living with has replaced their real partner. They may write letters to the Home Secretary and badger the police to find their original lost partner, and produce 'evidence' of trivial and slight differences in their partner's behaviour which shows that they are a different person. They will admit that the likeness is uncanny, and while being totally convinced that this 'new' person is an impostor, at the same time continue to live and share their bed with them. Sometimes such conditions move on to a full-blown schizophrenia, but usually remain in this *forme fruste*.

In another similar syndrome the patient may believe that strangers in the street are, in fact, his spouse, or perhaps some important person, such as the Prime Minister, disguised, so that here there is a false recognition.

Such people may become a menace by accosting strangers in the street and being unconvinced by their denial that they are who they are believed to be. On other occasions the patient may believe that some important person, perhaps a pop star or royalty, is in love with them, and pester them with letters and 'phone calls, convinced that such a person is about to come and sweep them away to be married. They will show evidence of correspondence with such a person to prove their point, often simply a formal letter, perhaps from the Prime Minister's secretary acknowledging receipt of their letter and some such phrase as the matter is being looked into, or similar piece of Civil Service jargon. This letter is carried around as proof of the eternal love of the Prime Minister for them! Such people not infrequently find themselves in the hands of the police through complaints eventually being made about their behaviour. These syndromes are known as **L'illusion de Fregoli**, and **De Clerambault's syndrome** respectively.

Another set of conditions which may come under the title of paranoia are the **monosymptomatic hypochondriacal psychoses**, where the fixed delusion, often sustained over many years, is that the patient is suffering from some type of physical illness they consider is being missed by all the experts. Often such patients become quite aggressive with medical advisers who try to reassure them that there is nothing physically wrong. This fixed delusional system must be distinguished from the less severe simple hypochondriacal phobia found in neurotic illness.

These monosymptomatic hypochondriacal psychoses may present in a variety of ways—for example, a delusion of skin infestation with insects or internal parasites or worms; a dysmorphic delusion, with a conviction of personal ugliness; or an insistence on the misshapenness or over-prominence of some bodily part, despite all evidence to the contrary. The same type of delusional body image disturbance may be seen in some cases labelled as anorexia nervosa, and in some cases of intractable chronic pain. Sometimes patients believe that they emit some sort of foul smell which others can sense, or that they give off some kind of sexual aura which is noticeable to other people near them.

While each individual syndrome is rare, the total number of cases suffering from paranoia is perhaps something around 5 per cent of all psychoses seen. The age range at presentation is very variable, the peak age for men seeming to be about 40 and for women about 60. Sex distribution is equal and the condition seems to be worldwide. Untreated, the condition can be very intractable and psychotherapy has no impact. Fortunately, pimozide given orally, or a delayed release injection, is now effective in many cases.

Residual Schizophrenia

Untreated schizophrenia in the past led eventually to a state of pseudo-dementia, which explains the old term *dementia praecox*. This was characterised by progressive deterioration of personality and intellect, with complete loss of drive, and emotional incongruity and flattening. This deterioration, combined with the inevitable results of long-term institutionalisation (the same kind of thing as has been seen in long-term prisoners in gaol in the past), led to a cabbage-like state divorced from reality, where the patients lived in a fantasy world following a simple organised daily routine, usually in locked wards with airing courts in which they might take exercise. By-products of such a state—for example, compulsive masturbation done publicly and lacking any awareness of social offence—led in some minds to the idea that moral degeneration was the cause rather than the effect of the illness.

B.S. had been a long-stay patient in a psychiatric hospital for some 27 years. Within the sheltered environment of the hospital she coped reasonably well though she tended to neglect herself if not constantly encouraged by the nursing staff and was somewhat eccentric in her behaviour. She had no interest in going out into town, nor in visits from friends or relatives. In discussion, if one kept to normal topics, little evidence of delusional ideation would be noted, but if one began to question her about her parentage she would reveal in a flat and unemotional manner that her father had been king of the world, and lived in Constantinople. She herself spoke all the languages of the world and had had 40 children to various members of the male staff about the hospital.

The incongruity of schizophrenic thinking is shown by the fact that while holding these delusional beliefs she was at the same time prepared to be in a psychiatric ward without demur and to cooperate with staff and to do small jobs such as washing up and helping in the ward kitchen.

Certainly for the 70 per cent or so who finished their lives in this state it was a disease to be dreaded by their relatives, and by patients themselves in the early stages when insight was retained. Like cancer, it condemned an individual to a terrifying end.

Advances in the drug treatment of schizophrenia and a recognition that chronic institutionalisation can be avoided by more sensible hospital routines (the latter can now be applied with control of the more acute symptoms which drug therapy has allowed) can prevent this progression into pseudo-dementia in the vast majority of cases. There remains an end result, however, particularly in those cases where frequent relapse has occurred, and in those more severely afflicted, which is now known as residual schizophrenia. This seems to be the end result of any type of schizophrenia, but especially of the hebephrenic variety. The acute symptoms delusions, hallucinations, etc. clear up, but the patient is left with a loss of drive and flattening of emotional response, which, after an individual attack, may take many months to clear. It is this aspect of the illness that responds least well to current drug therapy, and requires intensive rehabilitation to keep the individual in an active daily routine until it wears off.

The results of these disabilities are most keenly felt in the interrelationship of the patient and his closest friends and relations. Both will be aware of an inability to feel deeply on the part of the patient, and insensitive relatives or those who have not had the condition explained to them may read into the symptoms laziness, or lack of caring, on the part of the sufferer.

Indeed, the social environment of the schizophrenic both in and after discharge from hospital has been intensively researched. Deterioration and relapse after discharge from hospital can be countered by two factors—the maintenance of medication on a sufficiently long-term basis, and the support of the social relationships to which the patient returns. These two factors appear to interact, and it has been shown that relapse rates are greatest in families where degrees of emotional involvement, hostility and dominance are high in the relatives with whom the patient is living. This risk of relapse was greater if the patient's contact with these key people was high, e.g. over 35 hours a week.

Recordings of patients' psychobiological responses have confirmed the adverse effect of highly emotional families, with measurable changes in the metabolism of the schizophrenic in these circumstances producing increased cortical arousal. Thus the patient who returns to an emotionally charged environment and stops taking medication has a relapse rate of some 90 per cent, whereas those in an emotionally neutral environment who continue to take medication have a relapse rate of only 15 per cent. Those in a charged emotional environment but continuing to take medication had a 53 per cent relapse rate and those who, although discontinuing their medication, had an emotionally neutral environment had a relapse rate of 42 per cent. These figures are quoted by J. P. Leff, and are summarised in the *British Medical Journal* of 19 July 1980.

The implications of these statistics for the schizophrenic sufferer are that, where possible, a neutral environment should be achieved, and careful follow-up should attempt to ensure that the patient realises the need to continue taking medication even when feeling well, sometimes over a period of years. The real importance of this is that with each relapse the disintegration of the personality can become more profound, and the chances of full recovery that much less.

Treatment

The treatment of schizophrenia is basically the same for all varieties, and stems from the development of chemical compounds known as phenothiazines, the first of which was chlorpromazine, mentioned earlier. Chlorpromazine is of great historical interest as being the first of the phenothiazine drugs to be used widely and successfully in the treatment of schizophrenic breakdown. It has, however, a number of side-effects which are disadvantageous, its sedative effect being one of the most important. Sedation may be useful in the early stages of an acute episode but is certainly no help to the rehabilitation of the residual state. Its other main snags are a tendency to cause people to get excessively sunburnt when out of doors, owing to a photosensitivity, and its occasional production of jaundice as the result of a toxic effect on the liver. More recent phenothiazines do not have these disadvantages and may, therefore, be preferable. The intelligent use of the different varieties of phenothiazines is something which can only be acquired by experience, and the introduction of long-acting delayed release injections which can last the patient anything up to four or six weeks, and can be administered at out-patient follow-up appointments, allowing the individual to forget about his illness or tablet-taking in the intervening period, has been a great advance.

The **phenothiazine drugs** principally deal with the aspects of thought disorder which are found in schizophrenia, and the relief of delusional and hallucinatory experiences. The curative effect appears to relate to monoamine metabolism in the brain, and presumably the correction of abnormal metabolic pathways, the full significance of which is not entirely clear. Much of the research work has related to the findings quoted in that aspect of Chapter 5 on causation, and particularly on the relationship of such drugs to normal mono-amines found as neuro-hormones in the central nervous system, different ones controlling different aspects of brain function. It has also been the result of research on hallucinatory drugs such as mescaline and LSD, which again show similarities in function, and in the type of symptoms they produce, with that found in schizophrenia and the mono-amines which may be disturbed.

The phenothiazines have, however, been relatively poor at relieving the problems of reduced drive. More recently other groups of drugs, similar to phenothiazines, have been developed, such as the **thioxanthines**. These appear to affect a different mono-amine function in the CNS, namely **dopamine**, and appear to be more effective in improving drive and relieving the residual flattening of emotion which may occur. These are now also available as delayed-release injections.

The paranoid schizophrenias and paraphrenias do not, on the whole, respond quite so well to phenothiazine medication, perhaps because their nature is somewhat different. Another group of compounds, however, the **butyrophenones**, does seem to be more beneficial, particularly in the para-phrenic group, and again the intelligent admixture of such medication by experienced practitioners is likely to be the most effective method of restoring sufferers to their normal potential in the community.

This drug treatment is the mainstay of effective control of the condition and must be continued for at least a year after all symptoms have dis-appeared, and indeed some would argue that a small maintenance dose should be continued for much longer than this on the same basis as treating, say, pernicious anaemia, diabetes or epilepsy, where prevention of recurrence is obviously important if further damage to the individual is to be avoided. If the metabolic defect is going to be present for life, then the correction of it must also be continued on that basis.

In addition to drugs, however, electroplexy can still be very effective in those cases of schizophrenia where there is a marked emotional component or disturbance of behaviour—in particular, therefore, the hebephrenic and catatonic groups. In the past insulin coma treatment was employed with some success to relieve these acute manifestations of the disease, but this has now been replaced by electroplexy (ECT). A course of something like eight to twelve treatments, twice-weekly for some four to six weeks, is effective, in combination with the drugs mentioned above. Improvement is thus more quickly effected and the length of stay in hospital reduced.

Psychotherapy by itself is of no value in schizophrenia, and methods of behaviour therapy are probably only of use in residual schizophrenia, where relearning of social behaviour and removal of antisocial behaviour patterns may be desirable in helping the individual to be rehabilitated into the community.

Rehabilitation

What *is* vitally important, however, is to encourage the patient who is re-covering from such an illness to **re-establish social contacts** and to **re-establish work patterns** through **occupational or industrial therapy** projects and other types of rehabilitation, so that he does not, as happened often in the past, become institutionalised and accumulate a group of secondary problems which are just as debilitating in terms of full recovery as the original illness. To this end psychiatric units devote much of their time to such projects, which are as much a part of the treatment as the medication and nursing care itself. Furthermore, this care must be followed through into the community after discharge through day hospitals and social centres. Help may also need to be given to the patient's family to allow them to come to terms with some of the residual problems and to handle them sympathetically. Thus, the social services department, the general practitioner, the district nurse with psychiatric experience, the community psychiatric nurse, and the consultant psychiatrist in out-patient departments all have a continuing part to play if the morbidity of such an illness is to be reduced. Patients may find it easier in some cases not to live on top of their relatives, but may survive better in lodgings or hostel accommodation, where emotional expectations are less.

What has been achieved, therefore, in recent years, is that by acquiring control of symptoms with drug medication, the patient has been enabled to benefit from rehabilitative programmes which previously would have been impossible because of their disturbed behaviour. People should no longer need to feel fearful of this diagnosis, since treatment is now as effective as in, say, diabetes or pernicious anaemia.

Prognosis

The outlook in schizophrenia now for a first attack is good. It seems better in those with an acute onset, and where there is a marked affective component to the illness. It is less good in the gradually progressive hebephrenic or simple schizophrenia, with marked deterioration in drive and emotional flattening. While the residual symptoms may prevent an individual from returning to his full normal occupation, in most cases the use of long-acting intra-muscular injections of phenothiazines or related drugs, combined with a better understanding of the follow-up needs of such people, has made the outlook much more favourable. For those who do not suffer further attacks, restoration to their normal life-style within something like three months from onset is to be expected.

For the smaller proportion who do continue to suffer relapses, or who do not make a good response to initial therapy, the future is certainly much better than it used to be. Thus the new long-stay are only a fraction of those who required long-term care in the past. Some of this group may have to settle for less pressurised employment and for some degree of sheltered environment. The provision of day hospital and day-centre care, combined with local authority hostels and sheltered accommodation, has enabled many of this group to live now out of hospital, though they may need to come in from time to time for restabilisation.

There currently remain in psychiatric hospitals a nucleus of the older long-stay patients, comprising those who developed schizophrenia many years ago, before treatment was available, and who remain in hospital because they either continue to show residual symptoms which make it impractical for them to live in the community, or because of the effects of institutionalisation, plus the fact that over the years all their friends and relations have deserted them. Usually it is a combination of all three factors. For this group the rehabilitation energies of the hospital must still be put to work, in particular the use of such activities as industrial therapy, by which these disabled people can relearn a work routine with production incentives and active social rehabilitation.

This particular group is diminishing as the years go by, by virtue of the fact that we are no longer adding to it, except in very small numbers. At the same time such individuals are growing older within the hospital, and many are now past retirement age.

This reduction in full-time in-patient needs for schizophrenia in the last decade has resulted in suggestions by the Department of Health and Social Security, fuelled by somewhat naively optimistic reports from certain writers in the journals, that psychiatric beds can be run down to a total of some 0.5 beds per 1,000 population, and that the long-stay might all be housed in the community.

While a small number of these patients with residual problems would be able to survive, given plenty of community support, in some group home or hostel, the cost of providing and staffing all these small units or group homes is prohibitive. Furthermore, it is a dubious kindness to remove somebody who has been in a hospital community for many years, where he may have friends, security, colour television and three square meals a day, plus the social life which such an environment allows, and place him instead in the wider and ofter rejecting non-community of the local town. Here such people will have few of the facilities mentioned above and indeed many, while accepted in a more tolerant environment of a mental hospital, will stick out like a sore thumb, because of their residual eccentricities, when placed among so-called normal people.

Furthermore, we do not yet know what will happen to patients currently moderately controlled on medication over the years ahead. Will improvements in drug therapy and an understanding of the underlying problems and causes of schizophrenia allow treatment to progress, or will we see a number of patients later in life gradually getting out of control and requiring readmission as their families die off, or as they reach retirement age and become less able to support themselves?

Should this latter prove to be the case, then the current vogue for reducing psychiatric hospital beds to a minimum, which even now is making care and treatment difficult, will require rapidly to be reversed. The survey of what has happened to the discharged long-stay patients who have gone into the community in Middlesbrough, which is quoted in Chapter 22, must make sobering reading for those who feel concerned about this prospect.

Further Reading

Coppen, A., and Walk, A., *Recent Developments in Schizophrenia*, Headley Bros., Ashford, Kent, 1967.

Hemmings, G. W., *The Biochemistry of Schizophrenia and Addiction*, M.T.P. Press, Lancaster, England. 1980.

Hirsch, S. R. and Leff, J. P., *Abnormalities in Parents of Schizophrenics*, Maudsley Monograph 22, Oxford University Press, British Institute of Psychiatry, 1975.

National Schizophrenic Fellowship, *Living with Schizophrenics by the Relatives*, The Fellowship, 1975.

Schneider, K., *Clinical Psychopathology* (5th edn), Grune and Stratton, New York and London, 1958.

Wing, J. K., *et al.*, *The Industrial Rehabilitation of Long-Stay Schizophrenic Patients*, Medical Research Council Memorandum No. 42, HMSO, London, 1964.

Questions

1. What are the six characteristics of schizophrenia?
2. What is meant by paranoid?
3. What is the evidence for a genetic as opposed to an environmental cause of schizophrenia?
4. What types of hallucination are commonly found?
5. What is the mainstay of treatment in these illnesses at present?
6. What is residual schizophrenia?
7. If you know anyone who has or is suffering from a schizophrenic breakdown and have the opportunity, try to get the chance to talk to them and note the problems they may have in structuring their thinking.
8. Does your local hospital have an industrial rehabilitation unit?

11
Conditions Where Disorder of Affect Predominates

Summary

Affect may be defined as a continuing emotional state or mood. Affect encompasses mood disorders of depression, elation, anxiety and aggression or anger. In the affective psychoses the disorder of mood is on the depression –elation continuum.

Classification

Three principal types of affective psychosis are recognised. These are designated as unipolar depression, bipolar depression, and unipolar mania or hypomania. The distinguishing feature of the bipolar illness is the existence of both depressive and elated swings of mood in the same individual at different times.

Incidence

Incidence is in the region of 2 per cent of the population. Some 75 per cent of these are the unipolar depression type. In the milder case, distinction between this and neurotic depressive reaction can often be hard to make. Unipolar mania is rare.

Aetiology

As with schizophrenia, there is clear evidence of a genetic predisposition, which differs between the unipolar and bipolar groups, the latter having the stronger genetic factor. There is also evidence of biochemical changes within the nerve cell and in mono-amine metabolism in both groups. There is further evidence to suggest that the early and present environment may be relevant as a trigger to the condition.

Symptoms

As in any psychotic illness, in severer cases insight may be lost. The predominating symptoms are of mood change, within the depressive phase morbid thoughts and ideas of unworthiness, and in hypomania elation, euphoria and grandiosity. Concentration is disturbed. Further symptoms are irritability; sleep disturbance characterised by early waking and a diurnal mood swing; and loss of appetite, libido and general interests, with, in the depressive phase, hypochondriacal, psychosomatic symptomatology and either a retardation of thinking or an agitation with motor restlessness. In the hypomanic phase pressure of talk, flight of ideas and a motor restlessness are seen, often with fatuous punning and clang associations. In the depressive phase the risk of suicide is a particularly important factor to consider.

Treatment

Medication with anti-depressant drugs, for which a variety of kinds are available on the market, and with electroplexy to fall back on in severer cases, remain the standard treatment for the depressive phase. In the manic phase of illness phenothiazines or butyrophenone drugs, again with electroplexy for severer cases, are usually effective. For those with frequently recurring phasic bipolar mood swings the use of lithium products is sometimes of prophylactic preventive value. Psychotherapy is of itself no value in psychotic affective disease.

Outlook

The prognosis for an individual attack is now excellent, and the condition can be relieved in a matter of two to three weeks in the majority of cases. Full recovery and return to normality are to be anticipated, but with the possible exception of lithium, current methods of treatment cannot guarantee there will not be a recurrence at some stage in the patient's subsequent life. Some 50 per cent of cases have further attacks, which again can be treated successfully, and, as with many other diseases in medicine, the nature of the condition is that recurrence can be expected at certain times in the patient's life.

Description

Before considering the psychoses themselves, it is as well to take a look at the use of the word depression in more general terms. Depression is used in everyday language to describe a feeling of gloom or mournfulness as a response to some life event. In this context the word is being used to describe a feeling or symptom and not a disease. It is comparable to the word cough in that it describes something that is happening to the individual and not a cause or diagnosis. A cough may be a normal response to some irritant in the room, such as smoke. It may be a nervous habit, it may be from an upper respiratory tract infection, or from some more serious condition like tuberculosis or cancer of the lung. It may be possible to distinguish one type of cough from another by its sound, but to assess its seriousness other investigations may be necessary. Thus it is with depression. The symptom may be symptomatic merely of environmental pressures or imply some deeper underlying or internal dysfunction. The use of the term depression, as in depressive illness, therefore, is a thing to be avoided, since it immediately brings the response 'But doctor I have nothing to be depressed about'. Yet the patient with abdominal pain when told he has appendicitis is not likely to respond 'But doctor I have nothing to be appendicitic about'.

Thus we can classify depression as a symptom which is found (1) as a reaction of a healthy individual in environmental stress, e.g. bereavement, (2) as an over-reaction in a neurotic personality to the type of stress with which other people would probably cope (this group will be considered in the next chapter), (3) as a symptom associated with other organic disturbance or generalised bodily disease, in particular disturbances of hormones or metabolic defects such as may be found in myxoedema or from the effect of some drugs, and (4) as a common and often presenting symptom in the affective psychoses, unipolar or bipolar type. It is with the fourth group we are concerned in this chapter.

The disturbance of mood in the psychotic depressive state is often said by the sufferer to be qualitatively different from normal depression. It has a numbing effect on the whole person, and can be distinguished from the depressive reactions which they may have had in past times in their lives from other external causes. The depression in the affective psychosis arises inexplicably, and is of a depth and type which is not amenable to simple comforting.

Suicide

As Stengel has pointed out, two types of suicidal act may be distinguished. In the first type there is serious intent to produce death. Careful plans may be laid and often hints of the depressed person's intention dropped in the days beforehand. Such attempts are frequently successful.

In the second type, sometimes known as parasuicide, suicidal gestures in the shape of overdoses or self-mutilation may occur, often on the spur of the moment, and usually in the context of a neurotic personality with a depressive reaction or in an individual of immature personality. Usually such episodes are in the nature of a cry for help and do not usually produce death.

There is, of course, no completely clear dividing line. Accidents can happen not infrequently because the individual does not know the dosage of a tablet which is or is not lethal, and may make mistakes in both directions. Parasuicide is some ten times as common as the first type.

The serious suicide attempt is usually found in the psychotic illnesses, particularly where depression is present. Parasuicides are more frequently seen in the type of conditions that will be discussed in the next chapter, of depressive reactions associated with neuroses.

Death by suicide is a very real danger in the affective psychoses, and some 20 per cent of patients attempt to kill themselves during such an illness and some 10 per cent succeed. Successful suicide is somewhat commoner in men than in women, in contrast to parasuicide, which is the other way round. Rates vary to some extent with the availability of the means. Conversion to natural gas was followed by a reduction in the suicide rate, and the more careful control of barbiturate drugs has had the same effect. Nevertheless, some 60,000 suicide attempts are made in Britain per annum, which means that the average district general hospital will probably see upwards of about ten per week.

Suicide rates vary in accordance with the social circumstances of the community, and tend to fall during times of war or civil disturbance. They tend to be lower in predominantly Roman Catholic countries, which may reflect not so much the rate at which people kill themselves, but the tendency in such countries, where there is any doubt, for coroners to record a verdict other than suicide, particularly when the religious group considers such an act to have been sinful or illegal. It seems probable that organisations such as the Samaritans reach in general the parasuicide group, providing support for the disturbed personality but seeming to have little effect on the psychotic suicide, who is unlikely to contact them.

In Britain attempting suicide was illegal until 1961, and remains illegal for survivors of a suicide pact or for those who assist another towards committing suicide. In general, however, it would seem inappropriate for suicide attempts, which are usually the product of psychiatric disturbance, to come within the legal remit.

Methods employed in committing suicide vary considerably. Self-mutilation by cutting a major blood vessel is relatively rare in Western society, but may occur as part of a psychotic illness. Unless very determined, these attempts are usually unsuccessful. The fashion of cutting the wrist is rarely effective, since it is painful, and the blood vessels are deep and not usually large enough to cause lethal bleeding. Usually all the victim succeeds in doing is causing deformity to the hand, through damaging the nerves and the tendons supplying the muscles.

Self-immolation by burning has become more fashionable in recent years, a trend from the Buddhist Far East. Unfortunately, such deaths do tend to receive wide publicity in the press, and this can produce minor epidemics, as can such acts as jumping off high places.

Suicide by gassing has considerably decreased in Britain as a result of the conversion in recent years from coal gas to natural gas for domestic cooking and heating. Carbon monoxide poisoning from car exhaust pipes is still often used.

By far the commonest method is self-poisoning, through the taking of an overdose of tablets or drinking a liquid poison. The tranquilliser and sedative drugs are particularly popular in this respect, as are pain-relievers of the aspirin or paracetamol groups. Barbiturates, though more dangerous than the minor tranquillisers, have decreased as a cause of suicide since their dangers have become more clearly known to the medical profession, and voluntary bans on the prescribing of barbiturates have been enforced in many parts of Britain for some years. Most potentially lethal drugs are controlled through prescribing, but unfortunately aspirin and paracetamol, which have serious toxic effects on the kidney and the liver, are far more dangerous in the long term than many of the drugs available on prescription. The commonest drugs used for minor suicidal gestures tend to be the benzodiazepines, which fortunately are very safe.

The danger of suicide is one of the principal reasons for there needing to be a method whereby individuals with affective psychosis or other serious psychiatric disorder can be admitted compulsorily into hospital. The danger of suicide is a serious one in sufferers from affective psychoses, and since the disease is now fairly easily treatable in the majority of cases, this is a strong reason for being vigilant in order to prevent such unnecessary disasters befalling an individual who within a few weeks will have recovered, and will then probably be grateful for having been dissuaded from such an act.

Unipolar Affective Psychosis

Synonyms for this condition are endogenous depression, psychotic depression and the old term involutional melancholia, which described such a disease occurring around the menopause or after. Episodes of elation are not seen.

The incidence of the disease is somewhat difficult to establish in the absence of a conclusive identifiable test, but probably affects some 2 to 5 per cent of the population within a lifetime. The illness affects women somewhat more commonly than men, and there are peak incidences at times of hormonal disturbance in adolescence, following child birth, and at the menopause. In men the peak incidence tends to be in the early sixties.

Aetiology

A genetic factor of some 12 per cent is found in this illness in first degree relatives, with an increase of some 15 per cent between siblings, rising to some 80 per cent between identical twins. As in schizophrenia, this holds true whether the identical twins are reared together or apart, and the incidence holds remarkably constantly, regardless of the type of social, religious or political structure in which the individual lives.

Biochemical factors have been identified as associated with mono-amine metabolism in the brain. These are principally, first, a disturbance in the ratio between levels of salt and water within the cell and external to the cell membrane. In the central nervous system this balance is very important, the ratio of sodium to potassium within and without the cell membrane being the factor which allows normal nerve-cell conduction. An increase in intra-cellular sodium of up to 50 per cent has been found in these depressive conditions, which would certainly be enough in key areas of the limbic lobe to distort cell function. Second, alterations have been found at the point where one nerve cell links with another, namely the synapse, in parts of the brain concerned with emotion and particularly where dopamine receptors are involved. The chemical transmitter agent appears either to be broken down too rapidly or to be produced in ineffective quantity. This is the rationale for the use of anti-depressant drugs, to attempt to improve the function of the catecholamines at this point. It also seems to be one of the methods by which electroplexy is effective. Third, substances which induce elation, such as amphetamine, which at one time was used as a treatment for depression, are known to act by stimulating these chemicals at the synapse.

This is a rather simplistic explanation of what is in fact a very complicated metabolic structure within the brain of such mono-amines such as noradrenalin, serotonin, dopamine and other more recently discovered systems. What is clear from this research, however, is that distortions of production or function of these substances can certainly occur, and are certainly important in the control of mood states. It is not unreasonable to conclude, therefore, that when these findings occur together, there may be a cause and effect situation whereby chemical changes are linked with the presence of distorted or pathological mood states in the sufferer.

Minor epidemics of psychotic depression appear to follow such epidemics of acute virus infections in the community as influenza. This suggests an environmental trigger whereby a virus may produce distortions of mono-amine function for a short time in individuals who are prone to the disease.

The effect of environment has been carefully considered with regard to its possible role in the aetiology of depressive psychosis. Both circumstances in the early environment, which might predispose people to developing the illness, and the current environment, which might act as a trigger, have been considered. There is little clear-cut evidence to suggest that the present emotional environment of the patient is in any way causative in affective psychosis, although it must be stated that some sociologists have researched what they call life events, and seem to have shown an increase in stress, compared with the number seen in a control group. Such research, however, is full of pitfalls, and the explanations may point towards a different conclusion.

Research into traumatic life events has, however, been developed now both retrospectively and prospectively. Defining what is a traumatic life event is difficult. It is hard to establish whether the traumatic life event was the cause or the effect of a depressive episode in view of the slow onset of the illness and possible retrospective falsification of the event. What can be traumatic to one person may not be traumatic to another. The sad truth is that the vast majority of traumatic life events are unpredictable, unavoidable and occasionally do trigger off an episode in those who are prone to get such illnesses, thus it is unlikely that there is much one can do to guard against them.

Other research has shown that the death of a parent, particularly the mother, within the first few years of life seems to be found more commonly in individuals who in later life develop depressive illness, again compared with a control group. These, however, tend to be retrospective rather than prospective studies, and it is always possible that the reason for death in the mother was itself associated with depressive illness in the parent, when some of the deaths may be attributable to suicide.

Bereavement reactions in the normal individual may in the depression-prone individual trigger a psychotic depression, however, and in this case the timing is much more logical. Presumably bereavement in childhood might act through the basis of disrupting patterns of imprinting, and the grief expressed or repressed could conceivably set up some kind of circuit in the central nervous system which subsequently becomes irreversible. This interaction between the external environment and biochemical factors within the body is, of course, well known in psychosomatic disorders and could equally well apply in depressive psychosis.

Symptoms

The dominating and frequently presenting symptom in unipolar affective psychosis is the depression of mood. Untreated, the illness follows a characteristic course, which can be shown in graph-like form, as in Figure 6. The morbid mood and other symptoms gradually progress over a period of weeks until the maximum of severity is reached. The patient may then remain in this morbid state for some time before gradual improvement begins to

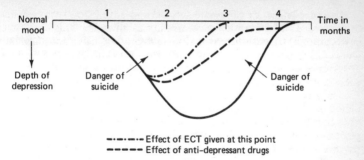

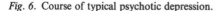

—·—·—·— Effect of ECT given at this point
————— Effect of anti–depressant drugs

Fig. 6. Course of typical psychotic depression.

occur, so that a U shape is formed on the graph, the patient over a period of weeks gradually returning to his normal self. The duration of such an episode varies from a few weeks to some months. In some 50 per cent of cases no further attack occurs, but in the rest a pattern is often seen whereby such an illness may occur in late adolescence, not infrequently having been mistaken for some other condition, such as school phobia, with eventual full return to normality. Years may go by, a recurrence perhaps occurring after on the birth of a child. Again years may go by, with perhaps a recurrence in the mid-forties at the time of the menopause. Thereafter recurrences may become a little more frequent, as shown in Figure 7, and perhaps fizzling out in the sixties.

As things currently stand, treatment can cut short the individual attack and relieve the symptoms until the condition completes its natural course. Neither electroplexy nor current anti-depressant drugs, however, are able to prevent recurrences in subsequent years. But if there are recurrences, each episode must be treated *de nouveau*.

The mood change, as we have noted, is one of morbid depression qualitatively different from normal sadness. The patient feels numb or blank, and is unable to respond emotionally to those of whom he is normally fond. The severity of the depression will vary from case to case, but in more severe episodes there will often be morbid thoughts, with ideas of suicide, delusions of self-blame, and nihilism, fears of death or bodily illness, belief of sinning, or that the patient is the cause of some worldly disaster. At such times insight is lost. The patient may seek a reason for his troubles, and

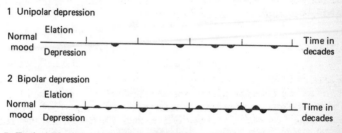

Fig. 7. Typical life pattern of affective psychosis.

blame some aspect of his environment, erroneously believing that he has lost all his money, that he is a failure at work or a failure within his marriage. Patients may take steps to remedy this state of affairs, and it is important that they should be advised not to make any important decisions until the depressive process has cleared, when they are likely to see things in an entirely different light.

A man of 52 presented at the clinic with a six-month history of increasing depressive mood. He had become weepy and could not concentrate. His work record had deteriorated. His sleep was disturbed, waking at 3 o'clock in the morning and being unable to go to sleep again. His appetite had dwindled as had his interest in his hobbies and his interest in the sexual side of his marriage. For the last two or three weeks he had become convinced, despite reassurance, that he was about to go bankrupt and that it would be better for his family if he were dead. He had, in fact, composed a suicide note to his wife but fortunately decided to go and see his doctor before making this final decision. He was admitted to hospital and responded well to anti-depressant tablets in approximately four weeks.

While the depressive mood state is commonly the most obvious symptom, and uncontrolled weepiness is seen, particularly in females, such depression may be masked by other complaints of somatic or bodily symptoms of psychosomatic type, which can confuse the issue and lead to much unnecessary investigation if the appropriate questions have not been asked. Men, in particular, may present with symptoms such as backache, general irritability or constipation, the underlying depression being missed by the unwary.

Besides depression, however, there are a group of characteristic symptoms which occur in the affective psychoses, and indeed may sometimes be more prominent than the depression itself.

Concentration becomes disturbed. The patient loses the ability to read a serious novel or do a crossword puzzle, and often becomes forgetful—for example, when doing the family shopping. Writing a letter or some such pursuit will become an effort. Along with this there is a general loss of interest in hobbies and social activities, the patient feeling that nothing is now worthwhile.

Irritability is another characteristic feature. There is an inability to cope with noise or stress, which often makes the patient, particularly if he is male, intolerant and mildly aggressive. Parents may become unable to cope with the normal chatter and activities of their children. Often in males this feature is more noticeable than the depressed mood itself, which is not always the dominant or presenting symptom.

Along with the loss of interest goes a loss of appetite. Thus food and drink become uninteresting, and the patient becomes anorexic. This often leads to constipation. There is a loss of interest in sexual activity, with a reduced libido, and patients may complain of morning nausea.

The characteristic pattern of **sleep disturbance** is seen, with early morning waking, in contrast to that seen in the depressive neurosis, where initial insomnia is the characteristic feature. The mood tends to be at its lowest in the early morning and improve as the day goes on. This is known as a diurnal mood swing. Thus the patient may wake at 4 or 5 o'clock in the morning feeling extremely low, and the risk of suicide at this time is at its greatest. The family doctor who may see the patient later in the morning will still see a picture which is quite severely depressed. By the time a specialist second opinion is obtained in the late afternoon the psychiatrist may be surprised to find the patient feeling much improved, and denying that there is anything wrong. By the following morning, however, the symptoms are as bad as ever.

A woman of 49 had a past history of depression, each episode lasting 3–9 months, the first was when she was in her late teens and secondly after the birth of her second child when she was 27. She had remained well in the intervening years but now at around the menopause was developing the symptoms of weepiness, agitation and disturbed concentration for which she could find no reasonable cause. She had visited her doctor and been placed on tricyclic anti-depressants but had not gained marked relief and had found the side-effects of dry mouth and blurring of vision unpleasant. It was apparent, however, that her symptoms were continuing to worsen after some three months and she was referred to the psychiatrist. An initial change of medication was not effective and she was admitted for a course of electro-plexy and made a full recovery after three weeks in hospital.

Hypochondriacal and psychosomatic symptoms are frequently found, with such things as headache, backache or palpitations, which again may lead the doctor on to the wrong track if the positive symptoms of depression are neglected.

In the severer cases insight is lost and patients develop a full-blown delusional system, with morbid ideas associated with sin, death or damnation. They may believe that they have murdered somebody, contracted venereal disease or are suffering from some severe wasting illness. They may believe themselves to be bankrupt and even hallucinations may occur, again of a morbid type: for example, visions of the devil or coffins or voices telling individuals that they have sinned. This depth of severity of depression is rarely seen these days because the family doctor is likely to initiate treatment with anti-depressant drugs at an earlier stage.

Two patterns of **motor change** may be seen. In one the patient becomes retarded in thought and speech, and emotion is flat, so that he may stand or sit for hours simply staring into space, saying nothing; this state, if untreated, leads to catatonia or stupor. In the other type the patient becomes increasingly agitated and restless, pacing indecisively up and down and unable to carry out any normal daily activity.

Treatment

The first priority is to establish the degree of risk of suicide, and to decide whether in-patient treatment is necessary or out-patient treatment will suffice.

Drug Therapy

Four types of medication have been found useful in the treatment of affective psychoses:

1. **Amphetamines.** These stimulant drugs are themselves mono-amines, and seem to work by activating the stores of catechol amines at the nerve-cell junction. They are of limited value in treating affective psychoses, since their effect soon wears off, there is a tendency to addiction, and in those with a tendency to schizophrenic breakdown the chemical action is liable to induce a psychotic state of this kind. Their use, therefore, has largely been discontinued, but the significance of their chemical action and the fact that they do relieve depressive symptoms on a short-term basis make them interesting from a research point of view.

2. **Mono-amine oxidase inhibitors.** As the name implies, this group of drugs acts by inhibiting mono-amine oxidase, which is an enzyme that breaks down the mono-amines after they have been released at the nerve-cell junction. This prolongs the action of such catechol amines as are present and, there-fore, in a different way improves the efficiency of the nerve cell within the limbic lobe.

3. **Tricyclic anti-depressants.** These drugs, so named because of their chemical ring structure, are now the mainstay of treatment of affective psychoses. Their mode of action appears to be to allow the increased availability of catechol amines at the nerve-cell junction, so that again they increase the efficiency of the cell mechanism. What we do not know yet is why the cell mechanism becomes deficient in its action in some people. However, although cause and effect cannot yet be adduced, we do know (*a*) that these mechanisms appear deficient in some affective psychoses, (*b*) that these drugs work in a manner which would improve the efficiency and (*c*) that they relieve the symptoms, which is, after all, the most important thing to the sufferer.

4. **Lithium products.** This group of substances is extremely interesting. Lithium salt has been known for many years and used for other purposes. When in the body in solution, lithium chloride like sodium chloride, breaks down into an ionic state. Sodium chloride, which is common salt, ionises—that is to say, the sodium develops a positive electrical charge and the chloride a negative one. The same happens with potassium chloride. These two substances are the main electrolytes, which are important in the conduction of the impulse down the nerve cell. It is the sodium-potassium balance that has been disturbed in affective psychoses. Lithium chloride, when it goes into solution, produces a chloride ion with a negative charge but lithium itself remains inert, i.e. it has no positive charge and is, there-fore, inactive.

The body processes sodium and lithium as if they were the same substance, so that if 50 per cent of the body's salt intake were to be lithium chloride, 50 per cent of the sodium ions in the body would be replaced, molecule for molecule and atom for atom, with lithium. In effect, this is replacing an active, positively charged atom, with an inert one and, therefore, in terms of the electrical potential, is reducing the amount of effective sodium within the cell. Since the level of sodium within the cell is abnormally high in some affective psychoses, and the result of this will be to interfere with nerve-cell conduction, the addition of lithium will restore the electrical activity more towards normal level. Again, we do not know the reasons for this sodium-potassium shift, but it is significant that lithium salts are very effective in preventing mood swings in some affective psychoses.

Anti-depressant drugs of the tricyclic type are, therefore, the mainstay of the drug treatment of affective psychoses. Their mode of action in terms of their effect on individual mono-amines in the central nervous system varies somewhat, and some anti-depressants have a more sedative or tranquillising effect, while others have a more energising effect. Thus, the type of anti-depressant best suited to the individual patient must be assessed and tailored to the individual need. All effective drugs in medicine can have side-effects, and one individual may react differently from another. Thus, if one anti-depressant proves not to be effective or suitable after a reasonable trial period, then another should be tried.

It is important to note that the tricyclic anti-depressants take up to three weeks before they begin to work, so that an improvement cannot be expected straight away. The patient should be warned of this. The main side-effects of the earlier tricyclic anti-depressants were of dry mouth, constipation, and some blurring of vision. These can often be avoided by increasing the dosage only slowly, and reducing again if the side-effects occur. Such problems were not serious, but were of nuisance value.

Some of the newer anti-depressants have attempted to reduce these side-effects by altering the basic molecule of the drug. New ones on the market include the tetracyclic compounds, oxazines, fluvoxamine and fluoxetine. More serious side-effects are rare. The drugs must be continued until such time as the depressive process would have burnt itself out, had the patient remained untreated. In practice this usually means somewhere around six months, after which, if the patient appears well, the drugs can be reduced and gradually withdrawn. This, to some extent, needs to be by trial and error, since the extent of the depressive process cannot be known in advance.

The mono-amine oxidase inhibitors are in general of less value in an affective psychosis. Their use will be discussed in the next chapter.

None of these drugs can prevent subsequent recurrence of the disease, any more than can aspirin prevent a further attack of toothache. The one exception to this is lithium, which has been shown to have a prophylactic or preventive effect in those cases where recurrences are excessively frequent or disabling. It is more effective in the bipolar affective disorders, to be discussed later. The dosage of lithium, however, needs to be carefully controlled through blood tests to assess the level in the body. If below the effective level, it will be of no value, and if excessively high, can cause serious side-effects, owing to the displacement of sodium by the lithium ion, with a resultant sodium deficiency which can effect the function of muscles and in particular the heart muscle. It is not a product to be given lightly, therefore, and should only be used for cases that have frequent recurrences, and the patient should be under psychiatric out-patient surveillance. Some out-patient departments run lithium clinics specifically for this group of patients. The treatment has been of immense value, and has revolutionised the lives of the small number of patients with cyclical recurrent depressive or bipolar psychoses who, until 20 years ago, would in all probability have been chronic long-term hospital patients.

Electroplexy

The mode of action and method of treatment in electroplexy has been discussed in Part 1. It is fair to say that electroplexy revolutionised the treatment of depression when it was introduced into general psychiatric hospital practice some 40 years ago. Many patients with the more chronic types of depressive state were enabled to leave hospital, and such conditions are now rarely seen.

Electroplexy remains the mainstay of treating the severer affective psychoses and those patients who have not made an adequate response to anti-depressant medication. A course of some four to eight treatments is given over a period of two or three weeks, and the effect is to cut short that attack of the disease and, in successful cases, restore the mood to normality. For many patients it is the safest and quickest method of treatment, though the temporary memory disturbance that may go with such a course can be a nuisance to some individuals. It is, however, much less of a nuisance than staying depressed, and, therefore, usually well tolerated.

Leucotomy

This again has been described earlier. Some authorities consider that for the chronic affective psychosis which has not responded, or has shown frequent relapses with other methods of treatment, the modified pre-frontal leucotomy operation offers the best method of permanent relief of symptoms. This is at present a controversial treatment, and very few such operations are nowadays performed.

Psychotherapy

Psychotherapy is of no specific value in the treatment of affective psychosis. This having been said, sympathetic supportive counselling by the therapist is of course valuable as it is in any other disease process, heart attacks and broken legs included. To attempt to treat affective psychosis, however, by methods which exclude anti-depressant drugs or electroplexy is in the author's view tantamount to negligence and certainly condemns the patient to a period of unnecessary suffering which could, in most cases, be quickly relieved by the application of physical methods of treatment.

Bipolar Affective Psychosis

The old term for this condition was manic-depressive psychosis. The incidence is much rarer than that of unipolar affective psychosis; it is seen in only about 0.1 per cent of the population and, therefore, constitutes about one in ten of the affective psychoses. Again, there is frequently a family history of the disease and the condition tends to breed true. A stronger genetic factor has been identified than in unipolar psychosis, and some 20 per cent of first-degree relatives are affected.

Aetiology

Again changes associated with electrolyte shift and the increase of intracellular sodium have been found. Again, also, changes associated with mono-amine metabolism are found and there is some suggestion that in the bipolar condition a different mono-amine system may enter the picture. This latter factor, combined with the different genetic pattern, implies that the underlying biochemical disorder probably relates to a slightly different enzyme disturbance, whereby the neurohormones are affected in a slightly different way, although the end symptoms as they present in the depressive phase appear much the same as those seen in the unipolar disease. The main difference in the symptomatology is the presence in the bipolar disease of phases of elated mood not seen in the other condition.

Symptoms

The previous personality of the sufferer from a bipolar illness is often that of a cyclothymic mood swinger with a pyknic (thick) type of body build. The first attack may occur in the late teens or early twenties, and usually comes without warning. Many years of symptom-free life may follow, with a recurrence perhaps in middle age. Attacks may gradually become more frequent (see Fig. 3) in later middle age, occurring every year or two and lasting, untreated, some three to six months. They may be hypomanic in character or depressive in character; this is usually a random event, sometimes hypomania merging into depression before a phase of normality again occurs. Usually by the late sixties the disease process has quietened down and subsequent attacks become rarer.

Occasionally, a patient's mood swings develop a regular cyclical pattern, with elation and depression alternating so regularly that they are almost predictable to the day by the calendar. These cyclical periodic psychoses are rare, but most interesting from the research point of view with regard to what is going on with the underlying biochemical disturbances.

In the depressive phase symptoms follow those of the unipolar depression described earlier. There is morbid mood, loss of concentration, irritability, loss of appetite, loss of libido, and the typical sleep disturbance, with early waking and diurnal mood swing.

The elated phase is identical to that seen in mania and hypomania, and will be described later. Again this phase will gradually increase in severity, reach a peak and then gradually recover over a similar period of time. Hypomanic episodes are on the whole less frequent than depressive swings.

A woman of 37 with a family history of bipolar affective disease in her father, had had a depressive illness at the age of 22. Some five years later a phase of elation and foolish over-spending had been noted with hindsight but had not needed hospital care. Over the last three years she had developed swings of mood, sometimes of depression and sometimes of euphoria, lasting some three months with phases of perhaps six months normality in between. Three of these had been severe enough to place her in hospital and the rest she had coped with at home on medication.

At this latest admission therapy with lithium was commenced and thereafter she remained more or less symptom-free for some four years. Discontinuing the lithium while on holiday at that point produced a relapse into a depressive state some two months after stopping medication. She was restabilised on lithium and had remained symptom-free at the time of writing for some seven years.

Treatment

The individual who develops an isolated attack of a bipolar affective psychosis will be treated in the same way as one with a unipolar depression or with a manic illness. Indeed, until the patient has had phases of both depression and elation, there is no real way of distinguishing whether the condition is unipolar or bipolar other than the presence of a typical family history. There is at present no confirmatory test which will allow one to make this distinction.

In the bipolar affective disorder, however, lithium salts are prophylactic in some 50 per cent of patients. Such preparations are at present the only available product which will prevent the recurrence of a psychotic episode. They are, therefore, of particular value for those who suffer from frequent disabling swings of mood, especially of the periodic or cyclical variety, and who 30 years ago would have probably become long-term hospital patients. The mode of action of these drugs has been discussed earlier, but we may reiterate that it is the replacement in the cell of excessive sodium ions which seems to restore this part of the central nervous system to normal functioning, and presumably it is this mechanism which—unlike anti-depressant drugs, which work at the cell synapse—gives it some preventive effectiveness.

It will be apparent, however, that unless relapses are occurring with sufficient frequency, the continued consumption of a potentially toxic drug, with blood levels needing to be carefully monitored to avoid the development of serious side-effects, would not be justified. It appears that during a psychotic phase more of the lithium is absorbed somewhere in the body stores, and the dose needs to be higher to produce the same effect. Once the psychotic phase is over, however, the dosage must be reduced or toxic levels may build up. For this reason, continuous monitoring by blood tests at a monthly follow-up clinic is desirable, and the patient must be aware of the potential side-effects and how they may show up, so that he or she can contact the doctor quickly if they appear.

The side-effects relate to the body developing a deficiency of sodium within the cell, and this shows as nausea, the development of muscle tremor, muscular weakness and, in severer cases, confusion and irregularity of heart beat. Lithium salts should not be used in individuals with heart or kidney disease. Occasionally a mild goitre can develop as a result of inhibition of iodine uptake. This is not of any serious consequence.

Lithium needs to be continued over some years if relapses are to be prevented, and it is necessary to persuade individuals who otherwise feel well to keep on with such treatment if further psychotic episodes are to be avoided. Unfortunately, these drugs are only effective in a proportion of cases, and other individuals may still need to be treated when the individual attack occurs by anti-depressant or anti-manic medication or electroplexy.

Puerperal Psychosis

Psychotic illness occurring within days or at most a week or two following child birth has been considered in the past by some authors as a specific syndrome in its own right. It has become apparent, however, that the types of emotional or psychiatric disturbances that may follow childbirth are in essence no different from those which can occur at other times in life.

The hormonal and environmental changes occurring immediately after childbirth would appear to act as a trigger in the individual susceptible to such a condition, but, once developed, the condition follows the pattern seen in equivalent illness in any other person, and the management to treatment is the same. Furthermore, such an individual may quite possibly develop a similar illness at some other time in their lives not associated with a childbirth experience. The puerperium, however, is a time of stress for all women and the symptoms of illness may be modified to some degree by the particular circumstances which occur at the time.

Older writers have identified the three particular types of presentation of puerperal psychosis, which may be either a toxic confusional state, an affective psychosis of manic depressive type, or a schizophrenic psychosis.

The toxic confusional state accounted for some 40 per cent of cases in the pre-antibiotic days. It was sometimes known as milk fever, but related usually to infection of the genital tract following trauma from the birth, and the confusional state was associated with fever and toxicity and comparable to a toxic confusional state from any other cause. Nowadays, with better hygiene and effective antibiotics, such conditions are very rarely seen, and account for only a small percentage of the psychoses found in the puerperium.

Puerperal schizophrenia again follows a pattern seen in schizophrenia at other times. The prognosis is worse, therefore, than for the affective psychoses, though it seems to respond better to treatment than the hebephrenic type of illness which occurs in adolescence. Often in the puerperal type of onset there is a more marked emotional disturbance, with more acute symptomatology, and response to therapy is quite good. Nevertheless, there is some liability to a recurrence with subsequent children, and since the more recurrences an individual has of schizophrenia, the more disabled they are likely to become, some would consider this grounds for advising against further children or even for termination should the patient wish it in the early stages of pregnancy.

The affective psychosis is usually depressive in character, though hypomanic attacks are not unknown. This is the commonest type of presentation of puerperal disorder, and sometimes there is a mixed emotional state, with symptoms of both hypomania and depression showing.

Protheroe showed in an interesting study in Newcastle that before the advent of electroplexy as a form of treatment the outcome of such illnesses was not good, many cases becoming chronic hospital problems with a not inconsiderable mortality. With the advent of electroplexy the cure rate and length of stay in hospital made a dramatic improvement, and with the later advent of anti-depressant drugs in addition, an even better response could be obtained, with the length of stay in hospital dropping further to an average of six weeks.

Slater comments that puerperal depression is particularly responsive to electroplexy, and since speed is the essence, this remains the treatment of choice.

For this problem many hospitals provide mother and baby units, where mothers who need in-patient treatment because of the potential danger to their baby, or the suicidally depressed or psychotic mother, may be nursed, and mother and child may continue so far as is possible to develop the appropriate bonding or imprinting relationship so necessary for good child rearing. The mother can gradually be helped to take over the increasing care of her child as her condition improves. Puerperal depression seems to be commoner in mothers having first babies, the incidence being something in the region of 1 in 40 births.

We must not forget that for many women childbirth and the puerperium are traumatic times, when learning a completely new way of life must be acquired. The hormone changes that take place after childbirth not infrequently produce a mild degree of depression known as 'baby blues', which in most cases does not herald serious psychosis. However, neurotic anxiety and depression are frequent in the puerperium, and require sympathetic counselling and help so that the mother can adjust to her new role.

Urgent admission was requested for a woman of 28 who ten days before had had her first child. For the first few days all had been well and she had returned home from hospital. Over the last five days there had been a relatively rapid onset of depressive symptoms with weepiness, and inability to cope with looking after the child effectively. There was a marked sleep disturbance with early waking at 4.00 a.m. and a feeling of hopelessness at the start of the new day. The woman had developed guilt feelings about her incapability of relating to the child and was feeling increasingly inadequate. She could not concentrate and found the crying made her very irritable. On the morning of admission she had left the child in the baby bath which had water in it and had run out of the house. She had walked down to the river, near the market town in which she lived, and considered throwing herself in the water. Instead she went to the police station and confessed to murdering her child.

The police hurried to the house and most fortunately found the baby gurgling quite happily in its bath.

The mother received a course of electroplexy and anti-depressant tablets and was well enough to have had the baby with her in the mother and baby unit in order to get used to it again for a week or two before discharge.

Unfortunately, the heavy hand of the law in this case handled the matter with some lack of understanding, the mother having been charged with attempted murder and required to appear in the local magistrates' court! There followed a legal wrangle, since even had the baby died the gravest charge could only have been infanticide, which is equivalent to manslaughter. There being no such charge as attempted manslaughter, however, and the local magistrates not being prepared or able to drop the hearing, the Child Welfare Department would not agree to the child returning to the mother's care until after the case had been heard. This harrowing situation was reported in the local papers and did little to help the woman's recovery. She was eventually acquitted in the Crown Court and has since lived happily ever after and had two more children.

Mania and Hypomania

Mania is a psychotic condition, whose main feature is a pathological or abnormal elevation of mood, hypomania simply being the descriptive term for the milder and more commonly seen form of the condition. Mania and hypomania most commonly are seen as part of a bipolar affective disorder in an individual who may also suffer from time to time from depressive attacks. Occasionally, however, a unipolar condition may be found. This is much rarer than unipolar depression. The incidence of mania and hypomania is some one person per 1,000 of the population.

Compared with unipolar depression, similar but grosser changes in the biochemistry are found in mania, whereby the shift of sodium into the intra-cellular spaces is 200 per cent instead of 50 per cent in the acute attack, with similar shift in body fluid. Thus lithium can be a particularly effective therapy. Similar hereditary factors seem to play a part, but other biochemical disturbances at mono-amine level may prove to be somewhat different to those found in the depressive phase. This remains at present a research issue.

In its milder form the mood change, characterised by pathological elation, is not always easy to define. Acute mania is a rarely seen condition, which generally occurs as part of an affective psychosis of bipolar type. Occasionally it is seen as an isolated incident, or may occur in African races as a condition described by Lumbo as African periodic psychosis, which is probably a genetically determined condition related to the affective psychosis we have described. Manic behaviour may also be seen in response to the toxic effect of stimulant drugs such as cannabis, or as part of a delirious state. But here we are considering mania as a symptom, just as we saw depression as a symptom which can be seen as part of an affective psychosis or as a result of other conditions and reactions to stress in personalities who are prone to such patterns of behaviour.

The more commonly seen condition is that of hypomania. In common with other psychoses, insight into the pathological state is commonly lost, so that patients are unaware that their mood and behaviour have become abnormal. Usually friends and relatives, therefore, are the first to spot that something is amiss. Unfortunately, whereas in the depressive states patients are at least aware of the feeling of malaise and gloom and know that they are not well, even if they misinterpret the reasons, patients with a hypomanic state may feel initially on top of the world, and state that they have never felt better. They consider their actions, often irrational and foolish to those close to them, to be sensibly motivated, and that everything they do will turn out right. Thus they fling wide the curtains at 5 a.m., open the windows and gaze at the rain outside before shaking the rest of the household awake, while singing 'Oh What a Beautiful Morning'! They will consider all who advise them to be fools, and are most unlikely to seek psychiatric help voluntarily. The danger in such cases is not that the patients might, as in depression, harm themselves—for instance, by a suicide attempt—but that their irrational actions may ruin themselves or their families financially or that they may endanger others by reckless behaviour rather than by deliberate aggressive intent.

It will be recalled that under the 1983 Mental Health Act patients can only be detained if they are considered to be a danger to themselves or to others by reason of mental illness. The risk of suicide would be clearly recognised as a justifiable cause for such detention. The application of the Act to an individual who feels extremely well can be ethically rather more difficult. Yet such individuals are often at considerable danger, and speed in obtaining help can be vital. Two examples may show the need for this.

An accountant who had history of depression some ten years before was noted by his family over a week or ten days to have become rather fatuously jolly compared with his normal self. He was waking excessively early in the morning and, although claiming to feel very well, his concentration and ability to remain on one topic of conversation had deteriorated. It transpired that during this short time he had sold a large number of shares and bought others extremely unwisely, and against the advice of his broker. As a result he had lost a considerable amount of money. He had been to a car dealer and bought a Bentley, new and quite outside his financial abilities to pay. He had put down a deposit and driven the car away, and before his family could do anything effective to stop him had taken the car for a spin, driving it recklessly and eventually put it into a ditch, causing nearly £1,000 worth of damage to the vehicle.

In this short space of time he had cost himself and his family in the region of £5,000. The car dealer could rightly claim that at the time of the purchase there was nothing to indicate that the buyer was not legally responsible for his actions and was, therefore, liable not only for payment but also for the damage to the car, which the dealer declined to have returned in view of the crash, and which the buyer was forced subsequently to sell second-hand at considerable loss.

In the second case, a lady with no previous history of psychiatric illness, who had been happily married for some five years, surprised her husband over a period of a few days by starting to spend rather extravagantly and to buy articles of clothing which were not to her normal taste. Matters came to a head when one evening a number of men called at the house apparently expecting to be entertained, not knowing of the husband's existence. It transpired that the wife had gone to a local pub during the lunch hour and had invited a number of complete strangers to visit her house that evening.

It is not uncommon for otherwise reputable people to perform minor criminal acts, or to become sexually promiscuous and, if unfortunate, become pregnant in the short time during which the illness is developing, and before they have been able to take the necessary steps to obtain treatment. This type of behaviour is not, of course, necessarily indicative of a hypomanic illness, and has to be taken in the context of the individual's previous personality and the other symptoms which suggest the development of a manic state. Apart from the mood change, which can be seen in one sense as an opposite of depression, many of the other symptoms of this type of affective psychosis bear great similarity to those seen in an affective disorder with a depressive content.

Furthermore, as has been mentioned, the biochemical changes underlying these psychoses, whereby there is a shift of sodium and fluid into the cell, are in the same direction as in the depressive phase of a bipolar disorder but more severe, with increase of sodium up to 200 per cent of the normal.

Thus, in this sense, manic illness would seem to be a severer stage of the same problem.

The other symptoms which are seen in the hypomanic state are as follows. Along with the elation of mood, which may extend to a frank euphoria, where everything seems a cause for rejoicing and the individual is artificially and fatuously jolly, there is sometimes a pompous irritability, which can become grandiose or aggressive if such an individual is crossed.

Over-activity and voluble rapid speech are seen, with what is known as 'flights of ideas'. Here, such an individual may switch rapidly from one theme to another during conversation, the associations being unclear and often the result of punning or clang associations, which suggest a new train of thought to the sufferer. If such a conversation is taped and played back slowly, the reason for the switch of ideas can often be seen, but during conversation the train of thought is very difficult to follow. Concentration is markedly impaired, as in depression.

As in the depressive phase also, sleep is disturbed, with early waking. The diurnal mood swing may be seen, with elation more prominent in the earlier part of the day. Loss of appetite may occur, but this is not so typical, and sometimes the appetite becomes ravenous. However, weight loss often occurs because of the over-activity. Loss of libido may be present, though the individual may become superficially exceptionally flirtatious, and have a high opinion of his or her sexual prowess.

In manic states the symptoms are even more grossly exaggerated. Thus the talk stream may become completely incomprehensible, being continuous but nonsensical. The over-activity may lead to such a degree of exhaustion, from the patient being constantly on the go and not sleeping, that physical harm can be done, particularly in those with any cardiovascular disorder, such as a history of heart failure, or respiratory diseases.

The mood becomes one of fatuous ecstasy, with constant punning jokes, singing or sexually improper behaviour making any attempt at a normal interview impossible. The patient is unable to settle to any type of activity, since the disturbed concentration makes him unable to stick to any theme for more than a few seconds. Attempts to check such behaviour may lead to aggressive outbursts.

Treatment

The urgency of admission to hospital for such cases has been emphasised. Drug treatment is now the mainstay of symptom control, and must be continued until the phase has cleared. Like the depressive phase of affective psychoses, the condition is self-limiting, given time, but drug treatment can ameliorate the symptoms and allow such an individual to return to normality much more quickly. The butyrophenones, such as haloperidol or droperidol, are most effective, but sedative phenothiazines, such as chlorpromazine, can be used. Lithium products, such as priadel, have been described earlier. Their mode of action is different from the other drugs mentioned, since they appear to reduce the excessive sodium levels in the cell. Thus lithium products can be effective in controlling the acute attack and also as a prophylactic, preventing the recurrence of subsequent attacks in many patients who otherwise might have frequent relapses.

A short intensive course of electroplexy is very useful in the more severe hypomanic or manic episodes, allowing a rapid return to normal mood, after which treatment can be continued on the basis of drug therapy alone. The effect of the electroplexy again appears to be to restore the disturbed intra-cellular and extra-cellular balance of electrolytes, possibly by direct effect on the cell membrane or through an action on the central nervous system mono-amines. The main advantage is rapidity of effect, compared with drugs, but ethical problems can arise from the absence of consent to treatment in those patients admitted under the Mental Health Act.

As has been indicated above, it can be most important to effect early control of the symptoms, and it has always seemed to the author that to withhold an effective method of symptom relief in such cases could reasonably be considered negligent on the part of the responsible medical officer. If a patient, because of loss of insight as a result of a psychotic illness, is unable or unwilling to give a valid consent to treatment which is designed to facilitate recovery or to relieve suffering, then some method must be adopted in any civilised community whereby someone can act in the sick individual's best interests. There seems no better way of doing this than an agreement between the next of kin and the specialist who is responsible for the patient's care.

The outlook for single hypomanic states is now usually excellent. The risk of recurrence when the illness is part of a bipolar affective psychosis is quite high, but since relapses are usually interspersed with years of good health, and since treatment of a recurrence is just as effective in this condition, regardless by and large of the number of attacks that have preceded it, one can now counsel every prospect of success to friends or relations who may be concerned.

Aggression and Aggressive Psychosis

A question we may initially ask ourselves is whether there is such a thing as an endogenous aggressive state. Certainly pathological aggressive behaviour can be seen as a result of brain damage, as part of an epileptic state, or as a result of the influence of drugs. Similarly, aggressive behaviour may be seen as a symptom of hypomanic illness, of schizophrenia, or in psychopathic disorders.

If we look not so much at hospital-geared psychiatry as at criminality, and research the inmates of our prisons, we shall find a not inconsiderable number of individuals who appear to have indulged in aggressive behaviour of a spontaneous kind, triggered off perhaps by the most trivial provocation.

The relationship of this sort of problem to personality disorders and to minor degrees of brain damage, with abnormal electrencephalogram tracings and some evidence of minimal brain damage, and perhaps a lowered intelligence, is statistically clear-cut. Furthermore, we can recognise at least four individual aspects of mood—namely, depression, elation, anxiety and aggressive arousal—and have seen that, in the first three of these, disturbances which go outside the normal range of emotional behaviour patterns can occur. These are seen as pathological, arising from within the central nervous system, presumably owing to some distortion of nerve-cell function, probably at a biochemical level. It would seem reasonable, therefore, to postulate—on the basis that all human functions can become disordered and that other aspects of thinking, emotion, memory and behaviour can be disturbed—that it is unlikely the mechanism mediating aggressive arousal cannot do the same.

Perhaps one reason that such cases are less clearly identified in psychiatric hospital practice is the way in which society chooses to deal with different patterns of disturbance in its members. Thus the illness model can extend readily to diseases where an obvious physical cause can be shown, such as a broken leg. As we move into the realm of diseases that affect behaviour, especially where the disturbance is some rather more subtle change in the internal milieu, then society's attitude may become more punitive. At least in the affective psychoses and schizophrenia the patient is seen to suffer, and society can extend some measure of sympathy. If the mood change is one primarily of aggression, however, this is liable to be turned outwards and impinge on society in a more direct way, since its members will be the sufferers or recipients of any aggressive outbursts directed against them.

It is, nevertheless, the author's contention that, if sought for, an endogenous aggressive psychosis should be identifiable. It is arguable whether society or, perhaps more particularly, the nursing staff of psychiatric hospitals should consider it appropriate to nurse such people rather than, as at present, adopting retributive punishment routines which, while depriving the individual of liberty, do little to correct the disturbance. Certainly, however, the advent of secure units where the abnormal offender can be both nursed and kept in secure conditions, so that society too may be protected, may help to achieve a more rational treatment for such problems.

Abnormal aggressive behaviour is in fact seen not all that infrequently and although the sufferer usually comes to be labelled as psychopathic, because such behaviour brings him into contact with the law and no other psychiatric illness can be identified, these individuals may themselves seek help, recognising that from time to time their mood becomes irritable and hypersensitive though not depressed. Furthermore, such problems may seem to occur to the individual out of the blue, and not be identifiably related to particular environmental stresses. For the rest of the time the individual is normal and has normal sensitivities, and thus does not show the psychopathic trends in general of amorality, a disability in forming relationships, or failure to learn from experience. Indeed, relationships are often quite strong and partners feel fully able to empathise with such a person during times when aggressive behaviour is not being shown.

Within work with the criminal, therefore, should this group be separated off as mentally ill? There will, of course, be a shading over, as there is with anxiety, into aggressive behaviour for other reasons; and cerebral dys-rhythmias, such as can occur in temporal lobe epilepsy, can certainly be worth investigating.

Treatment

What treatment can be offered for sufferers of such conditions? A full investigation of brain rhythms through the EEG, a search in the history for early evidence of meningoencephalitis, and an exclusion of other possible causes of violent behaviour, such as a manic-depressive affective psychosis, must be considered.

Drug therapy can be extremely helpful. Such butyrophenones as halo-peridol can be of considerable help in assisting the individual to control aggressive outbursts. Some of the quicker acting drugs, such as droperidol, are also useful. Curiously, the tranquillising drugs, such as the benzodiazepines, are often not helpful, since they may in fact, by reducing the natural inhibitions which anxiety can cause, allow the acting out of aggressive impulses that otherwise could have been kept in check. The most effective medication, in the author's experience, has been the use of drugs which are known to be effective in temporal lobe epilepsy, in particular carbamazepine.

Behaviour therapy techniques have also been tried in the control of aggressive behaviour. Some behaviour patterns may be amenable to such approaches either by positive reinforcement of good behaviour or by aversion therapy designed towards particular types of behaviour disturbances. On the whole, however, for those patients where an endogenous condition may exist one would not anticipate that this would be of great benefit.

Finally, brain surgery has been attempted with some success for particularly intractable violent behaviour, using leucotomy or thalamectomy or cingulectomy procedures. These are all very much in the realm of specialist research procedures, though good results have been claimed in some particularly severe cases.

Perhaps the opposite end of a continuum of aggression would be apathy, the eighth deadly sin of 'acedia' in the Ancient Church. While not characterised as an illness these days, there is little doubt that some patients may be seen and perhaps falsely diagnosed as suffering from depression, when apathy is the main and only symptom. No doubt they were those who made a good response to stimulants before such treatment was felt to be *de rigueur*.

Further Reading

Balmaker, R. H., *Mania—an evolving concept*, M.T.P. Press, Lancaster, England, 1980.

Baron, R. A., *Human Aggression*, Plenum Press, New York, 1977.

Brown, F., 'Depression and Childhood Bereavement', *Journal of Mental Science*, 107, 1961.

Coppen, A., and Walk, A., *Recent Developments in Affective Disorders*, *BJP* Special Publications No. 2, Headley, Kent, 1968.

Durkheim, E., *On Suicide*, Glencoe Free Press, Glencoe (Ill.), 1957.

Hare, 'The Two Manias—A Study of the Evolution of the Modern Concept of Mania', *British Journal of Psychiatry*, 138, 1989.

Sandler, M., *Psychopharmacology of Aggression*, Raven, New York, 1979.

Shopsin, B., *Manic Illness*, Raven, New York, 1979.

Stengel, E., *Suicide and Attempted Suicide*, Penguin, Harmondsworth, 1969.

Winokur, G. *et al*, *Manic Depressive Illness*, Mosby, St Louis, 1969.

Questions

1. What distinguishes the depressive affective psychosis from normal depression?
2. What is affect?
3. What distinguishes the suicidal gesture from the morbid suicide of psychotic illness?
4. How many suicide attempts are seen at your local hospital on average per week? How does your casualty department deal with these sufferers?
5. What are the problems relating to the treatment of manic illness?

12
Affective Disorders: The Neuroses

Summary

The principal affective change in the neuroses (or psychoneuroses) is that of anxiety. Neuroses are described as less serious psychiatric disorders in which insight is retained.

Incidence

Minor degrees of neurotic personality are extremely common. Women are more frequently affected than men. It is estimated that 25 per cent of attenders at general practitioners' surgeries show problems related to neuroses. In fact, some 10 per cent of the population suffer to some degree and some 5 per cent will require psychiatric hospital attention.

Classification

Symptom clusters without clear-cut boundaries are found in the neuroses. For descriptive convenience they may be divided as below:

1. Pervasive or generalised anxiety.
2. Phobic anxiety states:
   (a) Agoraphobia.
   (b) Monosymptomatic phobias.
3. Obsessional and compulsive neuroses.
4. Depressive neuroses or depressive reactions.
5. States of depersonalisation.
6. Hysterical neuroses.
7. Disorders of parasympathetic autonomic function.

As has been stated elsewhere classificatory systems are available (ICD 10 and DCM 3) which attempt to sub-divide neuroses into other than the traditional systems. In the author's view these new systems, although useful for statistical purposes, have yet to be proven valuable in clinical practice.

Aetiology

1. Possible genetic predisposition in some cases.
2. Influence of early environment—note Freudian analytical theories and Pavlovian behavioural theories.

3. Influence of present environment triggering repressed emotional material.

Treatment

1. Anxiety-relieving medication.
2. Various psychotherapies, ranging from superficial supportive counselling to full psychoanalysis.
3. Behavioural therapies.
4. Hypnotherapy.
5. Abreactive techniques.
6. Electrosleep.

Outcome

Two-thirds of acute neurotic episodes will have recovered within a five-year period, regardless of treatment. Treatment in such cases is designed to relieve symptoms or to hasten their disappearance, and prevent chronicity in the remaining third.

Description

In Chapter 11 we discussed the concept of affect, a continuing state of emotion. We considered the four main affective components of depression, elation, anxiety and aggression. We also considered disorders where morbid or depressed mood was the primary symptom, and disorders of mania or hypomania, where elation was a marked feature; and took a brief look at the possibility of aggressive psychoses or neuroses. In this chapter we shall look at a group of conditions traditionally known as the neuroses or psychoneuroses, in which the primary affective change is that of anxiety.

The neuroses are morbid states where there is a pathological change of affective state known as anxiety. Such states may be endogenous or reactive to the environment, and may be precipitated by present stress, though the individual has often been primed by early life experiences. The condition may be acute or chronic. Psychoneuroses may follow a typical pattern of symptoms. The neurotic personality is usually present. The condition may frequently be associated with a tendency to depressive reactions which supervene on an existing neurosis.

The incidence of psychoneuroses is hard to establish. Some authors have suggested that within everybody there is a degree of neurotic behaviour, environmentally induced. No individual can reach adulthood without receiving some stresses to which they respond maladaptively. Thus the seeds of neurotic behaviour are within us all waiting merely to be triggered. Similarly, it has been estimated that at least 25 per cent of individuals who approach the family doctor have a complaint which is basically neurotic or stress-induced, and in which anxiety is the predominant feature. If we restrict ourselves to the severer cases, those which are likely to come the way of the psychiatrist, then we are talking of something in the region of 5 per cent of the population.

Over-activity in the central nervous system, particularly in the limbic lobe and reticular activating systems of the brain, can be seen as a prime source of the symptoms we experience as anxiety. The underlying chemical and neuronal mechanism is similar for both fear and anxiety, defining the former as something which is experienced in response to a real or imagined threat. Anxiety thus may be normal in that it is appropriate in the particular circumstances in which the individual finds himself and, therefore, has a useful survival function in activating the autonomic nervous system and preparing the individual to make appropriate response. Pathological anxiety may arise from over-activity of these central nervous system areas, either from conditioned maladaptive over-reaction to trivial stress—that is to say, from external sources which have created a predisposition—or endogenously from an inbuilt over-activity or imbalance of neurohormones, and in this sense a disease. Theories as to the development of neuroses range from organic concepts, behaviourist theories of learning, and analytical theories arising from the work of Freud, Jung and others.

A wide range of treatment processes is available for the neuroses. This might be compared with the wide variety of treatments for baldness and the extensive existing crop of bald heads. One must look critically at treatments offered for neuroses to ascertain which give value for money. Neuroses are extremely common but have a natural tendency to remit, and the study of long-term results must, therefore, be compared with the high incidence of natural remission in any long-term survey.

Treatments may be considered under the following headings:

1. **Medication**, aimed at relieving the symptom of anxiety at a peripheral or central level.

2. **Behaviour therapies.** Treatments based on learning theory, whereby anxiety relief is attempted through the breaking down of maladaptive conditioned responses.

3. **Psychotherapy.** Here an attempt is made to relieve anxiety symptoms of neurosis through developing a relationship with the patient, whereby the underlying causes can be identified and talked through and insight obtained.

4. **Psychoanalysis.** A long-term method of treating the neurotic personality by analysis of early childhood influences through regression, free association and various other analytical techniques.

5. **Hypnotherapy.** Here anxiety relief is attempted through influencing the patient under hypnosis, whereby hypersuggestibility may lead to a resolution of symptoms.

6. **Abreactive techniques.** Repressed causes of free-floating anxiety can be identified and the emotional block believed to be causing the problem released.

7. **Physical methods** of treatment, such as electrosleep or carbon dioxide inhalation.

Some 70 per cent of cases of anxiety state will remit over a five-year follow-up period, regardless of the method of treatment. Treatment may be designed to cut short an acute attack or to attempt longer-lasting control of the neurotic personality. The psychological benefits of any anxiety-relieving technique depend largely on the confidence with which the patient is able to undertake the therapy.

The experience of fear or anxiety is a universal phenomenon with which all are familiar. The patient suffering from one or other of the neurotic states, however, is for a variety of reasons experiencing anxiety either at inappropriate times or to an excessive degree, even though there is some anxiety-provoking stimulus. The patient is hypersensitised to this.

As we shall show, neuroses may take a variety of forms but there is no evidence at present to suggest that we are looking at fundamentally different disease processes. We are seeing, rather, the response an individual makes to a stress situation, and which may then become a learned pattern of maladaptive behaviour.

In considering the manifestation of anxiety we must first look at the concept of the neurotic personality. Again, some would say that the presence of a degree of personality neurosis is also universal. This is based on the idea that a neurosis—a tendency to react to stress by manifesting some type of anxiety—results from early childhood experiences in which traumatic emotional experiences come to be repressed and pushed into the subconscious or unconscious parts of the central nervous system, where they remain and can influence subsequent behaviour patterns.

Some theorists would explain these concepts on behaviourist lines, using the model of learning theory. Many phobic states and obsessional neuroses can be seen in this light. A child may scald itself and develop a fear of kettles, a fear of steam, even generalising to a fear of all pots and pans, cookers and anything that looks like steam. As the child grows up, he may appear to overcome this fear, but it can be triggered off again by some situation which reactivates it, and a phobia develops. We have discussed the stimulus response theory elsewhere, and for a more detailed exposition the reader is referred to a companion volume, *Psychology Made Simple*.

Analytical theorists would explain the neurotic process on the basis of repression of instinctual drives, associated with failure of resolution of the Oedipal complex, and regression to an earlier phase of emotional development.

Regardless of the theoretical basis on which these concepts are developed, all are agreed that certain basic factors must be present. Some workers would postulate an **anxiety-prone personality**. This implies the presence of some prenatal influence on the individual, either genetically determined as an inherited factor, or conceivably associated with some influence acting on the foetus in the womb. Since all individuals in their youth will have had to cope with stresses and, depending on their severity and other coincidental factors, will have reacted in a more or less satisfactory way in coping with such problems, the basis for the development of neurotic patterns of behaviour is in this sense universal. In the anxiety-prone personality such stress situations are more likely to induce neurotic behaviour than in others, though the seeds of it are in us all. In addition to this predisposition there would appear to be the need in most cases for a trigger situation at some point later in life which provides the overt reason for a clear-cut neurosis to develop at some point.

Besides these environmentally determined factors, it seems probable, at least on a theoretical basis, that a disease process could affect the function and activity of those parts of the brain particularly associated with levels of arousal, fear and mood change. These are generally ascribed to that part of the brain known as the limbic lobe, including the nuclei of the hippocampus, amygdaloid nucleus, and associations with the frontal cortex, thalamus and other parts of the brain, including the reticular formation.

Circuits operating in these areas may get out of balance and the neuro-hormones, the mono-amines which we have discussed previously, may for endogenous reasons develop over- or under-activity, producing an endogenous neurosis akin to the affective psychoses and schizophrenia, where a biochemical disorder can be postulated.

To complete the picture, there is a well-recognised interaction among the level of production of hormones within the body as part of the normal biological rhythms, the association of disease processes, and the influence of the external environment. It will be apparent that the individual can indeed provoke an anxiety reaction quite deliberately at a conscious level by putting himself into an anxiety-provoking situation. Thus, a man who is nervous of heights can induce all the reactions of the autonomic sympathetic system simply by putting himself on the edge of a precipice. Monoamine over-activity will occur in the limbic lobe, and an increase in catechol amine production will be seen in the autonomic system, whose nerves will be stimulated, inducing sweating, increased heart rate and all the other signs associated with fear. This is induced for purely external reasons, but creates straightforward physical changes which are easily measurable in the body itself.

We can show the way this can function in psychosomatic disorders, where the anxiety is displaced on to physical symptoms affecting particular parts of the body. We have also seen that an alteration in the pH or acidity/alkalinity balance in the body (for instance, when lactate infusion is given) is apparently associated with the provocation of anxiety attacks in those prone to them. Similarly, the inhalation of carbon dioxide, which can reverse such processes, is of at least temporary benefit in alleviating anxiety.

We know, therefore, that environment can affect mood and we know that chemical changes in the body can affect mood. The interrelationship between these factors is complex, and some degree of neurosis is very widespread. Treatment can be directed at various levels and must take into account the likelihood that in a particular individual a variety of factors may be operating, and that not infrequently secondary anxiety can be induced in the neurotic personality by fear of bodily disease associated with the symptoms of the anxiety state itself. Thus, a vicious circle is set up where the patient fears his own fear-induced symptoms.

Symptoms

Because the primary condition of anxiety is mediated through the autonomic nervous system to all parts of the body, the symptoms of an anxiety neurosis can be very diverse. Particular syndromes seem to occur and seem related to this interaction between personality and the environmental triggers. Some symptoms, however, are very generally found in those where a high level of anxiety is present.

We are familiar with the normal effects of anxiety. A feeling of unpleasant tension sometimes described as 'butterflies in the stomach' is felt. There is apprehension about what may happen next. Headaches, which can occur, are often described as a tight band felt to be constricting the skull. The mouth may be dry and the pupils dilated. The skin is clammy and in many species pilo-erection occurs (hair standing on end). The heart beats faster and blood pressure will be slightly raised. In the acute episode there will be heightened awareness, an inhibition of micturition and sexual responsiveness. In the longer-lasting attack, frequency of micturition may be found, and the individual may need to make frequent trips to the toilet. Concentration after a while becomes impaired.

We are all familiar with what happens at the end of such a period of anxiety. We feel a sense of relief but a high level of physical weariness. This high level of tension or arousal is very tiring.

Thus, in the long-standing anxiety state a feeling of tiredness, poor concentration, lethargy and malaise is commonplace. An initial insomnia occurs, the patient cannot relax, and this, coupled with the anxiety, makes the patient complain of constant exhaustion. Two terms which are not now commonly used as diagnostic labels describe this type of general syndrome. One is neurasthenia and the other hypochondriasis.

In **neurasthenia** the prominent symptoms are weakness and exhaustion. A poor appetite may lead to some loss of weight, which adds to the misery. Thus the patient loses his drive and feels constantly wilted.

In **hypochondriasis** the emphasis is on the bodily manifestations of the process, and patients complain of constant aches and pains in various target organs. They are repeatedly seeking reassurance and fear they may be developing cancer, heart disease or some similar feared illness. Reassurance has but a short-lived effect, since the anxiety continues to manifest itself in other ways. Their constant complaining can become tedious to friends and relations, and lead to a deterioration in relationships, which adds to the patients' suffering.

Let us now look at these specific syndromes which we have listed in our summary.

Pervasive Anxiety

A generalised over-activity of the autonomic system which does not pertain to particular target organs may present as a generalised state of anxiety. There is not infrequently a history of neurosis in the family, though an inherited factor has never been clearly established. A predisposition is probably the most that can be identified, and an environment of distorted parental relationships of over-protectiveness, or the presence of separation experiences, is often found. A past history will show features of anxiety present in childhood and adolescence, such as night fears, bed-wetting, nail-biting or school phobia, feeding disturbances and so on. In other words, the evidence of personality neurosis usually goes back to the early days, although particular anxiety-provoking situations are often hard to identify because they have been repressed or forgotten.

Stressful life situations may then develop. They may be clearly identifiable or may not be apparent to the investigator, at any rate at initial interviews, but the symptoms of generalised anxiety at this stage become manifest. These are just as found in the normal fear or anxiety described above. The only difference is that there is no clearly identifiable cause the patient can understand, or the apparent cause is much more trivial than the average person would find reasonable in terms of the symptoms produced. There is a hypersensitivity on the patient's part to trivial stress. Furthermore, whereas the individual with an identifiable stress, such as an examination or interview, can see an end and can relax when the stress is over, the patient with the anxiety state is not in this happy position. There seems no end, and each morning when the patient wakes the same sinking feeling in the pit of the stomach proclaims that the symptoms are still present. This is perhaps the most wearing part of the illness.

A woman developed feelings of tension and anxiety related to pains in the right side of her head. It was probably significant that her father, to whom she had been much attached, had died a few months before having had such head symptoms before his stroke. The patient's symptoms generalised, however, so that at the clinic she presented with a four-month history of shakiness, loss of concentration, feelings of nausea in the morning and a feeling of fear gripping her stomach. She had difficulty in getting off to sleep and was irritable and constantly keyed up. In this case abreactive treatment using hypnotherapy combined with a period on tranquillisers allowed the symptoms to clear.

Phobic States

The anxiety associated with a neurotic state may be pervasive, as described above, or may crystallise upon psychosomatic symptoms. Not infrequently, however, the anxiety state relates to specific circumstances or events, and is not continuous throughout the waking day. Such anxiety is known as **phobic anxiety** and occurs in two common forms. These are agoraphobia and the monosymptomatic phobic states.

Agoraphobia in literal translation means fear of the market place. It has come to mean anxiety associated with crowds, travelling or situations where the opportunity to escape is limited. Often such patients fear that they may faint or vomit or in some way make themselves look foolish while in public. It is rare to find that this has actually occurred, but not infrequently the patient may have felt faint or may have known of others who have. The anticipation of such a possibility is the thing which provokes the fear. Such patients have to sit at the end of the row in the cinema or church or in a lecture hall. They cannot travel on buses or trains, and may develop quite acute anxiety even when walking along the street. Over a period of time the symptoms, untreated, may generalise, so that the patient becomes housebound and is fearful even to step outside. Relatives may to some extent connive with this by agreeing to do all the tasks normally performed outside, thus relieving the sufferer of the need to make such a sortie. While this is in one sense kindly, it is in another sense a recipe for disaster, since it reinforces the very pattern of behaviour which needs to be abolished for cure to be obtained.

As long as the patients are not subjected to these particular stresses, the level of anxiety is minimal. Unfortunately, if they react to a panic attack by running away from the fear-inducing stimulus and thus relieve their fear, they are, on the basis of learning or stimulus response theory, reinforcing the pattern of behaviour.

A woman of 38 had developed an anxiety about not being able to get out of places such as rows in the cinema or church or on a bus. This was in the context of a life-long neurotic personality who had been prone to develop anxiety reactions from childhood under circumstances of stress. The onset of her fear of being trapped, however, could not be related to any specific incident.

Over a period of months her symptoms generalised so that she became unable to go on to public transport or even into shops. She feared she might faint in such a situation though she had never done so, and tended to panic if placed in such a situation and to run out. By the time she was seen she was hardly leaving the house and had become what Roth describes as a 'housebound housewife'. She had managed to persuade friends and family to do her shopping and, although she functioned effectively within the home, developed a feeling of profound anxiety and terror if she had to go anywhere. Agoraphobia of this intensity merited hospital admission in order to break the cycle and to allow behavioural therapy to be effectively introduced.

Monosymptomatic phobias are much more specific than agoraphobia. The patient shows fear in the presence of particular situations, many of which are given fancy Latin names. Thus, **claustrophobia** is fear of enclosed spaces, such as lifts. Common ones are fears of heights or the dark, of insects, particular animals or snakes, or more subtle fears, such as fear of harming one's child or shouting out a swear word in church.

A woman of 27, somewhat depressed at the time, had the thought while pushing her toddler on a swing in the park, 'How awful if I were to hold a knife and it were to run into him as he swung back'. This somewhat bizarre thought became intrusive and preoccupied her mind to the extent that she became fearful of handling knives in the child's presence or of taking it again to the park. While she recognised the irrationality of the thought it would not go away and she became anxious that she might be going mad and might indeed carry out the action.

She could be reassured that there was no risk of this but nevertheless found the symptom quite disabling and was disturbing her relationship with the child. Behavioural treatment could here be initiated on an out-patient basis.

Some of these phobias are clear-cut and understandable in terms of life events, and some appear to develop with almost obsessional intensity for less obvious reasons. Many people suffer from mild degrees of mono-symptomatic phobias, which do not correlate with other psychiatric problems or with a tendency to more generalised anxiety states, and seem on the whole to be conditioned responses. Often their onset is traceable to specific events in childhood. The degree of disablement and the need or otherwise, therefore, for treatment depends largely on the type of fear from which the individual suffers. A fear of heights in a steeplejack or a fear of being in a car in a taxi driver would be highly disabling. A fear of heights in a housewife, however, would be of little consequence, and it would be easy for her to avoid this type of experience as long as she did not decide to take up climbing as a hobby.

Obsessional Compulsive Neuroses

An obsession refers to a repetitive thought which intrudes into consciousness. There may be the need to repeat in one's head a particular phrase or
snatch of a song over and over again, or thoughts of a more threatening
kind may persistently intrude into one's awareness, destroying concentration. Compulsions are the motor acting out of such behaviour, often in
a ritualistic manner, and particularly seen in checking rituals or tidiness.

The mechanism operating in obsessional compulsive neuroses is slightly
different from that seen in anxiety states. Wolpe has identified within this
group **anxiety-relieving** rituals and **anxiety-provoking** patterns of behaviour.
The mechanism of the former would appear to operate as follows. The
patient experiences a feeling of anxiety which is by its nature unpleasant,
and seeks to relieve it. Thus anxiety relief operates as a drive on the basis
of stimulus response theory as described in Part 1. A pattern of behaviour
which temporarily relieves this anxiety can be learned and repeated, and if
the anxiety itself is repetitive, then the learned pattern of behaviour is likely
to become a ritual. Thus people may need to check that doors are locked
before going to bed, and may find that they have to do this a certain number
of times. Clerks checking figures in an office may need to count the figures
not once but three times or three times three. An individual may need to
have everything straight, such as pictures on a wall or ornaments on a desk,
and may need to set out clothes in a particular style or pattern when going
to bed.

A mild degree of obsessionalism in a personality can be a useful trait.
It can make for conscientiousness and efficiency, and those with mild
obsessional personalities often find themselves in jobs demanding the careful
enumeration of items or checking of figures. If such symptoms become
associated with anxiety, however, and rituals which disturb concentration
and in fact reduce efficiency develop, then the problem can become more
serious and, indeed, in severe cases disabling.

Some obsessional thoughts, however, seem to have an anxiety-provoking
quality. Thus a woman may have a repetitive thought that she might murder
her child, or might disgrace herself in some way by, as one patient feared,
shouting a blasphemy in the middle of a church service. Such neurotic fears
are never acted out. The obsessional fears are not carried into action. But
the anxiety which they induce creates the same type of anxiety responses
seen in the other conditions described. Compulsive rituals may be used to
try to relieve this type of anxiety response.

A teacher, a male aged 32, was under some stress at his place of work. He
began to find that he had to check that doors were locked and taps turned
off. This took on a ritual pattern so that he was having to do this check round
twice before he felt satisfied that it had been completed. This applied whether
at school or at home and he then began to find he was having to do the same
when marking books or doing any kind of counting. If he failed to complete
the task satisfactorily then he had to go over the whole routine again. While
recognising the irrationality of this action he was aware of a distinct feeling
of tension and discomfort if he did not carry out the routine. Over a period
of months his rituals gradually became more elaborate and began to interfere

with the carrying out of his normal daily activities. Clothes had to be put down and folded in a certain way and washing had to be carried out for a specific length of time with two applications of soap and two rinses. By the time he came to the clinic's attention he was also showing quite marked depressive symptoms reactive to his obsessional state.

Neurotic Depression

In the previous chapter we discussed depressive symptoms in association with the affective psychoses. We stated, however, that depression was not infrequently seen as a symptom associated with neurotic states and, in particular, the various manifestations of anxiety. This type of depressive reaction, like that of pervasive anxiety, may develop without obvious external cause, or may seem to be an over-reaction or hypersensitivity to trivial trigger situations in the environment which to other people would not invoke this type of response. Patients with neurotic personalities seem particularly prone to develop reactive depressive swings, but their character is quite different from that of the affective psychotic state.

The mood of the neurotic depressive does not have the qualitative difference which those with affective psychosis comment upon compared with normal sadness. There is not the numbing sense of emotional nihilism. It is the same type of sadness of which we are all aware. It is simply the seeming inappropriateness of the cause or lack of an apparently adequate external stimulus which distinguishes it. Neurotic depressives can snap out of such a mood for a while if in stimulating company. When they revert again to dull normality, their worries flood back, but for a time they can lose themselves. This is rarely the case in the endogenous affective psychosis. Furthermore, in the neurotic depression the mood tends to worsen as the day goes on and the pressures build up. In contrast, in the endogenous depressive state the depression is worse in the mornings, associated with early morning waking, and improves as the day goes on.

The sleep rhythm also differs. In the patient with neurotic depression initial insomnia is the main problem. The cares of the day have piled up, they are tense and cannot relax, and, therefore, cannot get off to sleep. Once they do, they are liable to sleep through the following morning and miss the alarm.

While concentration may be disturbed, there is not the same pattern as found in the affective psychoses of loss of appetite, loss of libido, and general loss of interest in hobbies. These factors are much more variable and, indeed, over-eating may act as a compensation for the individual with a neurotic state. Sexual appetites follow no particular pattern, and often the neurotic feels better when engaged in some occupation, such as a hobby, which can absorb him for a while. As we shall see later in the chapter, response to treatment is also quite different in the two groups. Other features reflecting an anxiety neurosis and the personality that goes along with this state will be seen, whereas the affective psychosis often comes on completely out of the blue in a previously stable personality.

A lady of 28 was seen in the casualty ward after having taken an overdose of tablets. She had a history of neurotic reactions extending over a ten-year period and a history of three or four previous episodes of depression associated with environmental stresses. The precipitating problem was a breakdown in the marital relationship and the discovery of her husband's infidelity. She had for a few weeks, since the discovery of this episode, suffered from feelings of weakness and insecurity, and initial insomnia. Despite the depression she had gained some six pounds in weight and was aware of some compulsive eating. She felt nervous and anxious, and her concentration was impaired.

While the overdose was a cry for help the need to deal with the immediate after-effects required hospital admission. Tranquillising medication was unhelpful for her in the immediate weeks following the episode but this was better able to be discontinued as marital counselling, which both agreed to attend, became effective and the couple were reconciled.

Depersonalisation

It would appear that when subjected to stress over a long period the brain can sometimes, as it were, switch off and dissociate itself from the conscious environment. This is sometimes known as a **dissociative state**, and may take a variety of forms. Although mild feelings of unreality are quite familiar to most of us, there are not any words in common usage which can describe this symptom; but those who feel it frequently as part of an anxiety state know that it is present.

In **depersonalisation** the experience is of an altered awareness of one's own body image. Thus, when looking in a mirror, the face may seem unfamiliar or changed. It may not be recognisable as one's own. One's body may seem smaller or bigger or changed in shape, or parts of it may. Non-anxious people not infrequently get this type of experience when they are just going to sleep or just waking up and are in a twilight state.

In **derealisation** it is the outside environment that seems changed, or other people. Thus a familiar view may seem to the sufferer to be different, strange or unfamiliar. Other people may seem to be altered or unrecognisable, and, indeed, may appear threatening or in some way misshapen.

Thirdly, the emotional state itself may be affected by such feelings, so that the individual feels emotionally switched off. Thus, although physically he is responding, he is not experiencing happiness or sadness or any other emotional feeling at a conscious level.

Related to these feelings are other phenomena that may be seen in anxiety states or neuroses. *Déjà vu* phenomena describe the belief that something being experienced has happened before, even though logically it has not. Thus, a conversation may seem to be a repeat of something already said in the past, or there may be a false recognition of a place or situation: for example, where someone walks into a room and has the feeling they have been there before, although they know it is impossible for that to have been the case. Not surprisingly, people may interpret this kind of experience in a mystical manner, and give it some supernatural significance. The phenomena are easily explained, however, on the basis of false recall. Until the person has entered the room, there is of course no way he could describe what is inside; it is only when the perception has taken place that false recall can develop.

States of false recognition may occur as part of a paranoia. Paranoia has been described elsewhere and is usually thought of as a monosymptomatic psychosis.

States of altered awareness are commonplace as part of the picture of the anxiety neurosis. Such distortions of perception can, however, occur in other conditions, and the relationship between these phenomena and that seen in temporal lobe epilepsy is an interesting one, and has been commented upon as the 'phobic anxiety depersonalisation syndrome' by Roth, who noted the similarity between these symptoms and those seen in epileptiform phenomena affecting localised areas of the brain. Similar feelings are experienced as part of delirious states or as a toxic effect from some drugs, particularly the stimulants and hallucinogens. They may be found in a variety of physical diseases affecting the central nervous system. Finally, they may be found in other psychiatric conditions, in particular schizophrenia, where the distorted threatening type of derealisation phenomenon is quite common.

Hysteria

A not unrelated group of phenomena to those described in the last paragraphs is that subsumed under the title of hysteria. This interesting historical term has in general parlance come to mean something rather critical or abusive. In fact, the original word comes from the Greek meaning 'womb', since these symptoms, more commonly seen in women, were at that time ascribed to a wandering of the womb.

The hysterical personality, like the neurotic personality, describes a certain type of character structure which allows individuals to behave in a particular way when under stress. The hysterical personality will adopt symptoms which are psychological in origin but which mimic physical disease. As in anxiety states, these can affect any part of the body's function. The term is not correctly used in describing someone who loses control of himself and has an outburst of crying or disturbed behaviour. This type of acting out is, however, often called hysterical behaviour by the general public. On the contrary, in hysteria, a condition described by Janet as *la bel indifférence* is more normally seen, where the patient's attitude towards his symptom is surprisingly indifferent. This is, of course, not so surprising when one realises that the reason for the hysterical dissociative state is to remove from the patient at a subconscious level the need to act upon the anxiety-provoking situation.

Hysterical symptoms may affect motor function (as in the paralysis of an arm) or sensory function (as in the apparent loss of sensation to pain in a limb or loss of one of the senses, such as hearing or sight). Memory may be affected and a hysterical amnesia develop, with patients' total loss of recall of all information about themselves, without any history of head injury. There may be an occurrence of 'Fugue' states, in which the patient lives a double existence, for a while adopting an alternative identity; and this is seen in the extreme form of the Jekyll and Hyde type, where two complete personalities are apparently able to function at different times in one individual. Some transvestites may dissociate to the extent that they can take on the personality of the other sex when cross-dressed.

Virtually any symptom can develop for hysterical reasons. Hysterical fits may mimic epilepsy or disturbances of gait, or take on the tremor that mimics parkinsonism, and so forth.

The key to the diagnosis of such symptoms, which distinguishes them from organically determined states, is that there is no apparent physical cause, and no pathology to the affected part. For example, the patient complaining of loss of the use of an arm, with absence of power in the muscles and loss of sensation to pain or touch on the skin, will develop these symptoms in an area which is assumed to be the right one. Thus a glove-and-stocking type of anaesthesia usually occurs, but it does not, in fact, coincide with the nerve distribution that would result from nerve damage, nor the distribution which would be affected by damage to the blood supply. Nor is wasting of the muscles normally found, or alterations in the temperature to the limb. In other words, the symptoms just do not add up, and there is no appropriate history of injury or disease. Often there is, however, a history of emotional problems built up out of the development of the symptom, and a state of considerable anxiety may have been present until the symptom occurred, at which time *la bel indifférence* develops to the paralysis, which in the normal individual would be a highly worrying circumstance.

Arising out of this hysterical dissociation, secondary gain may develop, i.e. the effect of the symptom is such as to prevent the patient from carrying out some task which might be distasteful to him or from having to make some unpalatable decision. This tends to result in perpetuating the symptom, and it can often be very difficult to remove hysterical symptoms of this kind if a major secondary gain has developed. The incentive is not there.

The association between hysterical symptoms and hypnosis is an interesting one. In hypnosis a state of heightened suggestibility is produced through monotonous repetitive stimuli and the hypersuggestibility produced by the therapist. Under these conditions symptoms can be suggested to a patient, and he will then firmly believe in them and behave accordingly. If the subject can enter a deep enough trance state, then a post-hypnotic suggestion can be given, and the patient will act upon it even after being woken up.

Similarly, hysterical symptoms can often be removed under hypnosis or by using abreactive techniques. One way to treat such symptoms is to allow the patient to be brought to consciousness and act out the emotional feelings associated with repressed episodes of a traumatic kind with which the hysterical symptoms have originally been associated.

Not infrequently hysterical symptoms do seem to develop in association with acutely traumatic episodes, such as may occur during wartime or in battle, which the patient is unable to tolerate at conscious level. The memory of such an episode, therefore, becomes repressed, and for the patient ceases consciously to exist. It is completely forgotten. At a subconscious level, however, such memory tracings are not wiped out, and continue in some cases to cause distressing symptoms of a neurotic kind, for which the patient can then find no logical reason. With the abreactive release of such emotion, the patient shows a rapid generalised improvement. Unfortunately, these more striking cases are noteworthy for their rarity.

Hysterical symptoms seem to appear less commonly in our more sophisticated society, and nowadays anxiety tends to manifest itself in other forms. Hysterical symptoms are seen more frequently in more primitive societies. Freud felt them to be the product of repressed sexual or aggressive feelings, and at the time that he was in practice this was no doubt frequently the case, since sexual feelings, particularly in women, had frequently to be suppressed, but only at some cost to the patient's general stability.

One or two examples of hysterical symptomatology may illustrate some of the points mentioned above.

A single lady had to look after her aging and cantankerous mother. She felt very guilty when the mother fell in the garden one day and broke her hip. The daughter had often wished her away, and the old lady's admission to hospital seemed unhappily to have coincided with the daughter's less charitable thoughts. The daughter developed a paralysis of her right hand, no doubt the one she had thought of pushing her mother with. As it happened, this had the secondary effect of preventing the daughter from looking after her mother again when she was due to come out of hospital, since she was unable to do any lifting. The daughter seemed surprisingly unconcerned about this considerable disability, but the subconscious secondary gain made it difficult to eradicate the symptom.

In another case a young girl of rather outgoing personality was disappointed at being rejected for a nurses' training course when she left school. While under this disappointment, she was sliding on some ice with her younger brother when she fell rather heavily and banged her hip. She was taken in some pain to the casualty department, where a relatively inexperienced doctor, playing safe, decided to put the hip in plaster until the results of an X-ray could be seen by his senior the following day, since he feared there might be a fracture. When the X-rays were seen, it was established that there was no bone injury but simply bruising, and the plaster was, therefore, removed. At this point, however, the girl said that she was completely unable to move the leg or feel anything in it at all. A pin was stuck in her foot and she did not jump. The staff were worried that some injury might have occurred to a nerve, either through the result of the fall or the plaster having been applied too tightly. Examination, however, showed that, although she dragged the leg when walking and did not bear any weight on it, she could sit up in bed from a lying position, which movement requires the thigh muscles to act as an anchor. Furthermore, the distribution of loss of sensation would have had to be the responsibility of at least three different nerves, all following a different course in the hip.

Treatment in this case was partly by psychotherapy to uncover the underlying problems and the possible secondary gain which such a symptom was producing, but also by behaviour therapy, utilising the normal reflex responses that are present in both legs, and training her to move the good leg in response to a stimulus applied to the bad leg, eventually reversing the leads so that the bad leg was caused to move by a stimulus applied to the good one. Often some face-saving device is required to allow the patient to accept that the symptom is an hysterical one, so that they can avoid the accusation of friends that they were in any way malingering.

In a third case, a man was admitted to hospital complaining of total loss of memory. This is not usually found in concussion or head injury, where a loss of memory is as a rule patchy. This and the absence of any physical signs suggested a diagnosis of hysterical amnesia, and prompted the use of a pentothal interview in treatment. Here the patient, while under the influence of the drug, which is injected intravenously, is likely to be able to recall any repressed material. During this therapy session the man was able to reveal that he had recently come off a ship. Gradually the story was pieced together. The man had been benefiting from the attentions of a 'sugar mummy', who, in exchange for favours, had given him various gifts, including a car. The man's own family had been unaware of this relationship, but when in due course it had come to an end, the woman had demanded the return of the car. The man had refused because it would have put him in a very awkward position at home. The 'sugar mummy' had threatened to sue and, indeed, legal action was about to take place. This inevitably would have caused the man's family to find out about his liaison.

On his way to work that morning his memory for the past had become blotted out and he had taken a job on the crew of a ship travelling to the Baltic ports. He had been away just over a week, during which time his family had registered him as a missing person. When he had left the ship at the docks back in England, he had begun to walk up the road hitching lifts. At this point he could not recall anything about what had happened the previous week or about his former life, and he had reported to a police station complaining of this total amnesia and not even knowing his name.

This is a typical example of a hysterical fugue state. The loss of memory is associated with a stress to which the individual sees no solution, and once the memory has gone and such a person starts to live a double life, the secondary gain tends to perpetuate the memory disturbance.

A number of pentothal interviews may be required before the patient's recall returns to normal. Such therapy must be combined with supportive psychotherapy designed to help the individual to come to terms with the unpalatable reality.

Parasympathetic Over-activity

It may be that some neurotic syndromes are produced through over-activity of just one branch of the autonomic nervous system. We have seen how the sympathetic system can play a part in the production of anxiety and fear responses.

Over-stimulation of the parasympathetic system is less clearly defined. Syndromes associated with blushing, embarrassment, abnormal gut motility with diarrhoea and a development of some psychosomatic disturbances are probably associated with over-activity in certain centres of the limbic lobe through acetyl-choline, the mono-amine which mediates the cell activity in the parasympathetic system. It might be that treatment with acetyl-choline inhibitors would be a logical development for such syndromes. At present the more general inhibition of limbic lobe activity through benzodiazepines and the use of behaviour therapy techniques form a more practical method of treatment.

Differential Diagnosis

Anxiety is a very subjective phenomenon. One of the most accurate ways of measuring anxiety is simply to ask patients to rate how anxious they are. This can be given a little more scientific validity by the use of visual analogue scales. Objective measures of anxiety may use psychological rating scales, such as the Hamilton Anxiety Scale, or may attempt to measure anxiety levels directly by physiological tests of skin moisture, peripheral blood flow, or some similar technique. It is not always easy to correlate these results with the patient's own subjective feelings.

Anxiety is a very widespread phenomenon, and the possibility of an endogenous pathological anxiety state has been considered earlier in the chapter. We have noted that an infusion of lactate solution can induce an anxiety attack in those suffering from an anxiety neurosis, whereas such a response does not occur with the intravenous infusion of other solutions, such as dextrose or saline. This response is not clear-cut enough to use yet as a diagnostic tool. What is important is to distinguish between an anxiety state and some of the many physical diseases, which may present with anxiety symptoms and may, therefore, be confused with an anxiety state. This is, of course, again a reason for psychiatrists having a good grounding in general medicine before they specialise.

Many of the diseases that can be associated with anxiety as a symptom have been considered in our chapter on psychosomatic disorders. However, some stand out in importance, and, in order to avoid missing the occasional case, a careful physical examination, particularly of the nervous system, and certain screening tests, including tests of blood and urine, should be carried out.

Glandular disturbances of the endocrine system particularly often present with changes of mood. Anxiety is frequently seen. Thyrotoxicosis can mimic anxiety states. Pituitary disease or myxoedema, where there is a deficiency in thyroid hormone, can not only mimic neurasthenia but also depression and early dementias may be mistakenly diagnosed. Symptoms believed to be hysterical may show in disturbances of blood sugar levels, particularly with insulin-secreting tumours of the pancreas.

Temporal lobe epilepsy can produce symptoms similar to the phobic anxiety, depersonalisation syndrome mentioned above. Symptoms such as frequency of passing water or alterations in bowel habit may erroneously suggest urinary tract or kidney infection, or the presence of various types of bowel disease. Some types of anaemia, in particular pernicious anaemia, can mimic the symptoms seen in anxiety states or neurasthenia. One should always be careful about diagnosing anxiety states and in particular hysterical symptoms, without making a proper check. Such diagnosis should be made for positive reasons and not by excluding everything else in the book.

Finally, the possibility of other psychiatric illness should also be considered. Serious depressive illness may present initially with what appear to be anxiety symptoms, and obsessional symptoms are not infrequently seen in the early stages of a schizophrenic breakdown.

Treatment

A wide variety of treatment processes are available for the psychoneuroses. Their variety may suggest that no one treatment is particularly effective. Certain types of treatment seem more effective for specific syndromes than others, but in general terms the diversity of treatments reflects underlying theoretical viewpoints about the causation of neuroses—whether they are maladaptive conditioned responses that should be treated on behaviour therapy lines, deep-seated repressed complexes from early childhood that should be dealt with by psychoanalytical therapy, or physical disturbances in the limbic lobe metabolism, where medication and physical methods of treatment might be anticipated to be more effective.

Since psychoneuroses are not an homogeneous group, there is a diversity of cause and, therefore, room for a diversity of treatment. Important in the assessment of the cases, therefore, must be which type of the therapies available seems most appropriate, and this must take into account not only what might be ideal, but also, unfortunately, such economic factors as the time available, both the client's and the therapist's, and the practical business of what staff are available.

Mild degrees of psychoneurosis are extremely common, and to deal with all of them on the basis of analytical psychotherapy would demand the resources of a vast number of psychotherapists, which the country can certainly not afford, even if it were considered the most effective method of treatment in the first place. For the majority, therefore, the use of anxiolytic medication in the shape of tranquilliser pills is likely to be the most practical and, indeed, for short-term symptom relief the most effective treatment. Only the more serious cases can justify more elaborate methods, certainly within a Health Service context. Indeed, in many cases counselling and a few supportive sessions in which patients can express their fears are often anxiety-relieving enough. Dealing with such cases in more depth could, indeed, have negative consequences in making the patient too introspective and health-orientated.

Let us consider the various types of therapy in turn, indicating where their special usefulness seems to lie. Many of these treatments have been dealt with in a little more depth in Chapter 4. We need not elaborate further on some of these.

Drug Therapy

Until the advent of the benzodiazepine drugs a variety of sedatives had been available for the control of tension. These included the higher alcohols, and indeed alcohol itself, and sedatives such as the barbiturates. With the development of chlordiazepoxide came the availability of a new range of products, which acted more specifically on the limbic lobe and did not have the disadvantage of a more generalised sedative action on the central nervous system, and particularly the cerebral cortex. In the last fifteen years benzodiazepines have established themselves as a safe method of control of acute anxiety states. They have been widely prescribed and indeed many would say over-prescribed for any state of tension. They have proved themselves invaluable to those in need in the short term, but have tended also to be prescribed for those whose anxiety is environmentally induced and normal. In such cases it would be more appropriate to counsel the patient in his or her problems.

Unfortunately, the benzodiazepines, considered so safe in the early days of therapy, have been shown to create dependence and considerable difficulty during the withdrawal phase in a relatively small, but significant, number of people. It is now advised that such drugs should be used in the short term since dependency can develop within a few weeks in some cases. It has been shown that some of the newer non-benzodiazepine drugs such as buspirone and the new serotonin uptake inhibitors such as fluvoxamine and fluoxetine have a specific effect on panic states and probably on obsessional neuroses and are much less likely to create the dependence which has been shown with benzodiazepines.

The alternatives to drug therapy are not always easy to come by. Even counselling is sometimes a rare and expensive commodity and it is better to have aspirin for toothache, even though there is a hole in the tooth which needs filling, than to suffer unnecessary pain. Similarly, there is little to be gained by suffering unnecessary anxiety in the acute phase.

While some patients with neurotic personalities may need to continue medication on a maintenance dosage over very long periods, the majority can discontinue the preparation once the symptoms have come under control. A period of anxiety-free living allows such a person to build up confidence and makes the need for tranquillisers progressively less.

Some of the benzodiazepines induce a degree of drowsiness and act as muscle relaxants. Patients may become psychologically dependent on the product, and in rare cases there is a release of inhibition, which, instead of controlling tension, can allow the patient to act out and may produce paradoxical aggressive behaviour. These hazards need to be borne in mind, as does the tendency for these drugs to potentiate alcohol, which can lead to hazards, for example, when driving a vehicle if alcohol is taken while on such medication.

Since chlordiazepoxide was first developed, a number of new benzodiazepines have been introduced. The object has been to reduce side-effects or to increase potency, and a wide range of products is now available.

As an alternative to benzodiazepines in the relief of anxiety by drug therapy, small doses of the **phenothiazines** or related drugs may be used. Popular ones are trifluperazine, flupenthixol, haloperidol and pimozide. The profiles of these drugs differ slightly, some being more calming and others more effective in inducing improved levels of drive, for instance, in the neurasthenic type of anxiety state.

A drug of a different group is **chlormethiazole**, which is another alternative, acting at a central level. A new one is Zimovane (zopiclone).

Many of these preparations, particularly the benzodiazepines and chlormethiazole, can be used for the initial insomnia which often goes with neurotic conditions, and are used in this sense as sleeping tablets. The advantage that they have over the more conventional sleeping tablets, such as barbiturates, chloral, and the like, is their safety, since there is little danger from over-dosage because of their more specific action on the sleep centre and the fact that they do not depress respiration.

All the drugs mentioned so far have attacked anxiety at a central level in the limbic lobe or reticular activating systems. It is also possible to control anxiety, particularly when it manifests itself in psychosomatic symptoms, such as rapid pulse or attacks of palpitations, by using a group of drugs known as **beta-blocking agents**, which act peripherally at the nerve endings in the autonomic system. An example of such a drug is propanolol.

Finally, it is possible to control the symptoms of anxiety and neurotic depression with the **mono-amine oxidase inhibitor** (MAOI) group of drugs. These act by inhibiting an enzyme mono-amine oxidase which breaks down mono-amines at the synapse or nerve-cell junctions. We have discussed the theoretical implications of these drugs in an earlier chapter. Suffice it to say here that the ability of the MAOI drugs to restore or potentiate amines seems to be related to their effectiveness in phobic anxiety and neurotic depression.

There are two basic types of drug, one represented by phenelzine and the other by tranylcypromine. These drugs may take some four weeks to reach their full effectiveness, and are a nuisance insofar as certain dietary restrictions are necessary while taking them, in particular any foodstuffs containing tyramine, such as cheeses and concentrated meat extracts. Other drugs, such as those used to clear nasal congestion, may interact adversely and should not be used without medical advice. Such interactions temporarily raise the blood pressure and induce a migraine-like headache in susceptible people.

Obsessional compulsive states are considered to respond better to certain of the tricyclic anti-depressant drugs, in particular clomipramine. Some of the nervous habit spasms or tics which may go with neuroses, and are of hysterical origin, seem to respond best to such drugs as pimozide or halo-peridol. The acquiring of the necessary therapeutic skills to determine which drug will be most effective can only be gained with experience. The new specific serotonin uptake inhibitors such as fluoxetine may also have a specific effect.

Psychotherapy

The neuroses have been the traditional area in which psychotherapists of various disciplines have worked. On the assumption that neuroses represent repressed and unresolved conflicts dating from childhood, the psycho-therapist attempts by various techniques to bring out and resolve these conflicts. The field of psychotherapy covers a wide range from super-ficial supportive counselling, based principally on reassurance, to the depth-regressive analytical techniques of psychoanalysts working through Freudian theory, or other schools, such as those of Jung or Adler. These in-depth techniques are time-consuming and cannot be dealt with in great detail in a book such as this. The use of dream analysis, free-association techniques and similar procedures must be studied in a specialist book.

During psychotherapy the patient will develop a considerable rapport with the therapist, and transference reactions—the development of an empathetic relationship between patient and therapist, which reflects rela-tionships the patient may have had with key figures in early life—may develop and require working through. The interpretation of these relation-ships and the development of insight into the causation of the neurosis are the ultimate aim of such therapy.

Psychotherapy may be practised as an individual matter or can be dealt with on the basis of group psychotherapy. In the latter some six to eight people with broadly similar problems will develop a group empathy over a period of regular attendance through some months, and come to understand their problems better through the dynamics of the group experience.

Various techniques have been developed to try to speed up this psychotherapeutic process, which can otherwise be a time-consuming affair. Analysts would probably argue that these short-cut techniques reduce effectiveness, but to the author's knowledge there is little evidence to support this, and in any case one must work within the facilities available.

Hypnosis

This interesting technique was originally developed by Mesmer, and was expanded in the time of Charcot and Janet and taken up for a time by Freud himself. In its simplest form it acts as a process of relaxation and, indeed, many simple relaxation techniques, as taught at ante-natal classes, in yoga classes or meditation groups, use similar techniques. Simple relaxation can be of great help in the treatment of anxiety, and this in itself may be all that is required.

Hypnosis is simply an extension of this process, whereby a blocking of the middle part of the brain at the level of the reticular activating system is achieved, and the patient becomes hypersuggestible and can in some cases enter a deep trance state. Not all people are capable of this, and, indeed, not all therapists have the necessary experience to practice hypnosis at this level. Hypnotherapy can be utilised simply as an extension of relaxation, or in order to present the patient with post-hypnotic suggestions of a confidence-increasing kind.

Hypnotic techniques are perhaps used even more in the fields of dentistry and anaesthetics than in psychiatry itself. Childbirth can be made easier, and even operations can be performed without the need for anaesthetic in deep trance subjects. In psychiatry, however, it is principally of value in relieving phobias and various states of tension, and in the treatment of such neurotic side-effects as excessive smoking or drinking. As an extension to psychotherapy, however, hypnoanalysis can be practised. Here, the patient is taken back while under hypnosis to key areas of earlier life and enabled to relive some of these experiences, so that the repressed emotionally charged material is brought out and dissipated.

Abreactive Techniques

The enabling of a patient to relive repressed emotional experiences or to recall forgotten traumatic events, such as may occur in shellshock neurosis, a hysterical syndrome often seen in wartime, can be effected through hypnosis or through analytical techniques, but can be induced more readily and often equally effectively by use of drug-induced abreaction. Various techniques are available. Early treatment developed after the Second World War consisted of the inhalation of ether or ethyl chloride at levels insufficient to produce complete anaesthesia, but sufficient to cause a state of disinhibition and loosening of ego defences. The patient was then encouraged to relive the repressed emotional experiences.

Carbon dioxide inhalation was developed by Meduna, who also developed electroplexy. His technique was for patients to inhale 30 per cent carbon dioxide in a 70 per cent oxygen mixture to induce the same state of altered consciousness, a technique he found useful both as an abreactive procedure and as a generalised anxiety-relieving procedure in pervasive anxiety. The method was modified by La Verne, who used a rapid onset technique, with 70 per cent carbon dioxide and 30 per cent oxygen inhaled over a short space of time, which induced a state of relaxation much more rapidly.

In more recent years the development of safe, rapidly acting intravenous anaesthesia, with barbiturates such as thiopentone and other rapidly acting and rapidly wearing off drugs that have come on the market, has supplied a method which gives maximum control of the procedure, and enables the level of consciousness to be kept adjusted very easily and finely without all the preliminaries necessary in teaching hypnosis. Sometimes this type of injection can be combined with a stimulant drug such as methedrine, which reduces the level of sedation, or methedrine can be used alone as an abreactive procedure. The snag with methods that require the injection of a substance into the vein which in larger dosage works as an anaesthetic is that resuscitative equipment must always be on hand for the rare unforeseen reaction, and the patient usually needs a while to rest and sleep off the effects. With carbon dioxide inhalation the patient can get up more or less immediately after treatment is ended.

Hallucinogens such as LSD have also been used as abreactive drugs but the danger of precipitating a psychotic episode and the unpredictability of the effect plus the fact that these products are now mostly legally restricted has led to experiments in this field largely being discontinued.

Somlec

Relaxation and control of many aspects of psychoneurotic behaviour, in particular where pervasive anxiety is present, can be treated by a mechanism known as electrosleep (Somlec). This procedure has been widely used in continental Europe, though less so in Britain and the United States. In essence, a very low voltage pulsed current is passed between positive electrodes on the forehead and a negative one over the occipital area of the skull, inducing a monotonous rhythmic stimulus at the same frequency as that of the natural brain rhythms shown on the electroencephalogram during sleep. This produces an autohypnotic effect. The patient becomes relaxed and usually sleeps over the period of an hour or two that the treatment is administered.

The Somlec machines currently available can treat three or six patients at a time in a group manner. The treatment is pleasant and the patients usually feel relaxed and tension-free at the end of the session. A course is given, rather as in electroplexy, of some ten or twelve treatments. The technique seems particularly good for psychosomatic problems and insomnia. It can be combined with other anxiety-relieving methods of treatment, such as drugs, and group therapy can be utilised at the end of the treatment session to encourage, for example, those with phobic states to carry out tasks which they normally feel nervous about in the immediate post-treatment phase.

Behaviour Therapy

Behaviour therapy techniques based on learning theory have widespread application in the psychoneuroses. We have described the theoretical basis of this treatment in Chapter 7. If the patient with a neurosis is reacting with a maladaptive response pattern that has developed in childhood or early adulthood because of frightening experiences which have occurred, then the association of these responses with an anxiety-relieving process should be effective in extinguishing such a response. Thus, if a fear-inducing stimulus which normally produces the response of avoidance can be associated with something pleasurable which causes positive learning to take place, this will reinforce the pattern of behaviour which one wants to develop.

These techniques are particularly applicable in monosymptomatic phobic states, agoraphobia, and in obsessional behaviour patterns. The techniques used for relieving anxiety and the relaxation methods described above, or hypnosis itself, can be incorporated. Anxiolytic medication or the abreactive techniques can also be utilised as part of a behaviour therapy programme.

Wolpe noted that a variety of responses were anxiety-relieving, including sexual responses, physical exercise, and indeed psychotherapy itself. The behaviourists would suggest that techniques employed in psychoanalysis and more superficial psychotherapy have their prime effect by the anxiety-relieving process of the development of an empathetic relationship. Behaviour therapy techniques have been extended beyond the simple range of psychoneurotic anxiety to include sexual problems and many of the conduct and habit disorders seen more particularly by child psychiatrists.

Further Reading

Beech, M. R., *Obsessional States*, Methuen, London, 1974.

Hallam, R. S., Agoraphobia—A Critical Review of the Concept, *British Medical Journal of Psychiatry*, 133.314, 1978.

Hill, O. W., *Modern Trends in Psychosomatic Medicine* (3), Butterworth, London, 1979.

Marks, I. M., *Fears and Phobias*, Heinemann, London, 1969.

Rycroft, C., *Anxiety and Neurosis*, Penguin, Harmondsworth, 1970.

Shader, R. I., *Anxiety, Diagnosis and Management*, Raven, New York, 1980.

Silverstone, T., and Barraclough, B., 'Obsessional States', *Contemporary Psychiatry*, BJP Special Publications No. 9, Headley, Kent, 1975.

Smythes, J. R., *Studies of Anxiety*, BJP, Headley, Kent, 1969.

Snaith, P., 'Panic Disorder', *British Medical Journal*, 286.1376, 1983.

Questions

1. How widespread are neuroses?
2. Do you have a local branch of neurotics anonymous or an agoraphobia group?
3. What is the limbic lobe?
4. What is the role of psychoanalysis in the treatment of neurosis?
5. Does your local psychiatric unit have a psychotherapist on the staff? Do they have Somlec relaxation therapy available? Is hypnosis available?
6. What is hysteria?

13
Psychosomatic Disorders

Summary

Psychosomatic disorders may be defined as that group of conditions where a physical disturbance of bodily function has in its causation a clear-cut emotional or psychological component.

Such diseases may affect any of the bodily systems. Thus the cardio-vascular system, respiratory, genito-urinary, and gastro-intestinal, and the skin may all be affected in particular individuals. The target organ may vary, and the reason why one particular target organ more than another suffers in a particular individual is unknown.

Classification

1. *Gastro-intestinal system*
(a) Peptic ulcer; (b) ulcerative colitis; (c) irritable bowel syndrome.

2. *Respiratory system*
(a) Asthma; (b) hay fever; (c) allergic rhinitis.

3. *Cardiovascular system*
(a) Hypertension; (b) ischaemic heart disease.

4. *The skin*
(a) Eczema; (b) urticaria.

5. *Musculo-skeletal system*
(a) Rheumatoid arthritis; (b) torticollis.

6. *Genito-urinary system*
(a) Urinary frequency; (b) menstrual disturbances; (c) psychosexual problems.

7. *Metabolic and endocrine disorders*
(a) Migraine.

8. *Somato-psychic disorders*

No one speciality within the total concept of medicine can be considered in isolation. There is no clear-cut division of function even in a speciality such as obstetrics, where the delivery of a baby may require overlap with the skills of (1) general medicine, should the mother's condition be complicated by high blood pressure or toxaemia, (2) anaesthetics, should some emergency ensue during what was thought to be a normal delivery and a

Caesarean section be required, (3) neonatal paediatrics in the care of the infant from the point of delivery, and, indeed, even (4) psychiatry to care for those mothers who may develop psychotic states associated with their pregnancy or childbirth.

So it is with psychiatry that considerable overlap exists with the specialities of general practice and general medicine, with neurology and biochemistry. It also overlaps with non-medical skills in the field of sociology and social work, with a knowledge of pharmacology and a knowledge of statistics. The list could be expanded. It must be emphasised that many disease entities totally removed from psychiatry in terms of the primary pathology may produce disturbances in thinking, emotion and behaviour through secondary involvement of the central nervous system, and that a full general medical training is necessary in order to be able to pick up the relevance of such factors and identify them in any particular patient.

Certain general medical diseases, however, have an even closer affinity with psychiatry, in that there is a well-recognised association between emotional factors and the personality of an individual and the illness from which they suffer. Examples of this would cover some types of asthma, some types of skin disease, and peptic ulcer. Such conditions, where this association exists, are known as psychosomatic disorders.

The Autonomic Nervous System

A psychosomatic condition may be defined as one where structural changes occur in the body in relation to emotional factors. There is, however, a mind–body interaction between the soma and the psyche at all levels, and it is absurd to attempt to look at one or the other in total isolation. The key to such associations in terms of psychosomatic disease lies in the nerve supply governing the internal functions of the body, and known as the **autonomic nervous system**.

The brain, which is the central part of the nervous system, subserves a wide variety of functions. The **cerebral cortex**, divided into various lobes, is concerned with the conscious appraisal of situations, the coordination of incoming stimuli and outgoing motor activity, and intelligent thought. Below this level, however, are a large number of nuclei and ganglia which are closely interrelated. Another part of the brain, the **cerebellum**, is concerned primarily with coordinating movement and balance. Other special areas in the brain coordinate speech, sight and hearing, etc. It is not our brief in this book to review these. For an account of brain function at this level the reader must refer to books on neurology.

Underneath the brain, at what is known as mid-brain level, are a series of interconnecting tracts and nuclei which together go to form what is known as the **limbic lobe** of the brain (Figure 8). This is connected closely with the **thalamus**, with the **frontal lobe** of the cortex, which deals with emotion at a conscious level, and with various activating systems that pass down from the central nervous system into the spinal column and the nerves which supply all parts of the body.

The limbic lobe function is intimately associated with the control of mood states and what is generally called **affect**. The actual working of the nerves within these centres is dependent upon the mono-amines, described else-

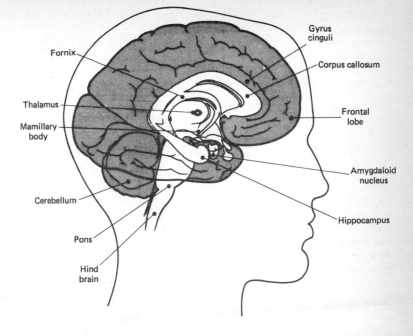

Fig. 8. The limbic lobe.

where, whose chemistry is thought to be distorted in various types of psychotic illness. These mono-amines are the catecholamines, such as noradrenalin, dopamine, serotonin and a number of other systems at present less well understood.

The effect of over-activity or under-activity of particular ganglia in the limbic lobe—the hippocampus and amygdaloid nuclei in particular—may be felt throughout the body. Furthermore, outside stimuli from the environment may provoke activity in the limbic lobe, as may be found in some anxiety reactions.

The effect of these changes is seen in the autonomic nervous system. This controls the internal and unconscious activities of body function, in contrast to the peripheral nerves, which are concerned with the perception of the sensations of touch, pain, etc., and the motor activity of muscles. The latter group act through the chemical mediation of a mono-amine known as acetyl choline, but the autonomic system is activated through other catecholamines.

The autonomic nervous system has two main divisions. The **para-sympathetic** outflow is concerned with glandular secretions, digestion, and a variety of other functions. The main outflow is from the spinal cord at the level of the neck and in the lumbar region at the base of the spine, with some also at the base of the brain. The nerves are distributed very widely to most of the internal organs. The **sympathetic** system is concerned with activating the body in response to danger or threatening situations, and thus the control

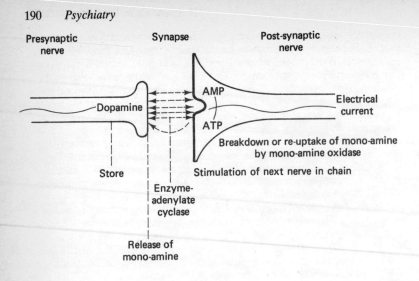

Fig. 9. The chemical function of the synapse or nerve cell junction.

of blood pressure, heart rate, and the outflow of the adrenal glands. The two systems work to some extent antagonistically, so that over-stimulation of one will produce suppression of the other.

Short-lived bursts of activity in appropriate circumstances, where the body can act upon the stimuli being received in a constructive and finite manner, pose no problems. It will be noted, however, that, should the environment pose a continuing threat or create indecisiveness in an individual, particularly where such a person sees no clear-cut line of action they can take to relieve such tension, the long-term over-activity of these autonomic systems might produce changes in the tissues which, over a long period of time, could be irreversible. This could arise from a genuine external threat, or from an individual previously conditioned who sees a source of tension where others would not. It would be innate—in that it is the way such an individual is made—or could result from early life experiences.

Again, such over-activity could arise from a malfunction of the various parts of the limbic lobe in the brain, where, just as in the thyroid gland or other endocrine systems in the body, an over-activity, under-activity or distorted hormone production could alter the balance of the system as a whole and provoke either a generalised anxiety state, or affect target organs in the body supplied by such systems. Finally, the mono-amines themselves at the nerve cell synapses or junctions might be functioning incorrectly and induce disturbances at a local peripheral level.

It is probable that in a complicated mechanism, such as the human frame creates, a number of these factors may operate, even though the end result may be similar. In the same way anaemia, rheumatism, or a cough may be the end result of a variety of pathological factors causing them.

The question of target organs is an interesting one in psychosomatic medicine. The dilemma can be stated thus. Why is it that physical symptoms apparently produced or worsened by emotional causes should affect one part of the body in one person and a different organ in another? Why does one person develop asthma and another a duodenal ulcer? What is the factor common to psychosomatic conditions and what makes them vary?

Some of the answers to these questions may lie in areas where research is as yet in its infancy. The action of mono-amines in the central nervous system is but vaguely understood. Another group of substances, the **endorphins,** is now attracting widespread interest, and may prove to be an additional group of factors which need to be considered in the aetiology of many disease processes. These chemicals seem intimately concerned with such factors as the perception of pain and the threshold levels at which people perceive sensations. This could be very pertinent to the conditions we are at present considering.

Certain personality factors do seem to be common to those individuals prone to psychosomatic disorders. These are a tendency to conscientiousness and obsessionalism, a relatively higher than average intelligence and an anxiety-prone personality. This seems to apply regardless of the target organ that is affected. Let us now look at some of the particular conditions in which psychosomatic factors are believed to operate.

Gastro-intestinal System

A clear-cut association between peptic ulcer and emotional factors has been recognised for many years. The mechanism for this seems more straightforward than some. The stomach produces acid as part of the mechanism of digesting food. Early experiments have shown that in states of stress the stomach mucosa, or lining, becomes a source of increased secretory activity, and this is mediated through the autonomic nervous system. Under certain conditions the mucosal lining can develop a small erosion, and the overactivity then produces a situation where the individual's gastric juices start to digest their own stomach lining.

Should long-standing tension induce constant over-activity, then a chronic ulcer can be produced. Thus a physical disease now exists which perpetuates itself and may continue, even though the original stress may have been resolved. Reducing autonomic activity by drugs or by division of the autonomic supply through an operation to cut these nerves can result in healing. So sometimes can treatment designed to reduce tension at a central level through the learning of relaxation procedures or use of the Somlec relaxation therapy.

Many people will recognise that when under chronic stress their bowel habit is changed and they develop a nervous diarrhoea. This again is mediated through autonomic over-activity, and similar factors probably play a part in the development of more long-standing disturbances of bowel function such as ulcerative colitis. Often operative intervention to remove areas of affected bowel may be the only solution once the disease is established. At an earlier stage use of drugs such as cortisone preparations may be effective, but it would be nice to think that such individuals could be spotted before the disease progresses this far, and some treatment aimed at reducing tension levels could be applied.

Respiratory System

Three common conditions in which emotional factors seem to be important are asthma, hay fever and rhinitis.

In asthma the small pipes within the lung, the bronchioles, have muscles within their walls which are controlled by mono-amines, in this case probably histamine. Other factors may also operate, and again such muscles are under autonomic nervous system control. A number of factors may exacerbate asthma, including, of course, allergens. This also applies to hay fever and allergic rhinitis. Nevertheless, there is a close interaction between the response of the body to allergy and emotional stress. In some asthma cases there seems to be a clear-cut allergic component, which can be identified, and in another the association with stress can be very obvious. This again has important implications for the type of treatment which should be employed.

A boy of 14 began to develop episodic attacks of asthma. A rather anxiety-prone child, he had a history of enuresis to the age of six and was a nail-biter. Tests for allergens failed to show any clear-cut relationship with common factors that might be involved, but it was noted that attacks tended to occur when there was friction between his parents whose marriage was going through a bad patch. Improvement began to occur when the boy was able to talk out what he had heard (his parents' conversation of separating) and some family therapy was able to be applied which fortunately could reassure him.

Cardiovascular System

The association between hypertension (high blood pressure) and stress is also well documented. An individual's blood pressure can rise simply under the anxiety of a physical examination, and this must be taken into account when the doctor assesses such factors. The emotion of anger seems to be associated more with some psychosomatic conditions than others. Perhaps we are seeing a different mechanism in suppressed anger, where particular parts of the limbic lobe may come into action and create a bigger emphasis on sympathetic or parasympathetic branches, depending on the individual case. However, again we see the operation of factors where an emotionally induced high blood pressure, if prolonged, can set in motion a chain of events in the body which then becomes self-perpetuating. The blood pressure can affect circulation and damage the smaller vessels in the kidney, or may promote changes which result in hardening of the arteries or atheroma.

Another way in which emotion may play a part in the cardiovascular system is in the development of ischaemic heart disease. There is some evidence to suggest that the small coronary arteries supplying blood to the heart muscle themselves, which are under autonomic control, can be made to contract during stress, and this can precipitate a heart attack in those in whom ischaemia is already developed.

Similarly, the heart rate is under the control of both sympathetic and parasympathetic systems, whereby the speed of the heart beat can be

regulated to suit the body's demands. Emotional factors can cause alterations to this rhythm which, when no physical exertion is needed, are
inappropriate, and can trigger off paroxysmal tachycardia.

The Skin

The skin is closely related embryologically to the nervous system. Skin
changes in many ways reflect emotional states. One obvious example is the
blushing that can occur with embarrassment, in this case probably a result
of parasympathetic over-activity. Individuals may go 'white with anger'
and so on. These are usually temporary changes but certainly show an
association between emotion and physical change.

The 'eczema, asthma, hay fever' syndrome is a well-recognised grouping
of conditions. Here, as in asthma, the eczema may be altered by the emotional
state of the patient. Thus some cases of eczema are certainly worsened by
emotional stress, and the same may apply in psoriasis. Another interesting
skin condition is that of urticaria, or nettle-rash. This again is associated
with a histamine release, can occur in response to allergy, and may be the
direct result of toxins injected under the skin by stinging. In a number of
well-documented cases, however, urticaria has occurred in response to
emotional states, and the presumed mechanism is that of mono-amine
activity. Dealing with the tension in such patients through psychotherapy,
relaxation therapy or anxiolytic medication may have a more beneficial
effect in the long term than simple treatment with antihistamines.

Musculo-skeletal System

The symptom of backache, hardly a disease in itself, is a common problem
among specialists in general medicine, gynaecology, rheumatology and
orthopaedics. Some cases may be due to congestion of the pelvic organs in
patients with psycho-sexual problems, but not uncommonly such symptoms
are found in depressive states. More significant has been the finding that
rheumatoid arthritis, thought to be a disease of collagen material in the
body, can relapse and remit in association with states of emotional tension
and their relief. This is not to suggest that the disease is entirely emotionally
induced but rather that personality factors and the patient's mental state
may influence the course and progress of the disease.

Genito-urinary System

Another common symptom with which people will be familiar is the need
to pass water more frequently at times of emotional stress and tension. This
is seen throughout the mammalian kingdom. If a simple test is done whereby
someone enters a field where there is a flock of sheep, the immediate reaction
of the sheep to this potentially dangerous situation is to pass water. In
states of chronic tension the individual may develop a hyper-sensitivity to
bladder fullness and feel the urge to empty the bladder more frequently
than is really necessary. The symptom of urinary frequency is commonly
found in anxiety states.

J.S., a woman of 35, complained of excessive frequency of having to pass water and a feeling of urgency when this arose. She had a past history of treatment for recurrent attacks of cystitis but pain on passing water was rarely a symptom and when urine tests had been done no bacteria isolated. She had, however, had a number of tests, including X-rays of renal or kidney function, and urethroscopy with cautery to the bladder neck.

When she was eventually referred for psychiatric opinion it became apparent that wider symptoms of an anxiety state were also present. Only when the problem of this neurosis was tackled did the urinary trouble gradually lose its significance and disappear as a symptom.

Disturbances of the menstrual cycle are also frequently seen in association with psychiatric problems. Excessive and frequent periods (menorrhagia and polymenorrhoea), pain associated with periods (dysmenorrhoea) and pre-menstrual tension are all seen associated with states of tension and anxiety, and in depressive-prone personalities. Unnecessary gynaecological operations such as hysterectomy may be carried out to control such symptoms, but more recent knowledge of the underlying disturbance of hormone levels, in particular oestrogen, progesterone and prolactin, has thrown more light on the causes and potential treatment of such problems. The conditions are intimately related with mono-amine levels, in particular dopamine, and over-activity in the limbic lobe can alter such levels quite dramatically.

Disturbances of sexual function are also often associated with levels of tension and with anxiety states. This is particularly the case in partial erective failure or impotence, and in orgasmic failure or frigidity in the female. The condition of vaginismus, where certain muscle groups go into spasm when penetration is attempted, is also commonly associated with the anxiety-prone personality. Treatment of the anxiety aspect of such conditions may be all that is needed to put matters right. There is evidence that menorrhagia has responded to hypnosis.

Metabolic and Endocrine Disorders

Most endocrine glands in the body, such as the thyroid, pancreas or adrenal glands and the gonadal sex glands, the testes and ovaries, are controlled by chemical stimulation through a feedback mechanism and regulation through the pituitary gland and hypothalamus in the central nervous system of the brain. They are also supplied through the autonomic nervous system, and the regulation of the hormone outflow from such glands is a complicated coordinated activity between these various systems. It would be no surprise, therefore, if emotional disturbances in an individual might produce changes in these hormone levels and, if the disturbance were prolonged, that an irreversible change in output might take place. Certainly there is some evidence to suggest that this may be the case in diabetes mellitus and in hyperthyroidism, where emotional crises in some persons' lives seem to be associated with the onset of these diseases.

In the condition of migraine we are on even safer ground. Here acute headaches are produced by disturbances in the muscles which control the passage of blood in the small arteries within the cranial vault, in this case probably mediated through the mono-amine serotonin. The association between migraine and the over-conscientious obsessional personality, and between environmental disturbances and the onset of a migraine headache, are well known.

It would be a mistake to think that the treatment of the psychosomatic conditions mentioned above could be resolved simply by sorting out the way such people react to stress. Bio-feedback techniques and the use of relaxation, psychotherapy and anxiolytic medication can certainly play a part but as a rule, by the time such an individual is seen, the physical disease process is already present and it is this disease which needs the primary attention.

Somato-psychic Disorders

So far we have been considering the psychosomatic aspects of general medicine. Psychiatry is also intimately concerned with somato-psychic disease—that is to say, symptoms, relating to disturbances of mood, thinking or behaviour, where the primary cause is a general medical condition and not directly concerned with a psychiatric disorder. A wide variety of conditions may come into this group. The specialists in psychiatric illness must be familiar with and able to recognise such conditions if they are not to be missed.

Endocrine disorders are particularly prone to present in ways which mimic anxiety states, the psychotic illnesses or a confusion like dementia. Thyrotoxicosis may present with symptoms very similar to that of an anxiety state. A shortage of thyroid hormone, as in myxoedema, can present with depressive symptoms or may induce a dementia-like state. Disturbances of insulin levels when the pancreatic gland is affected can produce a confusional state when insulin is deficient and the blood sugar rises, or when the reverse is the case, and insulin levels go too high, can produce hysterical symptoms which may be mistaken for a form of neurosis.

C.G., a woman of 28, presented with the typical symptoms of an anxiety reaction. She was tense and agitated, tended to be irritable with the children, and became nervous in company or when under pressure. She was more frequently weepy than normal, complained of palpitations and had a tremor.

She was noted to have mild enlargement of the thyroid gland in her neck and the eyes were perhaps mildly protruberant, both of which can be signs of an overactive thyroid gland. Confirmatory blood tests showed that indeed the thyroid was showing over-activity and the standard treatment for thyrotoxicosis brought the condition under control.

A.L., in contrast, a woman of 52, was admitted to a psychiatric hospital with a diagnosis of depression. She certainly showed a morbid mood with delusional ideas of unworthiness but also showed a marked retardation of her thinking and appeared slow in her speech and motor activity. Furthermore, her memory and grasp seemed somewhat impaired.

A number of screening tests were carried out since the mood change combined with the memory disturbance suggested an organic psychosis rather than a simple depressive state. Thyroid screening showed an extremely low level of thyroid function associated with myxoedema and therapy with thyroid hormone replacement produced an overall improvement in all her symptoms.

The pituitary gland, which controls many of the other endocrine glands, can produce psychotic or neurotic symptoms. Disturbances of the adrenal glands may present with nervous changes. Conn's syndrome may be mistaken for hysterical manifestations of a neurosis.

A large number of conditions which have a toxic effect on the body may produce psychiatric symptoms and in particular the memory disturbance that may be heralding a dementia. These include kidney failure from whatever cause, where the blood urea levels will rise, and liver failure, where toxic metabolites may poison the central nervous system.

Vitamin deficiency diseases can effect the function of the central nervous system and cause manifestations of dementia or psychosis. Particularly relevant is the disturbance of vitamin B12 levels, which is found in pernicious anaemia and used to go under the name of megaloblastic madness. Other types of anaemia can also present as neuroses, however, as can disturbances of vitamin C, vitamin D or other members of the vitamin B group.

A wide variety of toxins, poisons and alterations to the body's metabolism through high fever can induce delirious states characterised by confusion and sometimes hallucinatory experiences. The physical manifestations of such diseases are not always obvious, and infections of a more chronic kind, such as tuberculosis or syphilis or some virus diseases, can affect the brain substance directly.

Cancerous change in the body may induce some psychiatric changes, by a direct local effect from secondary deposits in the central nervous system, or from the metabolic disturbance. Carcinoid syndrome, which affects the bowel, is one such example.

The cardiovascular system can induce psychiatric symptoms if the blood supply to the brain or the ability of the circulation to carry adequate oxygen is impaired. This may occur after a stroke or a heart attack, or as part of a more general heart failure with circulatory disturbance. Hardening of the arteries (arteriosclerosis) is a common cause of dementia, and may be associated with other psychotic symptoms.

A number of metabolic disturbances in the body are important in inducing mental retardation. (This will be discussed more fully in Chapter 20.) Some disorders of this type, however, have been particularly interesting for historical or research reasons. One such metabolic disturbance, known as porphyria, is thought to have been the cause of the madness that beset King George III.

Chronic poisoning of the body with a variety of substances has also been of historical interest in the causation of psychiatric disorders. Lead poisoning, which can induce both pseudo-hysterical symptoms and dementia if prolonged, is a classic example. Many cases of lead poisoning have been accidental through contamination of water (or, in a famous case, of cider by lead storage casks), of water pipes, and through the inhalation of lead-containing products such as paint or petroleum. Other heavy metals can have similar toxic effects, including aluminium and mercury, the latter of historical interest in the production of 'hatter's madness', mentioned in *Alice in Wonderland*, a condition well recognised in the old days, when mercury was used in the hatters' trade.

Toxic side-effects from the drugs used to treat some disorders may present similarly. Bromide, which was used in sedatives, and arsenic, bismuth and antimony are but some examples.

This short chapter should serve again to emphasise the close correlation between conditions affecting mood, thought and behaviour—which is the province of the psychiatrist—and those of general medicine. This is what makes it so important that the psychiatrist must first of all qualify in general medical and surgical skills and get a broad view of what doctoring is all about before moving on to specialise. While this is true of any speciality it is perhaps even more important where the underlying disease may distort patients' own perception in such a way that they become a poor witness to their own symptoms.

Further Reading

Hamilton, W. B., *Psychosomatics*, Chapman and Hall, London, 1965.
Hill, O. W., *Modern Trends in Psychosomatic Medicine*, Butterworth, London, 1979.

Questions

1. What is psychosomatic disease?
2. How does the autonomic nervous system function?
3. How may disorder of the thyroid function present to the psychiatrist?
4. How does epilepsy relate to psychiatry?

14
Disorders of Personality and Behaviour

Summary

Definition

A group of problems faced by the individual and society as a result of failure to develop social maturity or the ability to empathise fully.

Classification

A heterogeneous group of conditions including:

1. Distortions of personality development.
   (a) Distorted personality; (b) inadequacy; (c) immaturity; (d) psychopathy.

2. Addictions.

3. Sexual behavioural anomalies.

Aetiology

1. Some evidence of genetic predisposition.

2. Minor degrees of brain damage.

3. EEG abnormalities.

4. Chromosome abnormalities.

5. Main factors: emotional deprivation in early childhood, broken homes, failure of imprinting of affection at critical age of development.

Psychopathy

A condition of persistently irresponsible or aggressive behaviour of such a nature or degree that it requires medical treatment.

Symptoms

1. Desire for immediate need satisfaction.

2. Inability to empathise with others or to make relationships.

3. Tendency to act on impulse.

4. Lack of foresight.

5. Lack of remorse or ability to learn from experience.

6. Inadequate and aggressive behaviour.

Treatment

1. Crisis intervention and support.

2. Psychotherapy—group therapy.

3. Use of drugs to control particular behaviour problems.

4. Behaviour therapy.

Outlook

There is improvement with aging, on later maturing of the individual, and 30 per cent improve with therapy.

Discussion

So far we have been considering disorders of mood and thinking, and these have followed fairly well defined disease patterns, or have been accountable for in terms of underlying biochemical disturbance or the results of environmental influences on a neurotic constitution. The group that we shall now consider is a rather loosely knit collection of problems faced by the individual and society as a result of the failure of individuals to develop along lines which allow them to fit in satisfactorily with the social structure in which they find themselves.

Environmental causes, coupled with possible minimal brain damage, often seem to be present in the aetiology, and there commonly seems to be an immaturity of response to stress, which may have to do with intelligence, since individuals at the lower end of the normal scale are handicapped in that direction. Indeed, Vineland developed a scale of social maturity, comparable to the I.Q. and known as an S.Q. or **Social Quotient**, which attempted to delineate the sort of handicaps this group of patients acquire.

Many people, including some psychiatrists, would argue that most of these problems are outside the proper realm of psychiatry. This, in the author's view, is to balk at the real issues. We have defined the psychiatrist's role as dealing with disorders of mood, thinking and, arising out of these, behaviour. There is little doubt that many individuals with personality problems seek help because of the disturbances of mood and behaviour to which their condition gives rise. Medicine, and particularly psychiatry, as a helping profession should surely not deny help to such people if its skills can be appropriately used.

Classification

Let us first of all consider how such a heterogeneous group may be classified.

We all recognise in our friends certain personality types. There will be those who are serious and conformist, and those who are outgoing and flighty. There will be the rigid, obsessional individual, the rather immature individuals who appear to be children at heart and often behave thus, and the less adequate souls who collapse in a heap when any kind of stress is imposed. There will be those who tend to be suspicious and always see a slight when none is intended, and those whose first reaction to an insult is to hit out. Equally, among one's friends, there could be those who are deceitful, take excessively to drink, have unusual sexual habits, take drugs, or land in gaol for committing illegal acts.

Do all these groups have anything in common? Is there some factor which allows the majority of the population to be stable enough to survive in almost any kind of society, but in a minority makes an individual who can only tolerate a sheltered environment? Or are the various groups hinted at above the result of a variety of causes?

Of course, the defects of a character mentioned above would be accepted by most people as within the normal variation of personality. Some are born that way, and there is no doubt in the minds of those who breed animals that personality can be just as much an inherited factor as can intelligence or the colour of one's eyes or skin. This should not be surprising, and variety is to be expected. There comes a point, however, where the personality traits outlined above become sufficiently different from those the majority would call normal for them to come to the attention of outside agencies, whether it be the social services, the law or the medical profession. A person's behaviour may be so inadequate as to need help from one or other of these sources in times of stress. An individual's drinking may become such a problem to his family and his friends that they recognise, even if he does not, that he is sick. A young person's behaviour may be so irresponsible, despite the fact that they are of an age when they should be more mature, that society needs to intervene. It will be seen, however, that the borderlines here are much less clear-cut and less delineated than most problems we have so far discussed.

There is a considerable bulk of evidence suggesting that early childhood experiences—particularly in the realm of emotional deprivation, separation from love objects, and the failure to develop normal imprinting patterns—are the common denominator in a large number of the problems which occur in late adolescence and early adulthood. It would seem that a possibly vulnerable inherited personality structure and environmental disturbances in the formative years are critical in provoking the kind of character difficulties which later show themselves. Many studies have drawn attention to the sometimes harmful causes of deprivation in children, and the author's book *Psychiatric Illness in Adolescence* reviews in depth the literature which has accumulated on the association between early environmental experiences and subsequent adolescent personality disturbance.

Distortions of Personality Development

We can group the personality disorders into certain types of problem for the sake of discussion. First, there are those **distortions of the normal personality**, such as excessive obsessional traits or an excessively suspicious nature, which have become so marked as to cause disruption to the individual's way of life.

Secondly, there are those who show an **inadequacy at coping** with ordinary stresses and strains. Usually such individuals are found to have had disturbed early upbringing of the kind mentioned earlier. They survive happily in a secure environment, which causes them no difficulties, but once responsibilities occur, they are liable to be unable to cope and develop a depressive reaction. They are often easily led, therefore, and land in situations such as extra-marital affairs from which they fail to extract themselves, and they go from crisis to crisis without the foresight that is necessary to guard against landing in trouble from such behaviour.

Thirdly, there are those personalities, usually seen in younger people, which are described as **immature**. Often there are associated EEG changes where an immature pattern is shown, and it may be that for some reason there is a delay in maturation of the central nervous system in such people. Usually, in time, they improve, but in the early twenties are liable to behave in a manner more appropriate to someone many years younger, although there is no impairment of their intelligence level. Immature behaviour is tolerated in children but becomes progressively less tolerated by society as the individual increases in chronological age.

Fourthly, there are those disturbed personalities who show **persistent irresponsible behaviour of an aggressive or petty criminal type**, combined with patterns of delinquency and possibly promiscuity. Such individuals may be known as **sociopaths** or, in severer cases, **psychopaths**.

The Mental Health Act defines **psychopathic disorder**, which is an extreme form of personality disorder as a **persistent disorder** or **disability of mind** (whether or not including significant impairment of intelligence) **which results in abnormally aggressive or seriously irresponsible conduct on the part of the person concerned**. It is a pre-requisite for admission that it is potentially susceptible to medical treatment. Under the 1983 Act persons may be detained in hospital on such a diagnosis if the disorder or disability is defined as persistent (in other words there must be signs that this disorder has existed for a considerable period before a patient can be classified as having psychopathic disorder), and it must also result in abnormally aggressive or irresponsible conduct. Treatability is no longer mentioned in the definition as it was in the 1959 Act, but the effect of Sections 3, 37 and 47 are that those with psychopathic disorder cannot be compulsorily admitted to hospital for treatment unless it can be stated that medical treatment is likely to alleviate or prevent a deterioration of their condition. This proviso is more stringent than the inclusion of the words 'requires or is susceptible to treatment' which was the definition in the 1959 Act.

Also in the 1959 Act there was an age restriction for the admission under the diagnosis of psychopathy in that it could only be used up to the age of 21, and patients could not be detained beyond the age of 25 under this heading. This implied that psychopathy would be alleviated with the passage of the years, and was a condition largely of the young. This is not entirely the case and this definition has been dropped out of the 1983 Act, the age restrictions no longer applying.

The definition also implies that it is the psychiatrist's job to attempt to treat such problems, and that such problems are treatable. Unfortunately, the severer personality disorders are often very disruptive in a social situation such as exists on a hospital ward or a community hostel, and thought must be given to the needs of the rest of that community and not just to the disruptive patient. Thus the management of such a problem may well require a special unit, and these are, by and large, not at present available within the Health Service setting. Furthermore, it is well recognised that such problems are difficult to manage.

The nature of the cause of these problems is such that the damage is done by the time the individual is seen, and the disruptive effect of early childhood deprivation is not in general fully reversible. This is a field for preventive medicine if ever there was one! Prevention, unfortunately, would imply some regulation of parental rights of a type which it is unlikely that our society would tolerate. There is much evidence to suggest that personality-disordered adolescents become personality-disordered parents, and in turn produce personality-disordered children, and the old Biblical aphorism that 'the evils of the fathers are visited even unto the third generation' certainly holds true in this kind of case. These are matters which must be decided by society as a whole, and cannot be imposed by one group of professionals whose job is basically to advise and help when asked.

Nevertheless, it is in the adolescent personality disorder that psychotherapy, either group or individual, is likely to have its most useful role, even though this type of patient, because of an inability to form strong emotional bonds, is often very unrewarding and liable to let one down time after time. It is of great importance that the medical, nursing and social work staff who are dealing with such individuals should understand the nature and cause of the patients' inability to develop a normal social conscience. At the same time, society itself needs some protection from the severer problems, and this requires the intervention of such services, even if the patients themselves are not fully cooperative.

Addictions

To continue our classification of personality disorders, we must now look at the group where there is the **development of a dependency or addiction to basically harmful substances**. We refer here to alcohol and the various drugs of dependency and addiction which are available in this country. These will be gone into in more detail in Chapter 15, but suffice it to say here that there well may be an addictive-prone personality, although, of course, many people may become addicted to something for other reasons, and one cannot include all this group as one homogeneous whole. Alcoholism, for example, may be the result of contact by an addiction-prone personality with the product over a period of time; it may be symptomatic of other underlying psychological illness, such as depression or anxiety; or it may be a reaction to environmental pressures which have become intolerable. There is even some evidence that some people have a genetic predisposition to develop such addictions, and avoidance to exposure is the only likely way of preventing such a situation.

Sexual Behavioural Anomalies

Finally, in our classification of personality problems, there is that of **sexually deviant behaviour**, or sexual behavioural anomalies. Sexual deviants also do not form a homogeneous group. There is a wide variety of patterns of deviance and a wide variety of possible causes. Nevertheless, it is convenient to discuss all these under the one heading.

Many of the laws concerning sexual activity in Great Britain and the USA are archaic in the extreme, quite out of touch with the realities of life. For this reason many of the referrals to psychiatrists concerning deviant patterns of sexual behaviour result from court actions or from fears of the possibility of such actions. Society also tends to show a very intolerant attitude to sexual behaviour outside of the norm, so that those whose sexual drives have developed, for one reason or another, in other directions are put into a position of feeling guilt, and become, in a sense, a persecuted minority. Much sexual behaviour of this kind is not remotely a medical matter, but at the same time it is spurious to suggest, as some do, that it is never a medical matter. It is the function of the psychiatrist in this respect to soothe people's fears and to counsel them where counselling is needed, or to offer treatment if this seems appropriate. This is a matter between patient and doctor, and the success of any therapy will largely depend on the motivation of the patient towards seeking such help.

If an individual is happy with his sexual behaviour and it does not infringe upon other people's sensibilities, then it is a matter solely for that individual. If, on the other hand, it brings the individual into conflict with society or the law, or can potentially do so, then counselling can be indicated. This may be to help the person come to terms with the particular problem and to learn to live with it, or, in some cases, to help such a person to extinguish the need for such behaviour and to enable him to establish patterns of behaviour which are acceptable to him and pose no threat to others.

In this chapter we are not concerned with detailing the types of sexual behaviour which may come to the psychiatrist's attention, but rather to consider it as one aspect of a personality problem. The majority of such cases are the result of the inability to develop mature, stable, heterosexual relationships on a one-to-one basis with a member of the opposite sex. There are degrees of failure to respond in this manner and degrees of regression. Thus an individual whose only sexual outlet is solitary through masturbation and sexual fantasies, or who has to resort to contact simply through, for example, anonymous exposing to other individuals in public, is exhibiting an immature pattern of response in terms of social relationships, and this is probably the key to the problem. The ability to relate more positively in an emotional manner to other adults will probably lead to a maturing of the sexual response also.

Homosexuality falls into a slightly different category. Here, again, there is not one homogeneous cause for the development of such behaviour patterns. It seems likely from research work done in many parts of the world that there is a small group of individuals in whom the homosexual pattern of behaviour is genetically determined, and that there are underlying hormonal differences which create this situation. In a larger group there is imprinting or conditioning towards homosexual behaviour as a result of the environment in which the individual is reared, and there is a third and sizeable group where the behaviour is the result not so much of a liking for one's own sex as a fear of relationships with the opposite sex. The need for a sexual relationship is there, but the individual cannot come to terms with such a relationship with a member of the opposite sex, and, therefore, may continue with adolescent patterns of homosexual activity at a level not so much of a love relationship as that of an exploratory mutual masturbatory relationship which is purely genitally orientated.

Any treatment offered will have to take into account these variations and seek to find what is in the long-term best interests of the individual by whom one is consulted. Often the motive for consultation is not a desire to change to heterosexuality but rather an attempt to escape from the pressures which society puts on what it might consider deviant minority groups. In recent years there has been much campaigning by socio-political groups and befriending organisations in an attempt to help minority groups who feel that they are at a disadvantage in society. It can often be more appropriate to bring these organisations to the attention of the patient than to attempt changes which may, in any case, be impractical.

Counselling organisations often take exception to the word 'deviancy' being used in homosexuality at all. This may be a semantic problem, but if a word causes offence to a group of individuals, then it is perhaps better replaced by a different word. It would seem, nevertheless, that homosexual orientation, where one individual develops a love relationship with sexual overtones towards another of the same sex, has a qualitative difference from heterosexual behaviour, and in that sense is not an example on one extreme of a normal range of distribution, such as we have applied in earlier chapters to height or intelligence or to such personality traits as introversion and extraversion. We use the word deviant, therefore, in the sense that homosexuality deviates from the pattern of behaviour found in the majority of the population, namely heterosexuality.

It must be noted, however, that Kinsey, in his report on sexual behaviour patterns in a large community survey done in the United States, found that a bisexual pattern of behaviour, whereby occasional heterosexual contacts may be made by those with a basic homosexual orientation and similarly occasional homosexual contacts may be made by those of a basically heterosexual orientation, was very common, and that some form of homosexual activity, using this in its widest sense, had been indulged in at some time or another by a large minority of the community. In this sense, therefore, sexual activity with a member of one's own sex is not outside what could be defined as the norm.

This argument, though it tends to make some people hot under the collar, is a rather sterile one. The important thing is to give help to an individual who seeks it, regardless of the problem, and to acquire the experience which allows that help to be of real value. These matters will be expanded upon in Chapter 18.

Psychopathy

Let us return now to a further consideration of some of the more important groups of personality disturbances that we have outlined above, and, in particular, **psychopathy**. There is evidence to show some degree of **genetic inherited factors** in personality disorders, but probably more important are a number of minimal factors producing minor degrees of brain damage or disturbance in brain function which may be responsible for preventing those who have a disturbed early environment from coping with it as well as others. Of these possibilities one must consider minimal brain damage at childbirth, due to episodes of deficient oxygen supply from delay at birth or delay in breathing. Furthermore, minor **chromosomal abnormalities** may be found, and, in particular, an additional extra sex chromosome in a few of these patients. As has been mentioned, the electroencephalogram often shows an immature or disturbed pattern, and occasionally metabolic disturbances, such as a lowering of the blood sugar level, may be found. By far the most important evidence, however, comes from early environmental disturbance, with a history of emotional deprivation.

In 1951 an account of the psychiatric aspects of delinquency was prepared by Bowlby for the World Health Organisation. Bowlby's study, *Forty-Four Juvenile Thieves*, is a classic. In this he describes the **affectionless character** and relates it to the emotional loss of a mother object during early childhood.

A League of Nations report as far back as 1938 stated: 'It may be regarded as an axiomatic principle of child care that no child should be removed from the care of an otherwise competent parent when the granting of material aid would make such removal unnecessary'. Goldfarb in 1943 also put his finger on the child's inability to make relationships as being the central feature from which all other disturbances sprang, and particularly on institutionalisation of a child, or a child being shifted from one foster mother to another, as being its commonest cause. Similar findings have been made in other personality problems besides delinquency—for example, in battle neurosis in soldiers and in prostitution.

It will be recalled that psychopathy is described in the Mental Health Act as 'a persistent disorder or disability of mind (whether or not including significant impairment of intelligence) which results in abnormally aggressive or seriously irresponsible conduct on the part of the patient, and requires or is susceptible to medical treatment'. Promiscuity and alcoholic abuse are specifically excluded in the Act in this respect.

The picture which the personality disorder presents is that of disruptive, mischievous or frankly aggressive behaviour. On the ward psychopaths may steal from other patients or threaten them. They may get staff into trouble and play one off against another. They have little moral awareness in this respect and find great difficulty, as Bowlby has described in his work on the affectionless character, in making empathetic relationships of any depth with therapists or even their friends.

A youth was seen in the local remand centre for a psychiatric report prior to a court appearance. He was 18 and came from an emotionally deprived background, having been deserted by his mother, who was unmarried, when he was some nine months old. He had been shipped around between children's homes and foster homes over the next eight years and had never been able to develop proper emotional bonding with anybody. He had spent a short period in Borstal in his early teens after malicious damage to his school premises. He now had a string of convictions for minor offences including theft and aggressive behaviour and for being in possession of drugs.

The legal authorities felt the boy to be on the slippery path and that prison sentences seemed unlikely to be a deterrent. At the same time compulsory detention in an adult psychiatric ward would probably have offered little. The ideal would have been a small, well-run specialist unit with a high staff–patient ratio where a group of such individuals could be given some training and behaviourally orientated group psychotherapy. Unfortunately, no such facility was available within the area.

There is thus a variable degree of amoral behaviour. The patient has a low social conscience and acts impulsively, without experiencing a sense of guilt. Thus, in those of criminal propensity shocking crimes, which normal people find impossible to comprehend, may be committed. Fortunately, this is rare. The psychopath does not learn from experience and thus may repeat antisocial behaviour in a rather foolish way, which almost guarantees being caught. As a result of this, they may consistently let the therapist down, even when he thinks that some stability in psychotherapy is being achieved. Their behaviour can easily alienate friends and relations, society and the police. It equally may easily alienate nursing staff.

A girl was admitted to the ward after cutting her wrist. She had been in and out of the psychiatric unit for the last five years and was now aged 23. The reason for admission was usually an overdose or some attempted self-mutilation resulting from some trivial environmental stress. She too had a disrupted early history and had lived for some years in children's homes. She had been taken into care as being in moral danger when she had indulged in promiscuous sexual relationships while under the age of consent. She was unable to form stable emotional relationships or to learn from experience and her mood was fluctuating but shallow. While in the unit she tended to be disruptive, assaulting staff or breaking windows or turning her aggression in on herself by burning her arms with cigarettes. She started to make better progress with the opening of a progressive care unit in the locality and the more vigorous attempt at social rehabilitation.

Treatment

It is important that the aetiology of such conditions is remembered. The individuals in question are often the throwouts of a deprived early environment, rejection in childhood being their personal tragedy. Psychotherapy must be intensive and prolonged in order to achieve any improvement, and must be started at as early an age as possible. Group work in therapeutic communities has probably provided the best results. Supportive care, however, in terms of regular psychotherapeutic interviews with a psychiatrist or other helping agency, may be sufficient to keep many patients going with the awareness that crisis intervention, with brief admission, as and when required, is always available. To keep the patients out of hospital when they themselves feel they should be in is usually to court disaster, with a 3 am phone call concerning an overdose! Equally, to compel them to stay against their will is to ask for a disrupted ward. Over a period of time the milder cases certainly do develop sufficient empathy with the therapist for real progress to be made, but it is in the author's view essential that such cases are caught young.

Estimation of intelligence is of little value in assessing the degree of psychopathy, though a low I.Q. will be an additional handicap to the patient. Punishment is likely to be of little value, since they do not learn from such actions. Usually the encouragement of positive patterns of behaviour by reward in a unit such as a token economy ward might supply is the most effective method.

Drug therapy can be only palliative and symptomatic, but personality disordered patients are more prone to develop depressive reactions, and can be treated with suitable anti-depressants at the time. They may, in addition, if there is any evidence of early minimal brain damage, be helped by anti-epileptic products, which may control aggressive behaviour, or by the butyrophenones such as haloperidol and benperidol, which have been mentioned earlier.

Fortunately, many personality disordered patients do mature to a more adequate social level, given time, and by the age of 25 to 30 may well have settled down. Yet the improvement rate in psychopathy is estimated at some 30 per cent only, despite treatment.

Some hospitals have developed the progressive care unit, where this type of patient may be treated over a three to six month period, if possible, of continuous care. The unit is run as a therapeutic community, with much group work. Rewards are given for positive behaviour, which may take the form of privileges or, as in a token economy unit, privilege tokens, which may then be exchanged for something the patient wants, such as items at the hospital shop. Basically, the patient starts in a no-privilege situation and is rewarded by a gradual increase of privileges as progress is made. Thus positive behaviour is rewarded but negative behaviour, as far as possible, is ignored. Punishment as normally thought of is avoided, though withdrawal of privileges gained could occur for anti-social behaviour. The final censoring is done by the group of one's peers, who, with the agreement of the staff, may as a last sanction expel the patient from the unit.

Within these units the patient is able to make empathetic relationships and develop a sense of responsibility within his peer group and not simply with authority figures. The patient with the psychopathic personality is liable constantly to let down those who befriend him or her, and this in the short term can be very unrewarding, and is liable to alienate staff. Using picked and experienced staff, however, the success rate in these units certainly seems to be better than any other method that has been tried.

Other Personality Problems

We have dwelt on the problem of psychopathy in a little depth. It is the ultimate problem within this group in terms of severity, and the causes, in terms of early environmental disturbances, social disruption, and failure of bonding, serve as a model for much sociological work.

The distortions of personality whereby normal traits, such as introversion or obsessionality, may become exaggerated beyond reason can merge imperceptibly into the milder schizoid personality through to a schizophrenic breakdown itself, or in the case of obsessional behaviour into the neurotic pattern of obsessional compulsive neurosis. Thus, if such traits become distorted to the extent that therapy is needed, it is likely to be psychotherapeutic or behavioural in type and follow the lines suggested for the treatment of neuroses.

The milder forms of personality disturbance subsumed under immaturity and inadequacy, and sometimes known as sociopathy, refer to those individuals who, while not disturbed enough to be labelled psychopathic, nevertheless show weaknesses in their personality structure which can usually be related to similar but milder experiences in their early history, of the same general type as is found in the psychopathic individual.

...opath will cope adequately in society, given a structured environ-
...out stress. In our complex society, however, where stresses related
... interpersonal relationships with a partner, or to the problems of
...ng up children, are increasingly met with in the absence of the type
o...upport which the nuclear family and the village community were able
to give in previous generations, such people are now increasingly thrown
on to their own resources. With the relative breakup of the family unit and
the freer movement of population related to work, minor crises within the
framework of a new town or highrise flat can loom large without the support
of aunts, grandparents, brothers or sisters, who are easily able to assist a
weaker family member. To bring a relative from another town when he or
she will have a job or social commitment of their own becomes a major
disruption, and the inadequate individual is more frequently put into a
situation of being unable to cope.

In such a circumstance, where the rest of us might hopefully muddle
through, the sociopath breaks down and requires the intervention of social
services or helping agencies, often using the suicidal gesture of the small
overdose as a cry for help. At such a point children may need to be taken
temporarily into care, starting a chain of events which produces further
disruption for the next generation. Within a totalitarian society such matters
are handled by the state services. In a free society, such as exists in most
Western cultures, however, it is perhaps the penalty we pay for individual
freedom that such people will fall by the wayside and those dependent upon
them may suffer through the absence of the ability to control their
environment.

The Adolescent Personality Disorder

The problems of adolescence will be treated more fully in Chapter 20 on
Child Psychiatry. The adolescent, however, goes through a period of change
between childhood and adulthood when the personality still is inevitably
inexperienced and immature. Personality disorders and crises in adolescence
are frequent but, fortunately, do not imply, in the majority of cases,
the development of more clear-cut psychopathic tendencies. Nevertheless,
suicide and delinquency are problems that loom large in this age group,
and stress the difficulties the adolescent has in coming to terms with society.

Suicide is the fifth commonest cause of death in adolescents, being 2.5
per cent of all deaths in this group: 12 per cent of total suicide attempts
are in the 15–19 age group, females exceeding males by 10 to 1, and the
ratio of non-fatal to fatal attempts is 50 to 1. A study in Sweden by Jacob
showed that only 4 per cent of attempted suicides had come from normal
environments. Most felt unwanted, and often there was aggression against
others and a hope of manipulating the environment in the suicidal attempt.
One parent was missing in 88 per cent of Jacob's survey, 25 per cent of the
girls were pregnant, and separation experiences in childhood were shown
to be very common.

Delinquency is a disease of epidemic proportions in adolescence. Cohen
suggests that the delinquent feels he has an inferior status to the wider
community, and the delinquent group restores his standing while at the
same time denying the values of the wider community. Bowlby states that

half those people found guilty of criminal offences in the courts have been under the age of 21 and over a sixth of the total under the age of 14. Of all age groups in the population, it is 13-year-olds who appear most often in court. Thus theft, like rheumatic fever, is a disease of childhood and adolescence, and, as in rheumatic fever, attacks in later life are frequently in the nature of recurrences! A survey in Newcastle showed that some 38 per cent of adolescents admitted to psychiatric units in that area had a diagnosis of adolescent personality disturbance. In most of these individuals the number of adequate relationships that they had managed to establish with others was significantly less than a control group's.

Supportive psychotherapy is the treatment of choice in this group, enabling the adolescent to develop a sense of worth or self-esteem. The type of therapy which seems most effective has been given the name of relationship therapy. Particular skills are needed in dealing with this age group, since the therapist must try to produce a supportive empathy without being over-intense or over-demanding of the adolescent's compliance. The adolescent must come to feel that the therapist is dependable rather than to develop dependence.

Further Reading

Bowlby, J., *Forty-Four Juvenile Thieves*, Bailliere, Tyndall and Cox, London, 1946.
Butler Report, Cmnd. 6244, HMSO, London, 1975.
Craft, M., *Psychopathic Disorders*, Pergamon, Oxford, 1966.
Haslam, M.T., *Psychiatric Illness in Adolescence*, Butterworth, London, 1975.
McCord, W., and McCord, J., *The Psychopath*, Van Nostrand, New York, 1964.
Whiteley, J. S., 'The Psychopath and his Treatment', *Contemporary Psychiatry*, BJP Special Publications No. 9, Headley, Kent, 1977.

Questions

1. What is psychopathy?
2. Where is your local 'secure unit', into which disordered offenders may be admitted?
3. Summarise for yourself the causes of personality problems and the concept of emotional deprivation, and the symptoms which can result.

15
Alcoholism and Drug Addiction

Summary

Alcoholism

The condition is defined as dependence on alcohol to such a degree that noticeable mental disturbance or interference with health, personal relations or social functioning occurs.

Approximately 1 per cent of population—between 200,000 and 400,000 in the United Kingdom—are known to be alcohol-dependent.

An addiction-prone personality is the cause in many cases, but variations in drinking patterns occur in different cultures and alcoholism may also be symptomatic of other stresses.

The following special syndromes can develop as a result of alcoholic excess:

1. Delirium tremens.
2. Wernicke's encephalopathy.
3. Korsakoff's psychosis.

'Drying out' is appropriate in early stages, with medication to relieve withdrawal effects. In the long term, psychotherapy and social rehabilitation are required. Aversion therapy is sometimes used.

Drug Addiction

It is defined as a state of psychic and physical dependence on a substance, characterised by a compulsion to take the drug, a tendency to need to increase the dosage to maintain the effect, and withdrawal effects on discontinuing it.

There was a rapid increase from about 300 in the 1950s to 3,000 registered by the 1970s. The number is still only 1 per cent of the number of alcoholics, however.

There are three basic types—sedating, stimulating and hallucinogenic—characterised as follows:

1. Mild sedatives—barbiturates, alcohol, tranquillisers.
2. Strong sedatives—morphine derivatives, opium, pethidine.
3. Mild stimulants—amphetamines, cannabis.

4. Strong stimulants—cocaine.

5. Hallucinogens—lysergic acid (LSD), mescaline, psilocybin, peyotl.

Alcoholism

We now turn our attention to the related topics of alcoholism and drug addiction, which we have suggested earlier can be symptomatic in many cases of an underlying personality disorder.

The World Health Organisation in 1951 defined alcoholics as **those excessive drinkers whose dependence on alcohol has attained such a degree that they show a noticeable mental disturbance, or an interference with their bodily and mental health, their interpersonal relations, and their smooth, social and economic functioning; or show the prodromal signs of such development.** This rather cumbersome definition attempts to embrace all problems, but Jellinec distinguished certain types of alcoholism: for example, the periodic bout drinker, the one who continuously over-indulges, and those who use alcohol in order to relieve symptoms of other psychiatric disorder. These different types are characteristic of certain personalities, and may vary with different social and religious groups. The end result of chronic alcoholism, however, with its attendant complications, is the same, whatever the type of drinking, if it continues long enough.

The treatment of alcoholism poses considerable problems for one particular reason. People are reluctant to admit to themselves that what they see as a weakness has got a hold of them, and has got out of hand. They usually, therefore, postpone seeking treatment for fear of the implications of their visit. It is, as a result, usually the relatives who suffer from such an addiction, since the patient begins to cause disruption to their social life through failure to cope with the normal day's work, spending excessive money on obtaining alcohol, and deteriorating standards with the drunken state.

Thus treatment in the early stages becomes very difficult, since in this kind of problem cooperation is an essential part of any rehabilitative process. Compulsory admission to hospital would often be a pointless exercise, even if it were within the legal terms of reference of the Mental Health Act, which, as has been stated earlier, it is not. The alcoholic can be admitted to hospital on a compulsory basis only if he is a danger to himself or others by reason of mental illness, from which alcoholism in the Act has been excluded. Admission may be arranged from time to time because of depressive phases, suicidal bids or serious self-poisoning as a result of excessive alcohol intake, but, apart from these circumstances, which only allow of a drying-out procedure, there is no means whereby the addict can be contained. The distress caused to the relatives by such a member within their midst, however, may quickly disrupt family relationships, which in turn sets up a vicious circle, since the alcoholic may drink more as a result of this disruption, and that causes further disruption.

Aetiology

The causes of alcoholism are varied. Some alcoholics have started drinking in an attempt to alleviate other symptoms, such as acute anxiety or depression, and some of the periodic drinkers appear to be those who suffer from a cyclical mood change, which is the disorder requiring treatment. Others have become addicted simply for social reasons, but there is evidence that certain people have a genetic predisposition to become addicts if exposed to the appropriate circumstances, whereas others do not. Equally, personality disturbances arising from early emotional deprivation experiences may play a considerable role in many cases.

Once chronic alcoholism is well established, certain characteristic features begin to appear, regardless of the type of drinking pattern the individual has practised. These include damage to the tissues as a result of long-term minor poisoning. In particular, the liver may be affected, since it is this organ which has to dispose of the poisonous breakdown products. In effect, the liver gradually rots, to be replaced by scar tissues, and, as a result, it ceases to perform its normal function. In the early stages this malfunction leads to a feeling of general ill-health, an increasing intolerance to the effects of alcohol, and may, in due course, cause disturbances in blood pressure, jaundice, and a variety of other generalised symptoms.

The other major organ which is affected by chronic alcoholism is the brain. There is a gradual deterioration in intellectual capacity and in memory, leading, in severe cases, to a dementia. This often shows itself in the early stages as memory blanks which occur after a heavy bout of drinking, commonly seen on a Monday morning, when the individual has no recall of what has happened during the previous 24 hours or so. Concentration becomes impaired and the ability to do a normal day's work begins to suffer. Social behaviour may become disturbed as a result of frontal lobe damage. Certain typical patterns of illness are seen as a result of alcohol, and these particular syndromes have received special descriptive names.

Delirium Tremens

The most familiar of these is probably delirium tremens, known as DTs for short. This condition usually follows a drinking bout, and is the result of over-excitement of the brain during the withdrawal phase of any kind of sedating product. It can occur with some drugs and with excessive use of sedatives. The individual becomes very agitated, there is a marked tremor, and often bizarre visual hallucinations and delusions of a paranoid kind. The individual may see insects crawling about and believe he feels them on his skin. He may see more vivid coloured hallucinations (which is where the pink elephants come in). He becomes suspicious and may believe he is being attacked. The condition usually needs treatment in hospital, where phenothiazine sedatives such as chlorpromazine, or benzodiazepines such as diazepam or chlormethiazole, may be used, along with high-potency vitamin injections, to control the problem for the day or two until it wears off.

A man was admitted to a general surgical ward for appendicitis. His appendix was removed and for 24 hours he made an uneventful recovery. He then began to be confused, mistaking the identity of people who were visiting or nursing him and becoming disorientated in a patchy manner in both time and place. He began to be visually hallucinated, seeing frightening moving creatures like large insects crawling around on the floor of the ward. His behaviour became disturbed and he became noisy and uncooperative.

At first the staff thought that this delirious reaction had followed the anaesthetic or possibly a chest infection but there was no raised temperature and no evidence on physical examination to suggest this.

The man had not given a history on admission of excessive drinking but it was subsequently learned from relatives that this had been the case for some time. It became apparent that his admission to hospital had resulted in his discontinuing an alcohol intake of almost a bottle of spirits a day. The withdrawal had induced a delirium tremens. He was transferred for further nursing and medical care to the psychiatric unit where he made a good recovery in a week with high potency vitamin injections and sedation with chlormethiazole.

Wernicke's Encephalopathy

Another condition is known as Wernicke's encephalopathy. This is a condition presenting with delirium, unsteadiness of gait, numbness and tingling in hands and feet because of a peripheral neuropathy, and sometimes paralysis of the eye muscles and disturbance of vision. It is the result of a particular vitamin deficiency (namely thiamine), produced by the dietary disturbance resulting from long-term spirit drinking. This condition can also occur in other states besides alcoholism where the diet is deficient, such as pernicious anaemia, cancer of the stomach and severe malnutrition from any cause.

Korsakoff's Psychosis

Thirdly, there is a condition known as Korsakoff's psychosis, so named because of the doctor who described it in 1877. Here there is a combination of the neuropathy with a memory disturbance, and a particular defect of memory characterised by a tendency to make up answers to questions even when these are contrary to the facts of the case. This is known as **confabulation**. Korsakoff's psychosis is seen as one of the end results of long-term drinking, and is often not completely curable but leads to various degrees of permanent dementia.

A woman of 62 in one of the hospital long-stay wards had been in the hospital for some 15 years. Prior to admission she had a history of some five years' heavy drinking both of wine and of spirits. Attempts at treatment had been ineffective through her lack of cooperation and her final admission to hospital had been precipitated by an acute delirium tremens. When this cleared, however, she was found still to show a marked memory impairment. Her state now was one of grandiose fatuous elation. She believed herself to be a millionaire but had no idea of where she was or why. She existed within the supportive environment of the hospital but her ability to learn new material was so grossly impaired that she could not recall after five minutes anything that had been said to her or which had taken place, such as what she had had to eat for a meal or who had visited her. The brain damage was irreversible but unlikely to progress since, within the sheltered environment, she did not have opportunity for further drinking.

Treatment for Alcoholism

The psychiatric hospital encounters the problems of alcoholism in a number of ways. The acute disturbance of behaviour caused by a heavy drinking bout or by the withdrawal effects of delirium tremens may necessitate urgent admission for drying-out procedures to be initiated. The individual may well become a danger to himself or others as a result of this state.

Alcohol causes problems partly by its direct toxic effect on both the central nervous system and other organs, such as the liver, where it acts as a poison, and also by its effect of reducing absorption of certain vitamins, in particular thiamine and the vitamin B group from the gastro-intestinal tract. The diet usually becomes deficient in these vitamins, since alcohol is used to replace food by the alcoholic, providing calories and energy but no adequate protein or vitamin supplements.

The treatment of the toxic effect, therefore, and the deficiencies that go with it, is the first aid measure which must be used to deal with possible delirium tremens and the more serious consequences of Korsakoff's psychosis and Wernicke's encephalopathy that can follow. To this end the delirium itself is treated with a drug which will allow the patient to work through the alcohol withdrawal and the associated hyperexcitability of the brain, which will occur for a few days as the sedative effect of the alcohol wears off, and control the confusion. Either a phenothiazine drug, such as chlorpromazine or thioridazine, may be given or a benzodiazepine may be used. More recently chlormethiazole has been shown to be most effective in controlling these withdrawal symptoms. At the same time high potency vitamin supplements are given, in particular thiamine in large dosage, should signs suggestive of Korsakoff's psychosis or Wernicke's encephalopathy be present. Delirium tremens usually settles in this way within a few days, but patients with a longer-term alcohol problem may develop residual degrees of dementia if thiamine treatment is given too late or the process has progressed too far.

Once the acute symptoms have subsided, and assuming that there is no marked underlying disturbance of intellectual function or memory, then a decision must be made in consultation with the patient as to what is to be done next. Unfortunately, the majority of sufferers do not wish to take 'the cure', and prefer at this stage to leave hospital, believing that they will, in future, be able to control their drinking habits more effectively. This is, of course usually a vain hope, and few alcoholics manage to cure themselves without assistance. Indeed, few manage to cure themselves without in-patient assistance, since the temptations of those still in the community in the early stages of going dry are more than most can cope with.

Nevertheless, the majority do discharge themselves from hospital against advice, and at present there are as a rule no grounds to detain them under the Mental Health Act. No doubt this is basically reasonable, since the individual in society has a perfect right to drink himself to death if he so wishes. The same argument against or for detention could be made in a variety of cases of self-inflicted health hazards, from smoking upwards.

Unfortunately, however, the chronic alcoholic usually affects others besides himself, and this means that society has to cope with the alcoholic whether it wishes to or not. Many social agencies, therefore, from the police to Samaritans and social services departments, may put pressure on the hospitals to do something, and, of course, the close relatives, who are the ones most intimately affected, may well plead for continuing care. The British legal and social system, however, is such that the individual can override these considerations and refuse to come in.

Aside from these ethical problems, what can be done to those individuals who do choose to stay in hospital and attempt to resolve the problem permanently?

After the drying-out phase, treatment must be conducted according to what the therapist feels to be most appropriate in the individual case. **An assessment must be made of the underlying causative factors which have created and are perpetuating the condition.** Psychotherapy may then be initiated in an attempt to deal with these factors, and this may consist of milieu therapy, counselling, and support through such groups as Alcoholics Anonymous, in which individuals who have themselves already conquered the problem offer individual and group support to new members in controlling their tendency to revert to alcohol drinking. Usually the alcoholic must try to give up drinking on a permanent basis, since it is rare that an individual who has once become an alcoholic can revert to social drinking without doing so to excess, though this counsel of perfection is seen by some as an unrealistically high aim.

While in hospital, psychotherapy can be conducted further on an individual or group basis, and a number of units have been set up to deal specifically with problems of alcoholism. There are regional centres in most parts of Britain. It is usually more appropriate that an individual attends one of these special centres than that he stays in the district psychiatric unit, since special facilities, and staff with a special interest in these problems, are usually able to help better than would equivalent treatment given in an ordinary psychiatric admission ward.

Drug therapy may be an additional aid in controlling such problems. Many of the phenothiazine drugs described earlier may be helpful in controlling agitation and anxiety, and are particularly useful in the withdrawal phase. Anti-depressants and anxiolytics may be valuable for those in whom alcohol addiction is secondary to other underlying emotional problems. Butyrophenones, in particular haloperidol, have been shown to have an anti-craving or an anti-addictive effect on the desire to return to drinking, which the individual may have for many months after stopping.

Useful additional aids are preparations such as antabuse and dipsan. These products are taken daily in tablet form, and are completely harmless as long as alcohol is not imbibed. What they do, however, is to block the breakdown of alcohol in the body at the stage where it has been converted to acetaldehyde. This is a rather toxic substance, and if it builds up in the body as a result of taking alcohol, it causes a feeling of marked malaise, nausea, a pounding pulse and vivid flushing of the face. The effect of this is certainly sufficiently unpleasant to deter the individual from doing it twice.

The advantage of such products is that the alcoholic knows that, so long as he is taking the tablets, he has good reason to avoid alcohol. He also knows that the drug takes a couple of days to wear off, and that he must, therefore, make a decision while cold sober whether to stop the tablets or to continue. He cannot drink for some 24 to 48 hours after making this decision, and one hopes that in this time he will have thought better of it or will have sought help. It thus gives a boost to the will power of the individual, but, of course, its value does depend in the long run on the willingness of the patient to continue with the treatment.

Finally, there is the method of treatment known as **aversion therapy**. This has been criticised by some groups on the grounds that patterns of behaviour are being altered in the individual in a way which prevents his freedom of will, and that coercion into such treatment is in effect a form of brainwashing. In discussions the author has had with individuals who object to such forms of treatment the argument has always seemed singularly fatuous. There is no doubt that aversive therapy can be effective in removing symptoms which the individual finds distressing and from which he requests relief. It would seem much more unethical to deny such treatment, knowing it to be effective, knowing that the individual is suffering from the results of his behaviour, knowing that other methods may not work so well, and knowing that he himself is anxious for such treatment and fully aware of its nature. Furthermore, the coercion which society imposes in requiring the individual to conform to some generalised norm of behaviour is not entirely to be despised. Any society requires a certain amount of unselfish consideration for its other members if its structure is to survive. A group of people living in a structureless environment are likely to find many more disadvantages than advantages. Moreover, the behaviour which one is assisting the individual to extinguish is not only antisocial to the group in which he lives but is harmful to the individual's health, both physical and mental, in the long term.

The technique of aversion therapy in the treatment of the alcoholic, which is very simple, is based on learning theory. If an individual has a certain need, say hunger, and a stimulus is supplied to that individual—in this example the presence of something edible—he will respond to this stimulus by eating the food. If this gratifies the need and the hunger is relieved, then this pattern of response will tend to be learned and repeated in similar circumstances in the future. On the other hand, if the consumption of the food did not satisfy the need, perhaps because it had an unpleasant taste or proved in some way to be inedible, then the need would not be satisfied and that particular pattern of response would tend to be inhibited on future occasions.

Thus learning takes place through the consequences of the response to a stimulus, depending on whether or not this is satisfying to the need experienced. Hunger is but one example of a need; there are, of course, many others which motivate human beings. Now the effectiveness of such a stimulus response system depends on the levels or strengths of the various aspects of it—the strength of the drive, the effectiveness of the stimulus inducing a response, the effectiveness of the response in reducing the drive, and so on. It has been found that patterns of response come to be associated with the primary response (in the example quoted, this would be things associated with the act of eating the food and its effectiveness in relieving hunger), and these associated factors also become incorporated into the learned response. Thus, if the release of hunger in this experiment were always to be associated with pleasant music, whereas the presentation of food which was unpalatable was always to coincide with a loud, unpleasant noise, it might well happen that in due course the loud, unpleasant noise would come to inhibit appetite, even in circumstances where the food was perfectly acceptable.

How is this relevant to the treatment of alcoholism? In certain circumstances people may satisfy a need, and thus induce a reduction of drive, with a consequent learning effect, in a situation which gives immediate gratification but which is, for various reasons, in the long-term harmful to them. Thus, the alcoholic produces relief of tension by the consumption of alcohol and develops a fixed pattern of response, even though he is intellectually aware that this immediate gratification is outweighed by the longer-term problems which result. Nevertheless, he is 'hooked', and is unable to give up the pattern of response because of the strength of the immediate gratification of need which is produced.

If a response to the stimulus of alcohol in this need situation which is in fact not gratifying can be produced, it should tend to inhibit the repetition of the learned pattern. Thus, if a situation which inhibits the tendency to repeat the pattern because of its unpleasant consequence can be associated with drinking alcohol, and if this response is stronger than the drive-reducing effect of the alcohol itself, then the individual will gradually come to drink less, since he will find it no longer satisfies his need.

It is, of course, equally possible that if something were associated with a drive-reducing situation, such as alcohol drinking, but its mildly unpleasant response was not as strong as the drive-reducing effect of the alcohol, then the alcoholism would not be extinguished but rather the mildly unpleasant response would tend to be incorporated into the drinking pattern as the result of association, without extinguishing it. This could result in an alcoholic who was also hooked on aversive shocks! Of course, in practical terms this is hardly likely to occur, if only because those carrying out the treatment know how to avoid such a situation. It could, nevertheless, be theoretically possible.

In practice, therefore, what is done in aversion therapy is to associate an unpleasant response with what has been the drive-reducing satisfying response which the individual has learned. In this chapter we are applying the principle to the treatment of alcoholism, but it can, of course, be used to extinguish other learned patterns of behaviour which have an immediate gratification effect but which are, in the long term, undesirable to the individual or to the society in which the individual lives. It is, of course, its use in the latter kind of situation which is questioned by some groups.

Originally, attempts were made to use an aversive stimulus in alcoholism by chemical means. In such therapy the individual received a preparation which induced vomiting, and this was given coincidentally with the consumption, in a controlled situation, of alcohol. The individual thus came to associate alcohol not with a need satisfaction but with subsequent vomiting and the unpleasant consequences which were produced. The timing in such therapy is, of course, crucial, and, using this type of technique, it was difficult to produce a reliable and consistent response which would satisfy the necessary therapeutic criteria. Subsequently, therefore, attempts were made to obtain more effective methods of aversive therapy, and the use of electrical aversive techniques was developed.

A small shock-box unit, often portable and worked by battery, can be attached to an appropriate place, such as the forearm of the patient. A small electrical shock can be delivered by pressing a button on the box, and this can be varied to increase the strength of the shock. If the strength is increased, the sensation becomes uncomfortable, and with a further increase frankly painful. The patient is required to adjust this to a level which he himself finds quite unpleasant without being so painful as to persuade him to discontinue the treatment altogether. The idea is to obtain a level which is aversive. The shock is applied initially by the therapist but later can be done by the patient himself at an appropriate time in the treatment procedure.

For alcoholism this would include a mock-up bar or, at any rate, the provision of the individual's favourite alcoholic beverage. The shock can be applied, for example, as the patient puts the glass to his lips and, of course, the procedure can be varied and made more sophisticated to increase its effectiveness. We are here only describing the simple theory of the technique.

Treatment sessions of about half an hour's duration must be repeated with some regularity over a period of a few weeks, under in-patient supervision, at any rate in the early stages, if the results are to be effective. Of course, the cooperation of the patient in such treatment is most important, since it is easy to cheat by not having the shock sufficiently strong to be aversive.

The technique has been used in alcoholism with varying degrees of success, but has not lived up to its original promise. It should perhaps be considered as one possible line of help for somebody afflicted with this problem, along with the other forms of therapy that have been described above. Whatever treatment is devised, the follow-up period must be prolonged, and there is always the risk of relapse if the patient does not remain vigilant against returning to a drinking pattern in times of stress. Most units which specialise in the treatment of alcoholics now tend to rely on dynamic group therapy in a therapeutic community atmosphere.

Drug Addiction

We now turn to drug addiction. Again, in this book, we are concerned simply with those manifestations of drug dependence which require psychiatric intervention. The social problems of drug-taking are outside our scope and will be touched on only briefly.

A distinction should be drawn at the start between drug dependence and drug addiction. The law recognises different categories of drugs, and it is those commonly known as hard drugs to which addiction is likely to develop. **Addiction is a state of periodic or chronic intoxication to a drug produced by its repeated consumption, and its characteristics include a compulsion to continue taking the drug and a tendency to increase the dosage.** There is development of psychological dependence on the effects of the drug as well as a physical dependence. The results are detrimental both to the health of the individual and, of course, to society. Drugs in this category include opium and the morphine derivatives, heroin and cocaine.

Drugs on which dependence or habituation can develop include a wide range of products considered by our society as relatively harmless. One could include tea and coffee, because of the mild stimulants which they contain. Alcohol may often produce habituation, as can certain types of sleeping tablets, in particular barbiturates, and some tranquillising drugs. Amphetamines and other stimulant drugs are particularly dangerous in this respect, and in such cases addiction can also occur. Normally in dependence or habituation, however, the desire is short of a compulsion, but there is a need to continue to take the drug, though no tendency to need to increase its dosage to produce the same effect. Some degree of psychological dependence will occur, but the physical dependence is not found, and the detrimental effect is usually on the individual only and not particularly on society as a whole. The effect of sudden withdrawal, however, even with these preparations, can be quite dangerous, particularly in the case of sedative drugs, where there may be a tendency to increased excitability of the central nervous system for a few days afterwards, with the possibility of inducing epileptic fits and a state of delirium tremens.

There is a third category of drugs which induce neither dependence nor addiction but are nevertheless potentially harmful and dangerous, and are, therefore, included under the Misuse of Drugs Act. Such drugs include, in particular, the hallucinogenic drugs, such as lysergic acid and mescaline, and stimulant drugs of the cannabis type.

Takers of drugs may see the psychiatrist for various reasons. They may seek help because they want to stop their drug-taking but find they cannot do this on their own; or they may have appeared in court as a result of drug offences, and a condition of attendance at a treatment centre may have been made under a probation order. For the psychiatrist, the more important reason for hospital treatment is, however, the development of a psychiatric illness consequent upon the taking of such drugs, and it is these problems that we shall now briefly consider.

Symptoms

Long-term habituation to **sedative drugs**, such as barbiturates, and, of course, to the more serious narcotics, such as opium, morphine and its derivatives, can produce a state of chronic lethargy, disturbed concentration and intellectual deterioration. Often the barbiturates have been taken initially for insomnia, and the patient finds that any attempt to discontinue the drug leads to a period of motor restlessness and complete lack of sleep, with unpleasant dreams if sleep does come. The picture thus seen can mimic neuroses and depressive states, and if the underlying cause is not recognised, can lead to inappropriate treatment.

The **stimulant drugs**, in particular the amphetamines and cannabis, and also cocaine, may produce a condition of motor restlessness when being taken, together with a delirious state in the intoxicated phase. More seriously, however, they can induce a psychotic illness indistinguishable from schizophrenia, particularly in those individuals who are prone to such an illness. It has commonly been found that individuals who are taking slimming tablets, which may contain amphetamine derivatives, and who have in the past suffered from a psychotic illness, may well develop a recurrence as a result. The possible reasons for this have been discussed in earlier chapters but relate to the fact that amphetamines are mono-amines, closely related to some of the natural catacholamines occurring in the central nervous system. It may well be that the disturbance of such systems induces the paranoid and delusional behaviour associated with amphetamine psychosis, which mimics schizophrenia. Such a psychosis can also occur, however, in individuals where there has been no such history in their own past or even in their family's. Sudden withdrawal of such drugs can equally induce a state of the delirium tremens kind, or a longer-term slowing of drive and flattening of affect, owing to discontinuing artificial brain stimulation.

The **hallucinogenic drugs**, such as LSD, are not, in fact, drugs of addiction. They can, however, be extremely dangerous, and indeed at present they pose a major problem on the drug-taking scene in some respects. The action of such drugs is to induce a state of altered awareness in the taker, with a heightening and distortion of sensory perception. Acute, bizarre hallucinatory states can occur, and the individual may develop a feeling of well-being and all-powerfulness which makes him believe, for example, that he can fly, and he may attempt to prove this from a high building. Equally, paranoid or depressive feelings can occur, depending on the situation in which the drug is taken. The dangerous part is principally its unpredictability. Furthermore, such drugs can be made fairly simply by chemical means, which poses a considerable problem of control. The drugs are extremely powerful and a very small quantity can produce marked effects. Furthermore, the drug is not detectable in the body once it has been consumed, so that only the patient can confirm whether or not the psychotic episode has been caused by such a drug.

A young man had taken LSD one week before and the experience at that time had seemingly been a pleasant one. On the evening in question he went with a friend to the local pub. There he consumed some four pints of beer. On the way home he began to feel strange. Sounds seemed much more acute and colours more vivid than normal. As they entered their digs he became convinced that his friend was about to attack him with a knife and picking up a walking stick in the hallway he battered his friend over the head with it viciously and killed him. No knife was found, nor was there any suggestion that this idea was other than delusional. The youth was charged with manslaughter and in the absence of psychiatric illness, since the flashback had cleared within a few hours, admission to a special hospital such as Rampton or Broadmoor was inappropriate. The youth was gaoled.

A girl had taken LSD at a party and experienced pleasant perceptual distortions for an hour or two. She returned to her own home but later in the evening became convinced that she could fly, all that was needed being for her to flap her arms. There was no question of attempted suicide. She went to an upstairs room, opened the window and proceeded to jump out, flapping her arms vigorously. This was noted by a passerby. Unfortunately, her belief was delusional and she fell to the ground, fracturing both legs and one wrist.

'Trips' are unpredictable. The fact that one has a good trip on one occasion is no guarantee that the next will be the same. A trip may produce thought disorder and bizarre experiences, and may recur in what is known as a 'flashback', even some weeks after the initial taking of the drug, perhaps provoked by consumption of alcohol or cannabis. There have even been suggestions of long-term genetic damage to the reproductive cells, which might make it particularly dangerous to young people who become pregnant or get someone else pregnant, with the possibility of foetal deformities.

The whole subject of hallucinogens makes an interesting study. Some types of these drugs were initially obtained by Mexican Indians who chewed peyotl, which is derived from cactus leaves. Mescal has also been used in drinks and is still obtainable in certain quarters, and may be combined with a distillate known as tequila. Other hallucinogens have been derived from ergot and from psilocybin, the active ingredient of teonanacuatl, a sacred mushroom used by the Chinatec in Southern Mexico.

The **medico-legal aspects** of drug-taking relate to the 1971 Misuse of Drugs Act, which replaced the earlier Dangerous Drugs Act. Under this Act possession is an offence, intent to supply is a more serious offence, and producing a controlled drug is subject to a 14-year maximum prison sentence. It is an offence to possess premises where drugs are knowingly used, and in Section 10 of the Act restrictions are imposed on any doctor who prescribes such drugs irresponsibly.

Treatment for Drug Addiction

Treatment of drug addiction follows a similar pattern to that of alcoholism. Gradual withdrawal of the drug under supervision, aided by phenothiazine drugs or chlormethiazole to alleviate withdrawal symptoms, is accomplished over a week or more. After this, intensive psychotherapy, usually of a group kind, is instituted, and treatment of any underlying psychiatric condition can then be started.

As with alcoholism, the National Health Service has regional drug addiction units where those patients who wish for help in dealing with their drug problem may obtain treatment. The primary treatment, however, will still fall on the district psychiatric hospital, which deals with the acute effects of drug addiction, the psychotic episodes and withdrawal phases of the drugs, as described above.

The essence of treatment is to tide the patient over the withdrawal phase, often replacing the drug of addiction with some less toxic medication in order to prevent acute symptoms, and then gradually withdrawing this as appropriate. The withdrawal of a sedative drug, such as heroin, is going to produce a rebound over-excitability of the central nervous system for a few days. This may produce a delirium, with episodes of acute fear and panic, visual hallucinations and a picture-like delirium tremens. Fits may occur. Often methadone is used as a substitute for a while in treating hard drug addiction of the sedative group. Phenothiazines can be used, and careful 24-hour nursing care is needed.

The effect of withdrawal of sedative drugs is similar to the effect produced by the ingestion of drugs of a stimulant group. When stimulant drugs are withdrawn, the brain will go into a phase of reflex under-activity in which the patient becomes sluggish and depressed. Again, this is felt as most unpleasant by the patient, and it is this fear of the effects of withdrawal that tends to keep the addict dependent on the drug. Furthermore, the body has adjusted to the absorption of far greater quantities of these drugs than the normal individual could tolerate, and it is this phase of re-adjustment which is hardest. In the withdrawal phase of stimulant drugs, therefore, anti-depressants or thioxanthines are often helpful.

Treatment of intoxication by hallucinogens, such as lysergic acid, is principally the same as for the treatment of schizophrenia, namely with phenothiazines or related drugs until the psychotic phase is over.

Often addicts approach the hospital not with the intention of treatment and cure but in order to try to obtain supplies. There is now a central drug addiction register where information on all known addicts is maintained, together with the up-to-date dosage that they are taking. New individuals wanting to be treated can either undergo in-patient care for withdrawal of the drug, which seems to the author the most appropriate thing for medical staff to be doing, or can apply to be registered as drug-takers, which entitles them to obtain supplies in a controlled manner from certain doctors who are registered to prescribe under the 1971 Act. Some would feel that for those addicted to hard drugs containment may be initially the only practical method of control, and certain registered centres are, therefore, prepared to prescribe controlled drugs within these regulations.

The same principles of treatment apply to drugs of addiction which do not fall within the hard drug category but where serious psychological dependency may have developed.

Any doctor may prescribe a drug which is potentially a drug of addiction for the control of acute disease. For instance, morphine derivatives may be used to control severe pain after an operation. Under the 1971 Act, however, only doctors with recognised experience in the treatment of drug addiction are registered to prescribe these drugs to addicts, as opposed to ordinary medical needs.

Further Reading

Emboden, W., *Narcotic Plants*, Studio Vista, London, 1972.
Hore, B. D., *Alcohol Dependence*, Butterworths, London, 1976.
'Misuse of Drugs Act', *British Medical Journal*, 2 October, 1971.
Subcommittee on Alcoholism, WHO Publication 42, 1951.
Watt, M. M., *Drug Dependence*, M.T.P. Press, Lancaster, England, 1977.

Questions

1. Where are the regional alcohol and drug addiction units in your area?
2. Is alcoholism a big problem in your area?
3. Why are cities likely to have a bigger alcohol and drug-addiction problem?
4. Do you have a local Alcoholics Anonymous organisation?
5. Do you have a local drug-addiction liaison committee?

16
The Elderly Mentally Infirm

Summary

The elderly mentally infirm occupy one-third of psychiatric beds, and one-sixth of the total hospital beds in the country. The population aged over 65 represents 12½ per cent of the whole.

Principal Diagnosis: Dementia

The problem is on the increase, and we shall consider the interrelationship between the services provided by the hospital psychiatric service, geriatric service, and the local-authority Social Services department Part III accommodation.

Three groups of elderly mentally infirm can be distinguished:

1. 'Graduate' patients who are psychiatric hospital long-stay, growing old within the hospital community.
2. Elderly patients with psychiatric illness of a type found in any age group.
3. The elderly with dementing illnesses:
   (a) Mild.
   (b) Severe uncomplicated.
   (c) Dementia complicated by other physical illness.

Social problems are compounded by the relative breakup of the closely knit family unit. Wandering, aggressive behaviour and incontinence are the main factors which cause relatives to give up looking after aging members of the family.

Day centres can be of considerable value in the care of the elderly.

Nursing care of the ambulant confused person requires special skills.

Description

The rising numbers of elderly in the community and the increase in life expectancy have brought into focus those degenerative conditions of old age, principally the dementias, which in former generations were less frequently seen, since many died of other conditions before reaching the age when dementia presents.

As the number of beds required for long-term sufferers from schizophrenia has diminished, so the number of beds required for psychogeriatrics has gone up. This group of sufferers, often no longer looked after by their families, as they were before the fragmentation of the family unit which industrialisation has produced, paid their taxes for many years yet at a time when they have become most vulnerable are relegated to what is a Cinderella part of the National Health Service. It would seem reasonable that greater resources should be devoted to facilities for making the final years of an individual's life at least more comfortable.

The demand for hospital beds is not, as some would suggest, a bottomless pit. The provision of adequate day-care facilities can do much to relieve what would otherwise be a burden for relatives, and home-help services can be provided, for example, for the occasionally incontinent elderly person in the shape of laundry facilities. Such matters require a high degree of cooperation between the local authorities, the geriatric services, and the psychiatric services which run psycho-geriatric facilities. Unfortunately, the allocation of funds from the Health Service for the provision of hospital facilities is often, as in mental retardation, motivated by the political implications of such financial commitment rather than the real needs of the dependent sections of the community.

In this chapter we shall be looking not at the specific diseases which may be found within the psycho-geriatric speciality but at the more general problems associated with the elderly mentally infirm. To this end some basic facts and figures need to be assimilated.

The Office of Health Economics publishes a series of papers on current health problems and trends. Its publication No. 26 on old age, published in 1968, gave projected trends, the validity of which are now being proved. In 1966 in England and Wales there were some 6 million people over the age of 65—about 12 per cent of the total population. Fifty years previously, the figures were 1½ million, which accounted for only 5 per cent of the population. At the same time, the number aged 85 and over rose from 50,000 to nearly 350,000. The increase from 1½ to 6 million has been much faster than the rise in other age groups. By the age of 75 there are more than twice as many women as men. Two-thirds of the women are widowed, a total of approximately one million. The death rate among persons aged 65 and over has fallen by about 20 per cent in the last 50 years, from 83 per 1,000 to 65 per 1,000.

The social circumstances of the elderly in the community have altered considerably in the last century. While the majority of the elderly live in private households, either with or near children or other relatives, nearly 2 million at the time of the survey were without a relative living with them or even nearby, and 1½ million lived completely alone. Some 300,000 lived in various types of institution, mainly National Health Service hospitals or local authority residential homes. Although those aged 65 and over account for only 12½ per cent of the population, they occupy some 35 per cent of the total beds within the Health Service. This is, of course, no surprise and emphasises the importance of this group.

Half the beds occupied by mentally ill females contained women aged over 65. While the number of occupied beds in psychiatric units has fallen considerably in the last 20 years, the number occupied by persons over 65 has increased by some 8,000. In non-psychiatric hospitals about 80,000 beds are occupied by those aged 65 or over, and in psychiatric hospitals some 52,000.

Research has suggested that the services provided in the shape of health and welfare for this group are by no means adequate. Kay, Beamish and Roth in Newcastle showed that only a small proportion of those aged 65 and over who suffered from psychiatric disorder were being cared for either as hospital in-patients or in residential homes. Equally, Townsend and Wedderburn showed that 25 per cent of those who could receive state help of various types did not apply.

The elderly with psychiatric symptomatology can be divided into three groups:

1. Patients who entered hospital for psychiatric illness before modern methods of treatment were available and who have grown old within these hospitals after many years there.

2. Elderly patients with psychiatric illness of a type that may be found in any other age group, such as depression, schizophrenia or the neuroses.

3. Elderly persons with dementing illnesses where there is a progressive degeneration of the nerve cells in the brain, leading to loss of memory, disorientation, and a general deterioration in the personality.

For practical purposes this last group can be subdivided into those where the dementia is mild and who are able to be looked after within the community; those where the dementia is severe enough to require hospital care but where there are no other complicating physical diseases, and the problem is, therefore, one of nursing the ambulant, confused person; and, thirdly, those with a dementia which is complicating or complicated by other significant physical disease. The latter is commonly chronic disease of the chest or heart or such organs as the kidneys.

The DHSS points out that

... proper assessment to determine the most appropriate pattern of care and treatment is a fundamental requirement. Wherever possible patients should be assessed at home in consultation with the general practitioner or failing that as an out-patient or day patient. However, there will be some whose needs can be satisfactorily assessed only as in-patients in hospital. Many of those with mental illness symptoms may be suffering from acute confusional states or from a complex mixture of social, medical and psychological problems requiring the collaboration of professional workers of different disciplines. The psycho-geriatric assessment unit can usefully serve as a focus where members of the geriatric, psychiatric, general medical, local health and social services may meet to consider the individual needs of each patient and to plan and initiate a treatment programme.

Those dementia cases that fall into the second category of the three listed above, namely, uncomplicated dementias that require hospital care, have steadily increased in numbers in the last two decades. They require a special type of nursing expertise and are more time-consuming than the longer-stay patients in the first group, because of the level of confusion with their often accompanying incontinence and disturbed behaviour. In the larger psychiatric hospitals they have gradually encroached upon wards previously designated for the younger, longer-stay patient as these beds have become vacated, and this has obviously led to some administrative problems.

In some of the newer district general psychiatric hospital units no provision has been made at all for such patients, nor have any figures been put out for the estimated number of beds that would be required for this group until years after the district general concept had been approved. The fact that such patients might well occupy the bed for some years, particularly when adequate community care facilities were non-existent, deterred consultants from admitting these people in need into supposedly short-stay beds designated for the treatment of the acutely psychiatrically ill. Once the bed was blocked by a patient with a dementing condition, then the expected ten-patient-a-year turnover in that bed was wiped out, and the bed could not be used for its proper purpose. This led to considerable conflict between the family doctor, community services, and the hospital, since all groups were placed in an impossible position.

Schemes such as that operating in the Netherlands would seem ideal, but require the provision of considerable financial outlay. There, large, well equipped blocks of flats for elderly people, allowing couples to continue to live together even when one member has become frail, have proved a considerable success. Within the flats complex there are in effect community hospital facilities and areas where those who are developing increasing dependence can be cared for by a warden with proper nursing facilities. Thus patients who gradually deteriorate can remain in familiar surroundings, and with their friends, a factor so important in dementias, where the ability to learn new material and orientate oneself in new surroundings is progressively lost. Flats for couples, single people's flats, and hostel or hospital designated areas are all within the same building. They are serviced and have pleasant gardens, and are in every way homely. Visiting is unrestricted and the range of freedom for the residents is, therefore, considerable, in contrast to the constraints of a hospital setting.

Unfortunately, such facilities are not available in Great Britain. The functioning of any service for the three groups of elderly persons with dementia depends on the relative availability of psychiatric hospital beds, geriatric hospital beds, and local authority Part III accommodation (which is accommodation provided by the social services departments in individual health authority areas for people in need of care, principally the elderly). The proper working together of these three groups can only be achieved if all have access to assessment, and if all have facilities for the proper disposal of patients who have been assessed and, if necessary, are undergoing treatment. The four possible disposal areas must, therefore, be available, as follows:

(a) the patient may return home, (b) the patient may require a supportive environment at a level provided by the social services department in a community elderly people's home, (c) the patient may require further care within a geriatric unit in a general hospital, and (d) the patient may require further treatment in a psychiatric hospital. If any of the three groups does not have adequate facilities to take up their appropriate share, then any system will fail, and the other groups will feel burdened by patients whom they see as inappropriately placed.

One of the early units, with which the author is familiar, was set up on these multi-disciplinary lines in Nottingham. The psycho-geriatric assessment unit could receive patients referred from the family doctor or social services department, and a joint assessment was made by both the geriatrician and psychiatrist specialising in the elderly mentally infirm, in most cases before admission was confirmed.

During their stay in the unit, which is normally limited to six weeks, a full assessment of the appropriate needs of the patients is made. Any necessary tests are carried out, and, at a regular joint meeting between the geriatrician, psychiatrist and social services department, along with the nursing staff, the most appropriate method of further care is worked out. This is then discussed with the patient and relatives, and before the six weeks is up appropriate arrangements will have been made. The three groups concerned—psychiatry, geriatrics and the social services—undertake to find appropriate facilities at the end of the six weeks, if it seems best that the patient's further care should come under one particular group. Equally, for the proper running of the scheme the relatives were required to undertake that they would receive the patient back home at the end of the six weeks if this seemed proper to all concerned.

Unfortunately, it has to be recognised that many relatives, if they have been under considerable stress from an elderly mentally infirm member over some period of time and have had little community support, find that the relief of having the person admitted to hospital is such that they subsequently refuse to have him or her home. In a properly conducted service this type of breakdown of communication between the patient's relatives and the helping services should never be allowed to develop.

By sticking to this format the Nottingham scheme worked well. Schemes which do not have adequate disposal facilities, or where some equivalent of the six-weeks rule is not imposed, rapidly find that their assessment beds cannot cope with undischargeable long-stay patients, and the unit ceases to be able to carry out its proper function.

Further facilities essential for the satisfactory running of such units are the day hospital and day centre. A day hospital is run by the hospital service and provides full hospital facilities, with nursing and medical cover, but the patient returns home at night and at weekends, thus retaining the links with the family but giving the family a break during the day, and allowing the patient who needs it to receive full hospital care during a 9.00 am to 5.00 pm period. This avoids the admission of many who would otherwise have to be full-time in-patients, and allows of earlier discharge, but depends considerably on the provision of adequate ambulance services for transport.

The day centre is staffed and run by the local authority social services department. It provides daytime activity and a stimulating environment, preferably with occupational therapy or other sheltered activities, and provides for those elderly people in the community living with relatives who perhaps go out to work during the day or need some free time to do shopping or visit friends.

A recent trend has been the development of the community unit for the elderly (CUE unit), which provides a community in-patient facility in a small hospital at district level. It is proposed that each sector of a district should have such a CUE unit which would provide in-patient facilities for those too confused to manage in the community itself. This is rather like reverting to the old cottage hospital, but is specifically designed to keep patients with dementing conditions as near as possible to their friends and relatives and their familiar surroundings.

Patients Who Have Grown Old in Hospitals for the Mentally Ill

We have already mentioned the dwindling group of long-stay patients. A reduction in the number of beds in psychiatric hospitals has been steadily achieved over the last 15–20 years simply because, with better methods of treatment, the numbers of patients, particularly those with a diagnosis of schizophrenia, who have required to stay in hospital over a period of years have been dramatically reduced.

Those who do continue to require long-term care, however, because their disease was too far advanced by the time treatment methods were developed and, therefore, still have residual symptoms, or those who have lost touch with their relatives and have nowhere to go, are now an aging population and, although dwindling, are becoming an increasing problem because of infirmity. Such patients are the residuum of those admitted up until the mid-1950s. Many, therefore, are now reaching their seventies or eighties and are becoming more a geriatric than a chronic psychiatric problem. The DHSS recognises the needs of such patients and states that 'every effort should be made to provide as full a life as possible for all such patients and to prevent them from being cut off from regular contact with people outside the hospital'.

Despite improved methods of treatment, a small number of patients are still becoming chronic in the sense that they require long-term hospital care. This group should not be ignored. Its size is somewhat difficult to determine, since we are in a time of change, when the number of long-stay schizophrenic patients is still dropping. It is always possible, however, that in spite of new advances in treatment the schizophrenic process may in some of these patients again break through in later years, and despite everybody's best efforts elderly schizophrenics who have been able to live in the community for many years may, as they become older, become less able to cope and by the 1990s be increasingly reappearing in hospital beds.

Furthermore, a few schizophrenics do still require long-stay care. The occasional severe personality disorder does not survive outside hospital, and a number of cases of dementia in younger people develop as a result of trauma to the brain, infection or some of the more slowly progressive pre-senile dementias. Thus, there is a slow accumulation of long-stay patients who in due course will finish up in this category.

Elderly Persons with Functional Mental Illness

Patients within this category, although elderly, are suffering from exactly the same problems as may occur in any age group, namely, depressive illnesses, schizophrenia and the various kinds of neurosis. They will be treated, therefore, on the ordinary admission wards just as elderly people with appendicitis would be on the same surgical ward as young people with surgical problems. It would not seem desirable to segregate by age under such circumstances.

Certain non-dementing psychiatric illnesses are seen more commonly in one age group than another. In the elderly, **paraphrenia** is particularly common. This condition, which has been described elsewhere, is akin to the schizophrenic process, though the personality remains more intact and thought disorder is not marked, perhaps owing to the stability of thought processes reached in this age group or to some different biochemical aetiology. The patient develops a fixed delusional idea, often associated with hallucinations, which may be tactile or olfactory, and often with a persecutory content. Thus, the elderly lady may believe that neighbours are in some way interfering with her, stealing from her, or some such thing.

Elderly Persons with Dementia

This group is characterised by some permanent impairment of psychological function as a result of a dementing process. Surveys have shown the prevalence of dementia to be some 10 per cent in persons aged 65 and over, though in many cases these will be mild and in the early stages, and the majority live at home.

The incidence of dementia rises sharply with increasing age. Those in the category of mild dementia have some degree of confusion and perhaps a tendency to wander and get lost, and may at times be restless or mildly aggressive if they misunderstand what others have tried to do for them; but they do not require continuous nursing care. It is in this group that the day centres and day hospitals play such a vital part.

If hospital care is needed for patients whose dementia is associated with other significant physical disease, a not insignificant group in the elderly, a decision must be made as to whether geriatric or psychiatric nursing is most appropriate. This will depend largely on whether the physical needs of the patient in terms of nursing care are predominant or whether psychiatric nursing care for the ambulant confused is most appropriate. Hence, joint assessment is important.

The bed requirements for patients needing to be treated in geriatric departments within this group are included in the 10 beds per 1,000 population aged 65 and over recommended for geriatrics by the DHSS. A double nursing qualification in both SRN and RMN by some of the staff is desirable.

Acute confusional states are usually associated with physical illness, often unsuspected infection. They tend to occur initially at night and are characterised by lucid episodes. Some disorientation and misidentification is common, and sometimes visual hallucinations can be frightening.

The largest group, however, will need to be in a community unit for the elderly or a more specialised district hospital or psychiatric ward for dementia, and would be those with a severe dementia but without other significant physical illnesses. The criteria whereby the need for hospital admission is decided are often social ones. Disturbed nights, a tendency to wander out of the house and get lost or be a danger on the roads, and incontinence are the commonest factors. Aggressive behaviour also rapidly causes relatives' tolerance to wear thin. To some extent these matters can be treated and controlled in the home, but often the mildly confused elderly person will refuse to take medication, even if this is carefully supervised by relatives. If sedation by injection is needed or if control of aggressive behaviour requires 24-hour nursing care, then obviously hospital admission becomes essential.

Some three beds per 1,000 for patients aged 65 and over need to be provided within the psychiatric services for this group. This is approximately 0.4 beds per 1,000 population of all ages, and is additional to the 0.5 beds per 1,000 recommended for psychiatric units in the district general hospital general psychiatry. In combination with the day hospital, and the provision of holiday beds so that relatives who are coping the rest of the year may have a break to go away, such a provision should be adequate for the needs of the type of community found in Great Britain at present.

Allowance must be made by relatives when an elderly person is admitted to a holiday bed for some worsening of the apparent level of confusion. This happens because disorientated patients, with no facility for new learning or immediate recall, cannot find their way around in a new place. For example, they do not learn the position of the toilet, which is probably familiar to them at home, and tend to become incontinent. A high nurse–patient ratio can do much to minimise these problems. Daily activities run by occupational therapy departments must also be geared to this feature of the memory.

Incontinence of urine may be a feature of bladder infection. Equally, it may suggest a gynaecological problem. In many elderly people, however, it is part of the social deterioration of dementia, and urinary and faecal incontinence are not uncommon in the severer cases. Easy access to toilets, the provision of incontinence pads, and special laundering facilities must be an important part of the planning for such patient groups.

Conclusions

1. Elderly patients who have grown old in hospitals for the mentally ill are a diminishing number. New accommodation is not needed, but improved conditions are needed, perhaps community based.

2. Elderly patients with functional mental illness are treated within the guidelines of 0.5 beds per 1,000 and 0.65 day places per 1,000 total population suggested for adult mental illness.

3. Elderly persons with mild dementia will be cared for at home or in local authority residential accommodation at the rate of 25 beds per 1,000 over 65 as suggested.

4. Elderly patients with dementia and other physical disease will be dealt with in geriatric units within the recommended planning guideline of 10 beds and two day places per 1,000 population aged 65 and over for the geriatric services.

5. Elderly patients with severe dementia but without other physical disease will require three beds and three day places per 1,000 population aged 65 and over, which is some 0.3 per 1,000 beds in the total population; this is additional to the scale of provision suggested above.

6. Elderly patients requiring joint geriatric/psychiatric assessment require an assessment unit of 10–20 beds per 250,000 total population, preferably sited at the district general hospital.

A major problem within the Health Service has been the appropriate placement of these various groups of patients and the easy transfer from one group to another. Often local authority, geriatric and psychiatric catchment areas do not coincide. The absence of joint assessment procedures makes the movement of patients difficult, and a situation can frequently develop where a demented patient, too big a nursing problem for the local authority hostels to cope with, is unable to obtain placement in a psycho-geriatric unit, while, at the same time, there are patients within the psychiatric or geriatric units that could be discharged from hospital to local authority care if such beds were available. The negotiation of direct swaps and the endeavour to place patients in community care as near as possible to their friends and relations taxes the ingenuity and tempers of the various professionals concerned. Furthermore, political expediency or the lack of a proper financial commitment to this group have meant that many author-ities are working on a shoestring, and are physically unable to provide the necessary scale of services to make these proposals work.

The problem is still a growing one. Roth showed in the units surveyed in Newcastle that admissions for the over-65s had increased in a two-year period by some 5 per cent, and, owing to the increased longevity, the numbers of over-65s in the units had gone up from 480 to 650, an increase of over 30 per cent in the same period.

Psycho-geriatric services have been, like mental retardation, a Cinderella area. In a government-financed service it is necessary to press for diversion of funds into these under-funded groups if proper treatment facilities are to be provided. The provision of community-based units (CUE units) has been mentioned earlier in the chapter. In the next chapter we shall go on to consider the dementias and other illnesses characterised by disturb-ances of memory and orientation in more individual detail

Further Reading

Arie, T., 'Management of Dementia in the Elderly', 1973, *BMJ*, December 8, 1973.
Arie, T. and Jolley, D. 'The Rising Tide (Mental Disorder in Old Age)', *British Medical Journal*, 286–325, 1983.
Chown, S., *Human Aging*, Penguin, Harmondsworth, 1970.
Dementia in Old Age, Office of Health Economics, London, 1979.
Happier Old Age, A, DHSS, 1978.
Kay, D. W. K., and Walk, A., *Recent Developments in Psychogeriatrics*, *BJP* Special Publication No. 6, Headley, Kent, 1971.
Office of Health Economics, Publication No. 26, London, 1968.
Post, F., *The Clinical Psychiatry of Later Life*, Pergamon, Oxford, 1965.
Services for Mental Illness Related to Old Age, DHSS pamphlet, 1972.

Questions

1. What percentage of health service beds are occupied by the elderly mentally infirm?

2. What is your local district percentage of beds per 1,000 population for geriatrics and psychogeriatrics?

3. How many day hospitals and day centres catering for the EMI are there?

4. How many local authority old people's accommodation units are there run by the Social Services departments, and how many total placements?

5. Is there a community nurse in your area specialising in psycho-geriatrics?

6. Does your local housing department provide adequate facilities for warden-assisted elderly people's accommodation?

17
Disorders of Intellectual Function

Summary

Classification

1. Organic psychoses.
2. Delirious states.
3. Dementias.
   (a) Senile.
   (b) Pre-senile.
   (c) Arteriosclerotic.
   (d) Syphilitic (GPI).
   (e) Others.
4. Epilepsy.

General Symptoms

Disturbance of consciousness, memory or orientation is present. Other symptoms include lability of mood, irritability, alteration of sleep rhythm, and disinhibited social behaviour.

Aetiology

A very wide variety of local or general disease, trauma or degenerative change produces a toxic effect or degenerative change to the nerve cell within the central nervous system.

Treatment and Investigation

There is need for physical treatment for the underlying cause, plus nursing care and rehabilitation.

Description

Another large group of conditions seen by psychiatrists is that where there is an **impairment of intellectual function**. In general, this means a **disorder of memory or orientation**, often coupled with confusion, which in the more acute cases can be associated with an alteration in the level of consciousness.

Much more is known about these groups of illnesses in terms of their cause than has been the case with many of the conditions described up to now. In general, the disturbance of central nervous system function is a result of the disturbance in function at the cell level, either because of toxic effects from more generalised disease affecting other parts of the body, or from a local disturbance of the blood supply or the metabolism of the cell itself.

Patterns of Disease

Three main types of symptom pattern are seen. First, there are those patients who show **psychotic symptoms**, with evidence of disturbed memory consciousness, often minimal. The picture may mimic a depression or schizophrenia, or hysterical state with features of anxiety, but the cause lies in some condition which is disturbing the balance of central nervous system function. These conditions may be as wide-ranging as, for example, severe anaemia, disease of the thyroid associated with a goitre, or a disease such as multiple sclerosis.

The second type is those acute disorders known as **delirious states**. Here a disturbance of consciousness is the most noticeable feature. The condition often occurs in association with acute infectious diseases, where the temperature rises very high or is associated with general toxicity in the body, such as is found in pneumonia.

The third group are the **dementias**. Here the condition is more chronic and the predominant symptoms are disturbances of memory, particularly for recent events, and a disturbance of orientation in time or place. These conditions often arise as a result of hardening of the arteries, or of a degeneration of the brain cells in elderly people, which is just one part of the aging process and is known as **senile dementia**.

Symptoms

In all these syndromes a certain pattern of symptomatology is found to a greater or lesser degree if the observer looks carefully enough for it. Symptoms can be listed as follows:

1. A disturbance of consciousness.
2. A disturbance of memory and orientation.
3. A disturbance of mood, characterised by easy swings from happiness to sadness, from weepiness to laughter and to aggression, which is known as **lability**.
4. Disturbance of sleep rhythm.
5. Irritability.
6. An alteration in social awareness, known as **disinhibition**, in the early stages of which the individual loses his awareness of other people's sensitivities and may become coarser than normal, often in association with toilet use and in sexual matters.

Let us look at some of these symptoms in a little more detail. First, let us consider the matter of **consciousness**. This may be disturbed to varying degrees from a mild disturbance of grasp and concentration, difficult to pick up unless one is looking for it, through to an acute delirious state, then to stupor, and finally to complete coma, where consciousness is lost and there is no contact with the external world. Any disturbance of consciousness found in what has otherwise been assumed by the doctor to be a functional psychosis must immediately make one suspect that there is some other pathology which has been missed, and demands a further thorough search.

Sleep may be disturbed in a variety of ways. The patient may be unable to sleep, and this may be either an initial insomnia or excessively early waking. In organic states, however, there is often a reversal of sleep rhythm, so that the patient tends to sleep during the day but is restless and awake at night. Often confusion is worse at night, and the patient may get up thinking that it is morning and roam about the house. Hypersomnia or excessive sleep may also be found, and in milder form often shows itself as excessive lethargy and drowsiness.

Two particular sleep patterns, known as **narcolepsy** and **cataplexy**, can also be seen. In narcoplepsy the individual shows sudden episodes of irresistible desire for sleep, quite often at inappropriate times, and simply falls asleep for a period, often during this time being unable to be awakened. This is commonly seen after acute virus infections of the brain, such as encephalitis. In cataplexy a state of sleep is induced by a strong emotional stimulus, which then follows the same pattern as above.

Memory may also be impaired in a variety of ways. In dementias the failure of memory is initially for recent events, because the brain is no longer capable of learning new material. That material which is already well learnt is retained, so that elderly people may be able to relate episodes occurring 50 or 60 years ago with great accuracy, but cannot recall, for example, what they had for breakfast that day. They may recount the same story many times and become a bore to their friends because they do not recall that they have told that tale already. This failure of immediate recall can become so pronounced in severer cases that such an individual can be told a fact, such as what day it is, and a moment later be quite unable to remember it.

Total loss of memory is more likely to be an hysterical feature in the context of some other psychiatric disturbance, but patchy memory loss, in which past and recent memory may fail, can be seen in the confusion of a more acute delirium. It is seen also in the more chronic disturbance of memory due to hardening of the arteries, as in an arteriosclerotic dementia. Sometimes there is a false recall, and sometimes patients may make up the answers they do not know, giving an incorrect answer with considerable conviction. This is known as **confabulation**, seen particularly in the type of dementia following chronic alcoholic problems and in severe vitamin B deficiencies.

In memory disturbances following trauma such as concussion, the loss of memory is a retrograde amnesia and affects only that time around the traumatic episode. The same may happen after an epileptic fit or after a coma induced by any kind of acute medical or surgical condition.

Orientation in time and place may also be impaired in dementias, and is typically very disturbed in the more acute delirious states. Sometimes when there is localised brain damage—for example, from a tumour—some of these changes may be quite specific, and one aspect of brain function is disturbed whereas others remain completely intact. The author, for example, had a case of a woman who had suffered from carbon monoxide poisoning and had a complete loss of immediate recall and some additional difficulty in calculating figures, but the rest of the brain function was completely normal and she learned to some extent to adapt to this defect, which, in fact, never fully cleared up.

The social disturbances which occur in the more long-standing states of intellectual impairment often pose considerable problems for friends and relations. The behaviour becomes disinhibited and often ceases to be acceptable, particularly when sexual matters are acted upon in an open manner, or the patient fails to make proper use of the toilet, leaving it with dress in disarray or person exposed.

Let us now look in a little more detail at the individual syndromes which we have mentioned.

Organic Psychoses

The organic psychoses are found in a very wide variety of medical conditions. Often when a patient comes into the hospital with a disorder in which such a diagnosis is suspected, a number of simple screening tests, such as blood tests, urine tests, X-rays and EEGs, can help to point the way to the type of problem which is presenting. In addition, of course, there will usually be other symptoms, which refer to the general medical condition, also present. Sometimes, however, such symptoms are minimal or are overlooked because the psychotic state dominates the picture. Such psychotic states may mimic schizophrenia or a manic-depressive illness. Apparently hysterical features may be present, or anxiety or agitation. Indeed, the whole range of symptomatology can be seen, but usually the experienced practitioner can spot that in some way the condition is not entirely typical. It is perhaps too mixed in character, and underlying it all there may be a mild degree of intellectual impairment or memory disturbance which makes one suspicious. This, associated with some unexpected physical finding, puts one on to the scent.

It is, of course, most important to pick these out from the general run of psychoses, since treating them without dealing with the underlying cause will result merely in a degree of symptom relief without putting right the real problem. It is for this reason that a number of screening tests are routinely carried out on a large proportion of patients admitted to hospital, and once in a while something unexpected is picked up.

Delirium

Delirious states are particularly common in children and in the elderly. They are less often seen these days as resulting from acute infections, since these are usually brought under control with antibiotics before such a stage develops. The majority of delirious states are seen on the general hospital wards, and are indeed best treated there, at any rate in the initial stages, until the underlying cause has been resolved. Sometimes, however, the state of delirium persists in a sub-acute form, even after the underlying cause has been corrected, and in these cases transfer to a psychiatric unit is often appropriate.

The symptoms are principally disorientation, with bewilderment, fear and terror, perhaps associated with hallucinations, which are generally visual and not auditory. The patient is unable to relate immediate experience to past experience, and is liable to produce paranoid interpretations of events.

A young man developed a high fever, the cause of which was initially unknown, and was admitted to hospital for investigation. During the night he began to shout and make a disturbance on the ward. Nurses who went to try and calm him down were fought off. The man believed he was about to be killed and was seemingly seeing frightening shapes moving about in the corner of the room. He was eventually able to be sedated but over the next 48 hours exhibited a fluctuating confusion with disorientation in both time and place and patchy memory disturbance. Psychiatric advice was sought for the treatment of the delirious state and in the meantime, the cause of the fever having been found, this was treated with antibiotics. Both physical and mental disturbance subsided with combined therapy over the next three days.

The mildest phase is a **difficulty in maintaining attention**, especially seen in the evening and night. **Emotional lability** ensues, with restlessness and **failure to grasp** and maintain a knowledge of events. **Disorientation** is more pronounced when the patient is moved to an unfamiliar place. Sleep rhythm is also often impaired. There is clouding of consciousness, and often a fluctuation in the level of consciousness and awareness, which varies from hour to hour.

A condition known as **organic vulnerability** may be seen in long-standing cases. Here the brain, under optimal conditions, is just managing to cope with the environment. Any slight worsening, however, of the brain's function creates a situation of memory disturbance and disorientation, with mild confusion noticeable to relatives. This may be triggered off by some inter-current infection, such as bronchitis, or by the effects of a mild heart attack, a slight stroke, or a wide variety of common ailments. There may be confusion only at night, the patient in the daytime appearing mentally intact. Nevertheless, there is often a history of the presence of some of the following symptoms: headache, episodes of depression or hypochondriasis, easy fatigue and mood swings. Emotional lability with petulant and demanding behaviour, a decreased tolerance to alcohol, and an obsessional attention to routine, may be seen. Commonly, there is a difficulty in finding the right word to describe things or in recalling names.

Dementia

A further stage in this chronic condition is the development of a frank dementia. This is the end point of a large number of organic disorders, and there is a slow but increasingly profound failure of intellect, and emotional and social adaptation.

In the diagnosis of an early dementia, from whatever cause, certain investigations are useful. Often the EEG shows a non-specific abnormality of a generalised type. Psychological assessment will show the degree of intellectual deterioration and, in the early stages, this often shows as a failure to cope with the formation of concepts, even though concrete learning is still relatively unimpaired.

Early assessment of possible dementias is vital, even in the elderly, since a small number prove to have a reversible and remediable condition, which may not be the case if the condition is left too long. Investigation in hospital may be very helpful in establishing the cause, even though the change in environment can temporarily worsen the confusion in some cases. In the short term, therefore, it is the diagnostic aspect of the case, leading to possible treatment of the underlying condition, which is the main concern of the psychiatrists. The long-term problems, however, are considerable, particularly in those cases where the diagnosis turns out to be a dementia of senile type or one due to hardening of the arteries, where cure is not at present practicable. These form the bulk of dementias in the elderly, and often long-term hospital care is the final result. Drug therapy can be used to delay the development of the condition and to relieve some of the symptoms associated with it. Thus drugs may be used to improve the circulation to the brain or to improve its metabolism, and drugs may be used to calm the patient who, because of confusion, is becoming agitated and difficult to handle at home.

Relatives may need considerable support if the patient is to be helped to remain in the community, and in the earlier stages local authority accommodation for those who have been living alone may be the answer. Nevertheless, about a third of the in-patients in the hospital will be composed of psycho-geriatric problems of this type, and it is usually the social difficulties associated with wandering or bed-wetting, or aggressive behaviour towards the family who are trying to help them, which eventually leads to the admission. Day hospitals for the elderly can delay this process.

Having talked in general terms of conditions where intellectual deterioration is found, let us now consider in more depth some specific disease entities which produce such an end result.

The dementias form a large and very important part of psychiatric hospital work. Dementias fill between 15 and 20 per cent of all hospital beds in the country. Furthermore, it is an increasing problem, since people tend to live longer and survive the physical diseases of old age more successfully with modern methods of treatment. Thus a patient with such a condition, even when admitted to hospital, may occupy the hospital bed, if the condition proves irreversible, for some years.

The amount of nursing care required for the confused, elderly, incontinent patient in terms of bathing and changing is very considerable. Furthermore, the job requires a dedicated nurse, since there will usually not be the satisfaction of seeing the patient steadily improve. The dementia patient is often admitted for social reasons, as has been stated earlier, and the number of beds required for such problems in a particular area will depend on the other facilities, in particular the number of geriatric hospital beds and the Local Authority Part III accommodation available.

There is at present a shortage of such accommodation, leading to waiting lists and forcing the elderly patient living alone or living with hard-pressed relatives to remain in the community when 24-hour nursing care is ideally desirable for them. It seems sad that so much money is put into acute hospital work but so little is given to those senior citizens who have spent a life-time working in and for the community and paying contributions towards the Health Scrvice, only to die sometimes in unattended squalor as a result of the failure of that community to provide for them in their senility.

The term dementia simply describes the end result of a large number of conditions and aetiologies. It is thus a descriptive term for a syndrome characterised by disturbances of memory, orientation, and immediate recall, and loss of social awareness, which go with the intellectual decline.

Many of the causes of dementia, however, are rarities. The vast majority fall into the categories to be described below. Of these, the commonest types are the dementias associated with hardening of the arteries, or **arterio-sclerosis**, and the dementia known as **senile dementia**, in which the brain cells themselves gradually deteriorate and die off.

By definition a senile dementia is one which starts over the age of 65. Below that age such a condition is known as **pre-senile dementia**, which is, of course, rarer. Often there is an inherited factor. Some pre-senile dementias seem virtually identical to the senile dementia, but others have a slightly different type of presentation, and the pathology of the nerve cells under the microscope is seen also to differ. Both conditions now tend to be known as Alzheimer's disease.

Senile Dementia

Senile dementia, even though its occurrence is in the late 60s, does also show a dominant inheritance. Of course, not all members of the family may show such a disease, since many may die of other causes before the condition would have developed. Some 4 per cent of the over-65s suffer from this condition, where there is a primary degeneration of the brain structure. The average age of onset is about 70, and it is steadily progressive. It is found more commonly in females than males, and there is at present no known way of curing the problem. The need for hospital admission will depend on social factors and the rate at which the disease progresses in terms of incontinence, confusion, and social deterioration. It will also depend on who is available to look after the elderly person, and what other community facilities, such as home helps and district nurses in the area, can be utilised.

Although there is no curative treatment, much can be done, particularly in the early stages, to help the elderly person with a dementing illness. The recognition and explanation to relatives that the old person can no longer learn new material and that his or her immediate recall is poor, though memory for past events may be retained, is helpful in the understanding of otherwise irritating behaviour. To maintain patients in familiar surroundings avoids the anxiety that they will have if suddenly finding themselves in an unfamiliar place. Perhaps they cannot find their way to the toilet, and thus become incontinent. Regular taking of the elderly person to the toilet, if hospital admission or new accommodation is essential, can prevent this problem.

Once those possible recoverable causes of dementia have been eliminated by suitable screening tests, than treatment with drugs may be helpful, in some cases in preventing further deterioration or at any rate slowing it down, and in improving mood and behaviour on a symptomatic basis. Thus, anti-depressants can be useful for the elderly person who develops depression as a part of this process, and phenothiazines, such as thioridazine, may be used to control behaviour which is over-aggressive or irritable. Anti-epileptic drugs may be valuable for those patients who, as a result of degeneration of nerve cells, develop occasional fits, a distressing aspect of the disease which may occur from time to time in the later stages. Finally, there are more specific methods of treatment now designed to improve the metabolism of the brain cell, such as cyclospasmol or hydergine, which may in the earlier stages considerably relieve the level of confusion.

A lady of 73 had been noted by her husband and friends, over a two-year period, to have a gradually increasing loss of recent memory. She had become forgetful and tended to mislay things around the house and lose them. Things that people told her she did not recall later and tended to be repetitive, telling the same story frequently to people who had heard it before. She coped, however, in the familiar environment until her husband's sudden death from a heart attack.

There were no children nor close relatives who were able to help and the woman's deterioration became much more pronounced now that her prop was taken away. It was realised that she had not been able to do the shopping nor cooking nor much of the housework and that her husband had dealt with or supervised these matters. It became necessary for her to enter a local authority elderly people's home and here in unfamiliar surroundings she was grossly confused, not being able to find her way to her room or the dining room, and frequently being incontinent as she was unable to find the toilet. Her behaviour also became increasingly disturbed and she required help with dressing. Eventually after some months she required transfer to an elderly people's ward in the local psychiatric hospital. The life expectancy with such an illness would be from 2 to 5 years.

Arteriosclerotic Dementia

In arteriosclerotic dementia, the basic problem is a degeneration in the blood supply to the brain as a result of hardening of the arteries, which causes a secondary degeneration of the arteries. In turn this leads to a secondary degeneration of the nerve cells, but the usual difference between this and other forms of dementia is in the progress of the disease, in that the arteriosclerotic dementia often progresses in a step-wise fashion, with periods of no change or slight improvement interspersed with occasional episodes of acute worsening. This may be due to a slight stroke, or the impaired circulation resulting from a mild heart attack, or something of this sort.

As a result, the failure of brain function is patchy, and the symptoms vary accordingly, depending on the site of the degeneration. The age of onset is about 60, and males suffer more commonly than females. In 50 per cent of cases there is evidence of high blood pressure, and the condition occurs not uncommonly in long-standing diabetes. Parkinson's disease, with its typical tremor, abnormal gait and slowness of movement, may also be present. The course of the disease may fluctuate, according to the availability of oxygen, in the same sense as that described under organic vulnerability. This will relate to such episodes as inter-current chest infection or kidney disease.

A man of 68 had a history of a mild heart attack at 61 from which he had recovered. Two years before he had suffered a stroke with loss of speech and paralysis down the right side which wore off after a few days and left him with only mild impairment. His blood pressure had been high but was controlled by medication. He noticed he was becoming forgetful and could no longer complete the crossword nor play bridge as well as he had done before. He suffered from headaches and on a couple of occasions lost his way in normally familiar surroundings and had to be helped home. He had transient episodes of visual disturbance and then woke one morning with slurred speech and weakness of the right hand. He was admitted to hospital where a more marked disturbance of recent memory and orientation was noted. He could not recall his home address, nor where he was at the time of questioning and for a few days was unable to recognise his sister who came to visit him. The symptoms gradually cleared but left him with a significant degree of memory impairment. He was able to return to his home environment but two months later had a further attack, this time affecting the left side, following which, although there was some recovery of movement, he was unable to walk unaided. Although able to recall events of his childhood and during the time of the Second World War, he could remember virtually no newly learned material and became emotionally labile, frequently weeping or becoming noisy for no very clear reason.

He remained in this state without further deterioration for some 18 months but was frequently incontinent and required continuing hospital care. At this point he had another more severe stroke from which he did not recover and died a few days later.

Pre-senile Dementias

There are four conditions usually described under the pre-senile dementias, whose onset is often in middle age. These go by the names of those who described them at the end of the last century: (a) **Alzheimer's disease**, (b) **Pick's disease**, (c) **Jacob Creutzfeld disease**, and (d) **Huntington's chorea**.

Although there are differences in the inherited factors and slight differences in the symptomatology of these conditions, owing to the type of degeneration that is occurring in the brain and the area in which it takes place, the first two are nevertheless superficially fairly indistinguishable from senile dementia, apart from the differences apparent from the younger age. Jacob Creutzfeld disease shows evidence of degeneration in the spinal chord, and thus abnormalities of movement, in addition to the dementia.

Huntington's chorea is an interesting though, fortunately, rare type of pre-senile dementia, which, because of its dominant inheritance (implying that 50 per cent of the offspring will contact the disease), has occasioned much family-based research. Most psychiatric hospitals have a few cases. The tragedy of the disease is that, since it does not usually come on until the late thirties or early forties, the individual is often married and may well have children. There has so far been no way of identifying carriers of the disease and, therefore, of advising on whether children should be produced. The underlying cause of the degeneration in the basal ganglia is still not known, and no treatment has proved to be effective. The disease is characterised by a progressive dementia, along with a typical type of abnormal movement known as chorea, which is due to degeneration of certain centres in the brain. It was described by George Huntington in 1872 and occurs in 0.04 per 1,000 of the population.

A woman of 34, an attractive housewife with two children, began to notice she was becoming clumsy and occasionally knocking over items of crockery on tables or spilling things. This appeared to be because of involuntary jerky movements which occasionally occurred in her limbs. She began to suffer from episodes of depression with weepiness and irritability. The family noted that she had become less concerned about her personal appearance and the cleanliness of the house and had begun to smoke, all out of character for her. Over a period of some two years there was a gradual extension of both the jerky movements and the deterioration of intellectual function and personality. A suicide attempt in a depressed phase brought her into hospital where the movements were noted and the family history was explored. It was discovered that a grandfather had died in his late forties of some dementing illness in which movements formed a part but his daughter, her mother, had died at 35, there being no way of knowing, therefore, whether she would have developed the condition. One presumed, however, that she would have been a sufferer and the diagnosis of Huntington's Chorea was made. The woman made a reasonable recovery from this depressive episode but over the next 12 months her intellectual deterioration continued and the jerky movements became more pronounced despite available treatment. She became very deteriorated in her habits and required permanent hospital care. Terminally, her muscles associated with swallowing became affected and finally she developed pneumonia, having choked on a drink.

There are a large number of other rare causes of dementia in younger people. Some are inherited diseases, some are metabolic abnormalities, and some follow infection or trauma from head injury. Dementia may follow meningitis or encephalitis, or may be the result of a tumour. Sometimes toxic products from diseases affecting other parts of the body may cause degeneration of nerve cells if the level gets too high, particularly in chronic poisoning with such substances as heavy metals, like lead or copper, or the results of chronic liver failure.

GPI (General Paralysis of the Insane)

One particular type of dementia has been of great historical importance in psychiatry. This is the dementia resulting from untreated long-standing infection with syphilis, one of the venereal diseases. If the causative organism, known as a spirochaete, gets into the central nervous system, a chronic meningo-encephalitis is set up, with gradual deterioration in brain function due to degeneration of the central nervous system.

The old name for this condition was 'General Paralysis of the Insane', known as GPI. Its effective treatment was the first great breakthrough in demonstrating a physical cause for an illness previously thought of as psychological, and led to the improvement and discharge of a considerable number of otherwise chronic asylum patients at the end of the last century. This discovery at a stroke raised psychiatry to a new respectability.

The first description of the disease was by Haslam in 1798. He worked as an apothecary at the Bethlem Hospital in London at a time when dementias were an ill-defined group of diseases, including GPI, the senile and arteriosclerotic dementias, and the later stages of *dementia praecox*, which, of course, was a pseudo-dementia, the result of long-standing schizophrenia.

At the end of the last century GPI accounted for 20 per cent of psychiatric hospital admissions. The causative organism was demonstrated in 1913 by Noguchi and Moore, but it had been noted before this that certain dementias improved dramatically when such fevers as typhoid or malaria swept through the old overcrowded asylums. As a result, methods of treatment were initially based on the idea that perhaps an organism was killed by high temperatures such as exist in an acute fever in the human body, and that inducing such an acute fever might cure the disease. This indeed proved to be the case, and patients were deliberately given malaria in order to induce fever. Later they were injected with tuberculin, which produced the same effect.

With the advent of penicillin and antibiotics, the treatment became very much more straightforward and, indeed, since the majority of venereal diseases are now treated in the early stages, this type of dementia now accounts for very few psychiatric hospital admissions. Nevertheless, the occasional case still does crop up unexpectedly, and for this reason blood tests to screen for this disease are routinely done in hospitals in any case of dementia.

One feature which often distinguishes GPI from other dementias is the grandiose nature of the delusional system which may develop: the patient may feel he is a millionaire or related to royalty. Confabulation may also occur.

A man of 63, who had been living rough, was admitted to the unit. He had been brought in by the police, having been found in a confused state in a derelict house. He expressed grandiose ideas—for example, that he was a millionaire and had won the pools, and that he intended to buy the hospital. His memory, however, was found to be disturbed. He was unable to give correctly the date or information concerning recent current events and was inaccurate about some of his life events which later were able to be checked.

On physical examination, he was noted to have changes in pupil reaction and reflexes consistent with some degeneration in the central nervous system and blood tests confirmed the presence of a long-term syphilitic infection. A second opinion from the venereologist confirmed the diagnosis of GPI. A course of penicillin was able to arrest the course of the disease and effected some improvement in his mental state, the delusional system being controlled with phenothiazines. Unfortunately a mild degree of dementia remained, even after three months, which was probably non-progressive but permanent. He was well enough, however, to be able to be discharged to hostel care.

Epilepsy

We now turn our attention to another significant problem in psychiatric practice, that of epilepsy.

Epilepsy connotes a wide variety of paroxysmal behaviours associated with altered consciousness and with cerebral dysfunction, and this is reflected by paroxysmal electrical discharges in the brain, which may be seen in the electroencephalogram. It is not a disease as such, but a symptom, since its mode of onset, course and prognosis depend particularly upon the conditions which underlie it, such as cerebral degeneration, encephalitis, etc.

The condition of epilepsy is generally the province of the neurologist, but it impinges on psychiatry in a number of respects. First, the incidence of epilepsy is higher in a psychiatric patient population than in the general population, because epileptiform seizures are found not uncommonly as a result of brain damage and brain maldevelopment, such as is seen in many of the patients at subnormality hospitals. Secondly, epileptiform seizures are found in degenerative damage to the brain, such as is found in the dementias, and thus fits are not uncommon in those parts of the psychiatric hospital which cater for the elderly psycho-geriatric group. Thirdly, there has been shown to be a slightly higher incidence of fits in patients presenting with schizophrenic-like conditions than in an equivalent control group. Fourthly, patients with straightforward idiopathic epilepsy, particularly when this has been long-standing and severe, may develop disturbances of thinking, mood or behaviour in which a psychiatric appraisal becomes desirable.

A second way of looking at this problem is to consider a group of individuals who suffer from epilepsy, and find out what kind of psychiatric problems they may themselves develop as a consequence of their epilepsy. Personality changes and neuroses are not uncommon. This is no surprise when one considers the effect which fits may have on the life-style of the sufferer, particularly in childhood. Schooling may be disrupted, and many activities are barred to the individual who suffers from epilepsy in terms of recreation and subsequent careers. Furthermore, people may be somewhat frightened of witnessing an epileptic fit, and the individual who suffers from such fits may, therefore, find it difficult to maintain a social life and retain companions. Often a rather paranoid personality develops, the sufferer feeling that people are against him, and this can on occasions progress to a frankly psychotic condition, not unlike schizophrenia itself.

The second problem is one of brain damage. Frequent and severe epilepsy, which is found difficult to control, may result over the years in a mild dementia simply as a result of the constant falls, blows to the head, and temporary lack of oxygen which have occurred as a result of frequent fits. Thus the individual may become a little like the punch-drunk syndrome of the professional boxer.

Finally, there are three conditions shown in epilepsy which may result directly in admission to a psychiatric unit. One is the **epileptic fugue**, where a loss of memory occurs in association with a fit, and where the patient may exhibit automatic behaviour or 'automatism', and, in fact, perform certain actions while not fully conscious and without recall of what has been done. This is rare, but if such action is aggressive in character, it may result in a court case, with legal arguments over the question of responsibility.

Secondly, one very occasionally finds that an individual who suffers from epilepsy may in the post-fit phase develop what is known as **epileptic furore**, when the individual becomes acutely disturbed and can become extremely violent and perhaps break up property. This sort of acute emergency may result in rapid removal under an order to a psychiatric unit for assessment.

A youth of 19 with a known history of epilepsy was at a friend's flat one evening. The first his friend knew that anything was amiss was when the youth uttered a cry and fell to the floor, his arms and legs thrashing about, and bit his tongue slightly so that blood appeared at his mouth. The friend was anxious and went to seek help, but when he returned he found that the youth, in a state of altered consciousness, had caused considerable damage to the flat throwing a television set straight through the window and causing some £600 worth of damage.

In order to recoup his losses the friend had to have recourse to the courts and the youth was had up on a charge of causing malicious damage. Although the act was unintentional while in a state of disturbance of mind when he did not know the nature of his actions, the youth was advised to plead guilty. Counsel suggested that a plea of not guilty could only be sustained if by reason of insanity, and that this might have caused the court to detain him under a compulsory hospital order for an indeterminate period.

Thirdly, there is that type of epilepsy known as **temporal lobe epilepsy**, where the individual, instead of having a full-blown fit of the grand-mal or major type, may exhibit episodes of altered consciousness, sometimes with hallucinations or feelings of altered awareness and depersonalisation, which are not superficially all that dissimilar from symptoms found in anxiety states. This association between some types of a phobic anxiety state and the curious symptoms found in temporal lobe epilepsy have been the source of some interesting research. The reason for the strange behaviour is that the fit or convulsive seizure in the central nervous system is restricted to parts of the temporal lobe of the brain which control these aspects of behaviour. This may be called a Psycho-motor attack.

A youth of 16 brought to the clinic by his mother had a history of two years' disruptive behaviour at school, inattention, and deterioration in work routine. He seemed to have lapses of concentration and was less able to cope with lessons. It was noticed during the interview that on two or three occasions the youth looked around the room in an exaggerated manner, stretched his arms above his head and yawned very obviously. At first this was put down to ill-mannered behaviour but the stereotyped pattern of it caused the therapist to enquire further and to establish from the mother that this had given offence at school and elsewhere and had become a frequent habit in recent months. Its repetitive character led the therapist to think along the lines of a temporal lobe disturbance, and further investigation with the electro-encephalogram established a temporal lobe dysrhythmia. When this was effectively treated with carbamazepine not only did these attacks cease but his behaviour became more normal and concentration improved so that he was able to function effectively in his schooling.

There are, apart from grand-mal or major epilepsy, other kinds of epileptic convulsion such as **petit-mal** or **minor epilepsy**, which is commonly found in children and may be an unrecognised form of behaviour disturbance in school.

Finally, we consider some of the **medico-legal complications** of epilepsy which may impinge on the psychiatrist. One such relates to laws concerning fitness to drive. An epileptic, for example, cannot obtain a licence to drive a motor vehicle unless he has been free of fits during the day over a period of three years whether on drugs or not. Commercial licences are completely banned to anyone who has suffered major epilepsy after the age of three. Nullity may follow a marriage where epilepsy in one of the partners had been undisclosed. Life insurance usually requires a higher premium. The British Epilepsy Association exists to assist people with regard to employment and the problems associated with epilepsy in sufferers.

The treatment of epilepsy is outside the province of this book, except as it relates to the control of disturbed behaviour in some individuals with personality disturbances in whom an abnormal EEG may seem to play a part. In these cases treatment with drugs useful in the control of temporal lobe epilepsy may be of value, in particular carbamazepine. This is often worth trying in such cases.

Withdrawal Fits

A final factor which may induce fits is sometimes seen on acute wards, and results from the over-rapid withdrawal of sedative medication. If the central nervous system has been under the influence of sedatives or tranquillisers in reasonably large dosage for a while, then the effect of stopping causes a temporary reflex over-activity of the nerve cells, and this can provoke an epileptiform type of fit in some people. This is a hazard with which all admitting doctors and nursing staff should be familiar, but, of course, the history does not always give one the necessary details, and a patient who has been taking sedatives illicitly may not choose to divulge this for his own personal reasons. The hospital does not have the opportunity, therefore, to wean the individual off such drugs, if this is deemed desirable, in a gradual manner. This effect may be produced by sedatives, such as barbiturates and other sleeping tablets, by minor tranquillisers of the benzodiazepine and other groups that have been listed in an earlier chapter, and also by alcohol.

Tumours

Another small but important group of conditions which must be considered in the investigation of intellectual deterioration is that of tumours arising within the skull or the brain substance itself. Depending on the site at which they arise, these may well present with a variety of bizarre clinical syndromes, having hysterical-like features or schizophreniform symptoms along with the intellectual deterioration.

Four per cent of brain tumours come to light in psychiatric hospitals, and 40 per cent of these are unsuspected; 70 per cent of patients with brain tumours show signs of psychological disturbance, though, of course, the incidence of tumours is rare and, therefore, constitutes a small number of the total seen with intellectual deterioration. In addition to the more general signs of intellectual deterioration, there are often signs of **raised intra-cranial pressure**. The symptoms are a lowering of alertness; altered consciousness; severe headaches, which tend to be worse when the patient is lying down and somewhat relieved when he stands up; and eye signs, which can be recognised by the doctor using an ophthalmoscope to look at the back of the eye. Tumours affecting the frontal lobe of the brain may be particularly difficult to spot. Psychological changes occur early, with headache and often a particular type of unsteady gait. Some intellectual deterioration is seen and a loss of sense of propriety, with sometimes a fatuous labile mood.

Head Injury

A further problem which may occupy the psychiatrist results from the after-effects of head injury. The acute episode of unconsciousness, concussion and retrograde amnesia is rare. Some forms of head injury, however, may leave bruising under the skull known as **sub-dural haematoma**. If this is unrecognised and enlarges, then psychological symptoms may appear. Furthermore, a simple dementia can ensue after severe brain damage. This can also occur in professional boxers and in severe epileptics.

Another problem that can occur following head injury is a hysterical condition known as 'compensation neurosis'. This relates usually to a minor head injury, and is characterised by headaches and loss of drive. The secondary gain which develops, usually as a result of the problems of accident compensation through insurance and the legal arguments that may follow, tends to perpetuate the syndrome, which is, in fact, commonly inversely related to the severity of injury. It is usually impractical to treat the condition successfully until the question of compensation has been settled by the courts one way or the another. Unfortunately, the courts are often unwilling to settle until the outlook of the disability becomes clear, and thus the thing can drag on for many months. This is obviously anti-therapeutic. Usually psychotherapy is effective in such individuals, but the medico-legal problems can be considerable. It is often difficult in cases like these to distinguish malingering from a genuine symptom of psychogenic origin, the distinction perhaps being the level of conscious awareness the patient has of the motivation for the perpetuation of such a symptom.

Organic Psychoses

Finally we shall take a brief look at those general medical conditions which primarily affect tissue outside the central nervous system but which can, nevertheless, present on occasion to the psychiatrist because of dominant symptoms either of intellectual deterioration or of a psychotic state mimicking the true psychoses. While such presentations are relatively rare, it is always important for the doctor specialising in psychiatry to have at the back of his mind a thorough knowledge and awareness of the possibilities. These may be classified as follows:

1. Organic psychoses may result from epilepsy, cerebral tumour or cerebral trauma, as have been discussed.

2. Psychoses may arise from infective or invasive inflammatory processes within the brain substance. These would include the conditions of encephalitis, where the central nervous system is invaded by a virus, and meningitis, where the vessels supplying and fluid bathing the brain substance are invaded by bacterial infection. These may be of an acute infectious type, as can follow many common infections, such as measles or influenza, or of the more chronic type, such as tuberculosis and syphilis. The brain substance may also be invaded by helminth or worm infestations, such as cysticercosis.

3. Disorders of a degenerative kind such as Parkinson's disease and Huntington's chorea may affect the basal ganglia. One might also include in this group the pre-senile dementias.

4. Inherited degenerative conditions such as Friedreich's ataxia and some cerebellar degenerative conditions.

5. Motor neurone disease.

6. Multiple sclerosis, disseminated lupus, and other collagen disease.

7. Then there are a large group of metabolic and endocrine disorders where a diagnosis of anxiety state, psychosis or dementia can be mistakenly made if the underlying condition in the early stages is not recognised. These include such things as serious malnutrition, a lowering of the blood sugar, as found in tumours of the pancreatic gland, and a raised blood sugar, as found in diabetes. Vitamin B12 deficiency, as found in pernicious anaemia, can present with psychiatric disturbance, as can illnesses affecting the thyroid gland, either where too much thyroid hormone is being produced, as in thyrotoxicosis or Grave's disease, or where too little is being produced, as in myxoedema.

Addison's disease, a condition affecting the adrenal gland, and Sheehan's syndrome, where the pituitary gland is affected, may also produce disturbances of mood and apparently hypochondriacal or hysterical symptoms.

A raising of the urea levels in the blood, as found in renal failure (disease of the kidney), and an increase in toxic products in the blood stream from liver disease may also produce a picture not unlike early dementia. A number of other metabolic peculiarities, such as porphyria, severe electrolyte disturbances, and some tropical diseases, may also need to be considered.

8. Some chronic infectious diseases may, because of the variability of the symptoms, including malaise, headaches and pains in various places, be misinterpreted as part of an anxiety state. Apart from syphilis and cysticercosis, already mentioned, one must consider brucellosis and endocarditis.

9. Intoxication from drugs may be an important source of malaise or confusion, and this is not always admitted by the patient if he feels he is dependent on some product to which he does not wish to confess. Common ones already mentioned are alcohol and barbiturates; but bromides, which used to be contained in many sedative medicines; and some of the rarer poisons, such as lead, thallium, and carbon monoxide, which can result from a leaky exhaust pipe in a car, constantly giving the regular driver or passenger a small dose of blood poison; need also occasionally to be considered. The common addictive drugs, such as amphetamines, cannabis and LSD, in addition to the more serious hard drugs, such as opiates and cocaine, may also be an undisclosed source of apparently bizarre symptoms.

Encephalitis

The condition of encephalitis results when a virus infection spreads to the central nervous system. In many cases this is mild, and full recovery takes place. In some cases it is severe, and death may ensue. A small proportion of cases, however, continue to have lasting evidence of minor intellectual deterioration or personality change, and some go on to develop Parkinson's disease in later life. The development of schizophrenia-like psychoses in these conditions has frequently been reported, and also a number of adolescent behaviour disorders have appeared to relate to an earlier history of encephalitis in childhood. Of particular interest is the epidemic of **encephalitis lethargica** which occurred in England at the end of the First World War. Many subsequent problems arose from this particular epidemic, and most psychiatric hospitals still have a sprinkling of long-stay patients dating from the after-effects of illness incurred at that time.

Thyroid Disease

Diseases of the thyroid gland are particularly important in psychiatry, since a mildly over-active thyroid may easily mimic an anxiety state or depressive reaction. It is important, therefore, to eliminate by appropriate examination and blood tests this possibility in those cases that do not seem to respond satisfactorily to conventional anxiolytic treatment. Secondary anxiety can, of course, arise from an underlying condition of this kind. When the thyroid gland is under-active in the condition known as **myxoedema**, the patient becomes slow and lethargic. This may present as an early dementia because of the intellectual deterioration or may be confused with a retarded depression in the elderly, in old books known as **myxoedema madness**. It is most important that these underlying problems are identified, as they are easily treatable.

Hypoglycaemia

Another condition of interest is that of **hypoglycaemia** or lowered blood sugar, which occurs in some diabetics and in those with insulin-producing tumours of the pancreatic gland. The symptoms of hunger, restlessness and weakness may progress to aggressive behaviour and automatism, with altered awareness and, in effect, a delirious state. Usually the diagnosis can be recognised by the fact that the symptoms come on after a period of going without food, and the blood sugar level is, of course, low at this time if it is taken. Administering glucose can banish the symptoms, and this often gives a clue to diagnosis. Otherwise, the condition may be confused with epilepsy, or simply with a behaviour disturbance possessing hysterical features.

Myalgic Encephalomyelopathy

This entity also known as post-viral syndrome has been known for very many years. It may often mimic depression or hypochondriacal illness and can be confused with it. Indeed patients with ME often complain of morbid mood, but the key symptom is that of muscle weakness and excessive tiredness after even minimal energy activity. It is believed to be the result of the continued activity of certain types of virus which remain active in the body and particularly affect muscle metabolism. There is a proven association with a tendency to get this condition and a past history of depressive illness and treatment is largely symptomatic, avoiding excessive exercise and getting plenty of rest. Trials using anti-viral agents, and gammaglobulin injections have been mounted.

Pernicious Anaemia

This usually presents with disturbances in the blood which are recognised as anaemic. Sometimes the spinal columns are affected, and weakness and alteration in sensation in the limbs may occur. Occasionally, however, the initial presentation is due to the deficiency of B12 vitamin in the central nervous system, and then neurotic symptoms, depression, and mild evidence of intellectual deterioration may occur. This has gone under the name of **megaloblastic madness** in the older textbooks, the word 'megaloblast' referring to the type of blood cells seen under the microscope in pernicious anaemia.

Bromide Intoxication

This also has an interesting historical connection with psychiatry, since the drug was used extensively as a sedative some years ago. The drug is excreted slowly, so that a toxic level can easily be built up over a period of weeks, and symptoms of bromism begin to develop. These show as irritability and a loss of concentration and grasp, leading to restlessness and confusion. The skin becomes dry and there is a tremor, and sometimes delusions and hallucinations supervene. Attempts in the old days to treat this mistakenly with further sedation, using bromide, completed a vicious circle and a perpetuation of the syndrome. Bromide is still contained in a few medicines, but has been replaced by more modern preparations in the vast majority of cases.

Lead and Mercury Poisoning

Finally, let us look briefly at heavy metal poisoning. **Lead poisoning** may occur in an acute form in children from the ingestion of lead from paint sprays or lead toys, but is of more consequence to the psychiatrist in its chronic form, which may result from the repeated ingestion of small amounts of the heavy metal through perhaps lead piping or, as in a famous case, from cider that had been kept in lead-contaminated casks. In chronic lead poisoning patients show a loss of appetite, abdominal cramps, headache and constipation, and this may be not unlike a depression or early dementia. There is often apathy, but a delirious state may supervene. The cause of such vague symptoms can easily be missed if the problem is not thought out, but it can be diagnosed by appropriate blood tests when it is recognised.

Other heavy metals can also produce symptoms of this kind. A famous one is that of mercury, which is probably the explanation for the Mad Hatter, since in the old days hatters used mercury in their trade, and sufferers developed Hatter's shakes or **Hatter's madness**. Lewis Carroll's Mad Hatter's tea-party no doubt was a case of chronic mercury poisoning!

Manganese poisoning can mimic the condition of Huntington's chorea, because of its action on the basal ganglia in the brain; and thallium poisoning and arsenic poisoning may also need to be considered, since, once in a while, chronic poisoning which is not always accidental may occur. Because of the psychiatric symptomatology, such instances may appear on the psychiatric ward, and the underlying reasons can be overlooked.

Investigation and Treatment

This brief survey of the ways in which general medical and surgical conditions may present to the psychiatrist must inevitably be incomplete. Otherwise, this book would turn into a mini-textbook of medicine, in addition to its current purpose. Nevertheless, the interrelationship between medical and psychiatric disease is so close that admixtures of the two may finish up in a variety of departments in a hospital, depending on the presenting symptoms. To this end any person who enters a psychiatric unit and in whom there may be symptoms suggestive of underlying general organic disease should, where there is any doubt, be subjected to certain standard screening tests, which will in most cases eliminate at least most of the commoner general medical conditions fairly simply.

One can consider these screening tests in three groups, the first attempting to eliminate common conditions, the second slightly less commonly seen problems, and the third specific but rarer abnormalities.

First line screening normally includes a standard urine test for sugar, protein, and blood, which will eliminate diabetes and diseases affecting the kidney and renal tract. A full blood count is carried out to estimate haemoglobin levels, the white cell count, and the sedimentation rate. A normal red cell count will eliminate various anaemias. A normal white cell count will eliminate generalised infections of the body which would cause an increase in the various types of white cell. A normal sedimentation rate will eliminate generalised infection and also inflammatory conditions, such as might be caused by the rheumatic diseases or collagen diseases. A WR (Wasserman reaction), if normal, will eliminate the possibility of syphilis. Finally, a standard chest X-ray may be appropriate to eliminate respiratory diseases, including tuberculosis, carcinoma of the lung and other lung and heart diseases.

These few simple tests can do much to clarify the picture, particularly where the question of an early dementia may be raised. Should some test be abnormal in this group, or should there be further cause for doubt, then second line testing will be initiated.

Second line testing may include blood tests designed to estimate liver function, thyroid function (which may suggest myxoedema, or thyrotoxicosis), blood electrolyte levels, blood sugar, vitamin B12 levels (to exclude pernicious anaemia) and possibly further tests of kidney function. X-rays of the skull, together with electroencephalogram or brain scan, may be required to eliminate disturbances within the central nervous system, such as tumour, pituitary disease, or epilepsy.

The third line testing would depend upon the leads that had been obtained in these first two batches. For example, a lumbar puncture might be indicated, or more elaborate blood and urine tests for particular rare diseases.

Treatment of the conditions listed in this chapter under the heading of generalised disease will be two-fold. First, and most important, the underlying general disease must be treated if the psychiatric developments secondary to it are to be controlled. Thus, it may well be appropriate for transfer to be made to another department within the hospital group.

At the same time, however, symptomatic treatment of the particular psychiatric symptoms associated with a delirious state or a toxic psychosis must also be considered, in order to alleviate the patient's suffering quickly. This will usually amount to some temporary tranquillising drug of phenothiazine or benzodiazepine type, or the use of chlormethiazole to control agitation and confusion. Appropriate night sedation must be given to help sleep without increasing the confusion. Barbiturates, and in the elderly benzodiazepines, are often not suitable for use, tending to increase night-time confusion and produce daytime drowsiness. Chloromethiazole or a small dose of one of the sedative phenothiazines, such as thioridazine or promazine, are usually better.

Further Reading

Herrington, R. N., *Current Problems in Neuro-Psychiatry*, BJP Special Publication No. 4, Headley, Ashford, Kent, 1969.
Post, F., *The Clinical Psychiatry of Late Life*, Pergamon, Oxford, 1965.

Questions

1. Distinguish delirium from dementia.
2. What are the typical features of senile dementia? How does it differ from an arteriosclerotic dementia?
3. What is epilepsy? What psychiatric problems can be associated with it?

18
Psycho-Sexual Disorders: Partnership Dysharmonies

Summary

Classification

1. Arousal or erective failure.
2. Orgasmic failure.
3. Ejaculatory disturbances.
4. Vaginismus.

Aetiology

1. Anxiety about performance fears leads to vicious circle of inhibition of parasympathetic autonomic response and over-stimulation of sympathetic autonomic system.
2. Lack of interest in partner.
3. Poor technique by partner.
4. Physical or organic causes include neurological disease, peripheral neuropathy, and hormonal disturbances.
5. Psychiatric disturbance—depression.
6. Secondary to medication given for other purposes.

Treatment

1. Sensate focus programmes in three stages—non-genital pleasuring, genital pleasuring, and intercourse.
2. Counselling and psychotherapy.
3. Drugs, such as hormones, aphrodisiacs, and anxiolytics.
4. Sexual aids.

Description

Problems of sexual dysfunction are commonly found in psychiatric referrals, and indeed a survey in York in 1972 showed that some 20 per cent of patients referred to ordinary psychiatric out-patient clinics had a psycho-sexual problem, either as the presenting complaint or comprising a major part of the need for referral.

Psycho-sexual problems are, in fact, extremely common and a number of helping agencies may take part in dealing with them, including the family doctor, marriage guidance clinics, family planning clinics, gynaecologists, social services, and so on. A vast number are also dealt with on a postal basis through advice columns in magazines, and an even larger number will fail to seek help at all, owing to embarrassment or a feeling that the problem is not one that can be usefully presented to a helping agency. Fortunately, the pattern is changing, and a number of areas have introduced clinics specifically to help people with psycho-sexual problems, both within and outside the Health Serivce. Many of the Health Service clinics combine the services of psychiatrists, clinical psychologists and social workers, and are occupied in joint therapy along the lines outlined by Masters and Johnson in the United States. It is useful to have a clinic specifically for these problems, since they are time-consuming and, to some extent, separate from the general mass of psychiatric problems, even though there is often a large psychiatric component. A clinic for such problems is likely to obtain cases that would not have been referred to an ordinary psychiatric out-patients' department and thus reaches a slightly different population source.

Psycho-sexual disorders fall into two main groups. There are those dysfunctions which are primarily **partnership problems**, such as impotence and frigidity, and there are those which are often considered under the umbrella heading of 'deviancy', where the sexual problem is that of an individual distortion of sexual response, and which we shall call **sexual behavioural anomalies**.

Some authors have attempted to classify psycho-sexual disorders on the basis of the degree of capability of the patient of engaging in a mature sexual relationship. At one end of the scale will be those people in whom any kind of relationship with another human being of a sexual nature is impossible. Resort is made to sexual fantasies, where the need for communication is minimal. Such people would, for example, include those who indulge solely in masturbation as a form of relief.

Another group consists of people where a limited participation with another is possible but the degree of contact is minimal. Here we see such conditions as exhibitionism, voyeurism and frotteurism.

A third group comprises those people where a relationship of a relatively impersonal kind is tolerated but where special conditions are attached to the type of behaviour which gives arousal. This would include prostitution, and deviant practices, such as sado-masochistic pursuits, bondage and such things as rape fantasies.

In a fourth and separate category comes homosexuality, in which the relationship is a full one but not heterosexual in nature. This group includes those to whom a normal heterosexual relationship is possible but where deviant behaviour tends to occur within this situation, such as might be found in types of fetishism. Finally, there would be a group where normal heterosexual relationships existed but where the capability of one or other partner, in terms of the ability to achieve normal satisfying orgasm for both, was lacking. In the present chapter, we shall be looking at this final group. The sexual behavioural anomalies are dealt with in Chapter 19.

Male and Female Problems

Partnership problems can be subdivided in terms of the particular type of dysfunction found.

The first group are those in whom there has been a loss of libido or sexual interest associated purely with a failure of interest in the partner— that is to say, the prime problem is not a sexual or indeed psychiatric one at all but is a 'falling out of love' of the two people concerned. Any sexual dysharmony, therefore, would be purely secondary to the prime problem.

Apart from this, three types of problem are found in males: there may be a failure of erection, a failure to achieve climax, or a premature ejaculation. Three similar problems can occur in women: a failure to achieve sexual arousal, a failure to reach climax or a condition known as **vaginismus**, where there is a failure to tolerate penetration.

Sexual arousal in either sex develops as a result of a variety of stimuli. It may result from erotic thoughts or visual images from, for example, a sexy film or reading a sexy book. It may result from provocative sexual behaviour on the part of one's partner or from stimulation during foreplay. There is probably some culturally determined sex difference here, in that men tend to be aroused by a visual stimulus, and in terms of partnership relationships this is likely to be the coquettishness of the female, her manner of dress or her invitation towards a sexual approach. The woman tends more to be aroused by the actions of her partner in response to this behaviour. In other words, she is aroused by the awareness of arousal in her partner, and her partner's activity in caressing her or kissing her as a result of this. This is, of course, not a hard and fast rule but is generally the pattern.

An individual may fail to reach a satisfactory orgasm, even though sexual arousal has been adequate. There may be a variety of reasons, but the usual ones are failure of adequate stimulation by the partner or some psychological hang-up which prevents the full development of feeling in intercourse. There may be fears concerning pregnancy and so on, but more commonly it is simply a failure on the part of the partner to appreciate the other's needs and how to satisfy them. This is usually due to a failure of communication, often initially through shyness, but the relationship may deteriorate and result in barriers being put up between the two.

Failure to reach orgasm, however, may quite possibly be due to a failure to develop arousal in the first place.

Mechanism of Arousal

In the male, sexual arousal is manifested by erection of the penis, which depends on stimulation of the appropriate tissue mediated by the *autonomic nervous system*, and in particular a group of nerves known as **para-sympathetic nerves**. It is these nerves that also control the quieter functions of the body, such as digestion and the secretion of various internal organs to do with internal body functions. If stimulation reaches a sufficiently strong level, another mechanism which produces the orgasm, and in the male the ejaculation of semen, comes into play. This is controlled by another set of nerves within the autonomic nervous system known as the **sympathetic nerve**

supply, which in other parts of the body also controls reactions to external stress, such as fear, resulting in an increase in pulse rate, blood flow and blood pressure, increased blood supply to the muscles, widening of the pupil and various other factors seen in defensive situations.

These two aspects of the autonomic nervous system are both under the control of that part of the brain which deals with emotional state, the limbic lobe. In general, they operate antagonistically to each other. Thus 'chewing the cud' mechanisms and 'preparation to defend oneself' would interfere with each other. When operating, one tends to suppress the other.

Translated into sexual problems, it would be inappropriate to maintain an erection when running away from a bull in a field. Similarly, it would be inappropriate to be in a state of defensive readiness when in the arms of one's lover—as a rule!

The snag occurs where anxiety develops. Anxiety is a type of fear response mediated through the sympathetic system and can occur easily through fear of failure after an episode of impotence. Orgasmic failure in the female can similarly quickly induce anxiety. This suppresses the para-sympathetic system and reduces arousal or erectability even more, and in the male may trigger premature ejaculation before full arousal has been effected. A vicious circle is quickly set up, where more anxiety stimulates higher sympathetic stimulation and more para-sympathetic suppression, arousal fails increasingly, and anxiety gets higher and still more failure results.

In the female, sexual arousal is shown by the development of an erection in the clitoris, which developmentally is the female equivalent of the penis, though smaller and not carrying a passage way from the bladder within it. In addition, there is the development within the vagina of a flow of lubricating fluid which allows of easier penetration, and there is some erection of the tissues of the inner labia and the vaginal walls, which become more spongey and sensitive.

Failure of arousal may be due to a wide variety of conditions. The commonest is that the female in question has ceased to be erotically interested in her male partner. She may have lost respect for her man or is no longer 'turned on' by his advances. A second and very common cause is poor technique on the part of the male partner, who may falsely believe that the female is stimulated principally by vaginal excitation, and, owing to inexperience or thoughtlessness in his foreplay, fails to arouse the woman sufficiently before penetration occurs. Many women are, in fact, much more aroused by clitoral stimulation than by vaginal, and the position adopted during intercourse may, in these cases, fail to provide the necessary stimulation or give the clitoris adequate time for orgasm to occur. If the man climaxes prematurely and ceases at that stage to stimulate the female, even though her climax has not been reached, then failure may occur. Initially, this will result in orgasmic failure only, but after a while, with continuing dissatisfaction, failure of arousal may also occur—another vicious circle! The lack of arousal will produce a lessening of sensation, since the vaginal walls will be dry, and the clitoris, as it is not enlarged, will not receive the same stimulation as it would in the erect state. If this situation continues, a total failure of libido can result, and the woman may indeed develop an aversion to being touched at all by her partner, since this implies a likelihood of the situation developing to intercourse, with the frustrations that this engenders.

Other reasons for failure of orgasm in the female may be a loss of sensitivity following childbirth, or a failure of oestrogen secretion at the menopause. Oestrogen lack can cause dryness of the vagina, and atrophy of the tissues, which makes the whole business sore. Sometimes after childbirth a tear may have occurred in some of the ligaments inside the pelvis. Again the pain which this produces on intercourse, known as dyspareunia, may be sufficient to decrease arousal and prevent full enjoyment. An imbalance of certain sex hormones, such as proclatin, may also be identified.

A number of physical conditions may produce a loss of libido and failure to reach climax in both sexes. Commonly found are high blood pressure, diabetes and illnesses which affect the central nervous system, such as multiple sclerosis. In addition, psychiatric illness and, in particular, endogenous depression can often present with a failure of the libido.

Drugs may be an important cause of loss of sexual function, in particular the anti-depressants. Indeed, the delay in achieving ejaculation which may occur during treatment with anti-depressants has been put to good use by giving this medication in attempts to treat premature ejaculation. Other drugs in common use which can produce failure of arousal are some of the phenothiazines, in particular those with a piperidine side-chain, such as thioridazine, and hypotensive drugs used in the treatment of high blood pressure, such as methyl dopa. The contraceptive pill may also induce a failure of libido.

Erective or Arousal Failure

The terms 'impotence' and 'frigidity' are best discarded as insufficiently specific, and tending to have different meanings for different people. Furthermore, they have come to be used as terms of abuse. The frigid lady is the one who will not go to bed with the man who wants her to! In any case, mechanisms of arousal are more similar between the sexes than they are different.

Erective or arousal failure may be primary or secondary, total or partial, i.e. the dysfunction may exist from the very start of the individual's sexual activity or may come on after a period of some years of normal functioning. Equally, the condition may exist at some times and not at others, or, indeed, with one partner but not with other partners. The same situation applies to either sex, and has, of course, implications as to cause.

The common reasons for failure of arousal in either sex are lack of interest in the partner or anxieties about competence in the sex act. We have looked at this in general terms in our discussion on cause. Performance anxiety often becomes a secondary feature quite rapidly, even though some other factor caused the original problem. Primary total arousal failure in males is extremely rare and usually implies either some organic physical problem with regard to the development of the genitalia or the nervous system that supplies it, or deep-seated psychological worries. Physical examination is always essential. Sometimes a disturbance in sexual orientation may be found, the individual being latently homosexual.

A young man in the army in Singapore went out one evening with a group of his friends who all picked up women in the local bar. This was not really the young man's scene but not wishing to look foolish in front of his friends he eventually found himself in an experienced lady's bedroom. He felt embarrassed and was a little anxious that he might catch something nasty and developed an erective failure when he attempted intercourse. The lady, disappointed, did not mince her words about his potency and competence. He avoided such situations during the rest of his stay but towards the end of his tour of duty fell in love, became engaged and eventually married a local girl. In the absence of anywhere to go on honeymoon the corporal of his platoon invited the couple to use a spare room in their house for a week's holiday. The couple did not attempt intercourse until the first night of the honeymoon. A combination of his previous unfortunate experience, the presence of his immediate senior and his wife on the other side of a partition wall, and the wine at the reception combined to cause him to fail again when his bride's hymen proved to be intact.

In the two or three failures which followed his anxiety increased with fantasies that he might be homosexual or permanently disabled. He became depressed and his new wife was unable to understand the cause of his problem. Erection was normal until penetration was attempted. He eventually sought medical advice and a local army psychiatrist was able to counsel the couple and sort the problem out using a sensate focus procedure.

In the female, arousal is not always so easily recognised by the individual who is inexperienced, and sometimes poor technique on the part of a partner during the early sexual encounters explains the build-up of a resistance, in the absence of enjoyment. If arousal is present and normal on at least some occasions, or, in other words, the condition is partial, then this more commonly implies a psychological problem.

Failure of arousal coming on after some years of normal functioning may again imply disturbance in the relationship or may imply the development in middle age of some disturbance of an organic nature. The latter may be a disturbance of hormonal type, the development of some physical disease which affects the autonomic nerve supply itself, the onset of some such psychiatric disturbance as depression, or the side-effects of some of the commonly used drugs which are needed for the treatment of other medical conditions.

In the last case, the drugs used to treat blood pressure, psychotropic drugs which affect mono-amine functions, such as phenothiazines or antidepressants, and hormones, including the contraceptive pill, are the commonest offenders. Patients needing to go on any of these drugs should be warned of the occasional complications in terms of sexual function that can crop up.

Orgasmic Dysfunction

Again problems here may be primary or secondary, total or partial. In the male, orgasm is usually coincident with ejaculation, and tends to be looked upon as the same thing, although technically the two processes are determined by different nerve supplies. The timing, however, of the ejaculatory mechanism is fairly complicated, and occasionally may be disorganised separately from orgasm. Thus it is possible in the male for non-ejaculatory orgasm to occur, and equally possible for ejaculation to take place without the experience of climax, though these situations are rare. The mechanism of orgasm in the female is basically the same as in the male, though there is no ejaculatory process, of course, and the muscular contractions within the vagina probably function at a physiological level to encourage the passage of sperm into the uterus or womb.

By primary total orgasmic failure we mean that an individual has never experienced orgasm by any means, i.e. not by heterosexual intercourse, nor petting, nor a homosexual act, nor self-induced through masturbation or a sexual dream. Since the majority of individuals experiment with masturbation at least at some time during their lives, usually in adolescence, it is unusual, particularly in the male, where the genital organs are exposed and available, for an individual never to have experienced orgasm by any means. Again the implication is of a low libido, possibly from physical causes. Occasionally, however, indviduals brought up in a sexually repressive or inhibited atmosphere, with strong moral strictures against such behaviour, may have developed an incapacity to respond for psychological reasons.

Primary orgasmic failure is somewhat more common in the female and again may result from inhibition of sexual expression or from inadequate love play by a partner. Total orgasmic failure secondary to inadequate arousal is, however, a common problem in the inexperienced younger person, particularly with females, and usually responds to counselling.

In the older male a gradual decrease in the capability of orgasm of the same frequency as that found in the younger man is commonplace. Similarly, the strength of erection diminishes. These are not problems within a good relationship as long as both partners recognise the cause and do not attempt to push matters beyond what is practical for the individual. It is when performance anxieties develop that problems can occur.

The same argument applics to partial secondary orgasmic failure as to arousal failure. Thus the problem may be of diminution of libido for psychological reasons or loss of interest in the partner, or may be a result of physical or organic disease of gradual onset.

Some drugs, particularly anti-depressants, may interfere with the ejaculatory process of males and, of course, following a prostrate operation, ejaculation may be retrograde into the bladder, and thus orgasm apparently takes place without the production of an ejaculate. Some serious abdominal operations, such as ileostomy, may damage the nerves to the sexual organs, and produce disturbances of sexual function which can be permanent. In this case sometimes supportive aids or prosthetics may be helpful to the couple, allowing them to continue a reasonably normal sex life.

A woman of 30 with previously normal sexual appetites found that following a period of depression and treatment with imipramine that she became non-orgasmic even though she was able to maintain a normal level of arousal. It seemed probable that this was drug-induced since the depression would more likely have caused a generalised loss of sexual interest. A change to a non-tricyclic anti-depressant fortunately restored sexual functioning to normal since it was too soon for her to be able to discontinue anti-depressants entirely.

Ejaculatory Disorders

These are of course confined to the male. Retarded ejaculation or failure of ejaculation is rare. Sometimes ejaculation is possible outside the vagina with masturbation but not during intercouse itself, and this implies a psychological problem. The total failure of the ejaculatory process occasionally results from maldevelopment of the genitalia. Secondary ejaculatory failure can occur following operations which affect the genito-urinary tract.

Premature ejaculation is, however, extremely common and is usually part and parcel of the anxiety-induced erective failure—the two branches of the autonomic nervous system, sympathetic and parasympathetic being put out of balance by the development of the fear response, as explained earlier. A vicious circle rapidly develops: performance anxiety causes partial erective failure, with premature ejaculation due to activation of the sympathetic part of the autonomic nervous system, and this failure of performance induces more anxiety, which in turn increases the problem. The anxious male, therefore, can rapidly get into a situation where a very premature ejaculation, even before penetration can be attempted and without even the normal orgasmic response, may occur if heterosexual intercourse is attempted. Often response is normal if intercourse is not attempted—for example, during masturbation.

Treatment through graded desensitising exercises utilising the partner as therapist, and as described under Masters and Johnson's sensate focus techniques later in the chapter, are normally very successful. Control is gradually attained by increasing levels of genital pleasuring, initially manually and later by means of what Masters and Johnson describe as the squeeze technique, moving on to intercourse, with the female superior position being used. This allows the female partner, who is acting as therapist, to have control over the speed at which things are moving along, and the male is relieved of the responsibility of having to decide when penetration occurs, this often being the time when anxiety induces ejaculatory response.

Vaginismus

This condition, confined to women, describes the situation where the female is unable to tolerate penetration. Sexual arousal is normal and orgasm can be obtained through petting if the partnership is a satisfactory one. When the male attempts to penetrate, however, the muscles which cross the floor of the pelvis, known as the pubococcygeus muscles, go into spasm, producing a tight block around the vagina about an inch from the opening. This has nothing to do with rupture of the hymen, which is usually found to be absent by the time a patient comes to the clinic complaining of penetration failure.

The usual reason for the muscles going into spasm is the fear, on the part of the female, of being hurt, though sometimes more deep-seated psychological fears about penetration are uncovered. The spasm of muscles is outside the patient's conscious control, and attempts by the male partner forcibly to overcome it lead, in fact, to further pain on pressure on these muscles, which in turn increases the female's anxiety and increases the muscle spasm. Thus another vicious circle is set up.

Fortunately, again, this condition is easily treated in the right hands. The method of treatment is to teach the patient to relax the muscles in question by consciously learning how to control them with the aid of vaginal dilators of graded sizes, which develop confidence in this control. Once the patient has confidence in the ability to insert the largest of dilators, she may then attempt intercourse in the female superior position, which allows her again to control the speed of entry.

A woman of 24 had been married two years. The marriage had never been consummated although the couple had a good relationship and enjoyed stimulating each other in foreplay and to orgasm. There was no problem unless penetration was attempted when the wife became anxious, arched her back and tightened up all her muscles. A physical examination by a gynaecologist had shown that the hymen was no-longer intact and there was no physical abnormality that might cause problems. The woman, however, felt very inadequate and the couple were anxious to start a family which had provoked their further request for help. An explanation of the condition was given to the couple in behavioural terms with the use of diagrams and reassurance. During the latter part of the treatment session the woman was examined and the smallest of a set of six vaginal trainers was inserted. She was then encouraged to handle this herself and to remove and reintroduce the training aid, a small, glass, blunt-ended tube about the diameter of a thumb, until confident with it. She returned home to practise and become confident with this and over the course of the next three sessions her confidence was gradually extended with increasing sizes until the number 6 was achieved. She was then encouraged to return home and treat her husband as a number 6 dilator that happened to have a man on the end using plenty of lubrication and the female superior position. The husband had, in the meantime, been primed as to what was to happen and all he had to do was to lie still and try to maintain an erection without ejaculating. The couple succeeded at the second attempt and the problem was resolved.

Management of Partnership Dysfunctions

Psycho-sexual problems of impotence, frigidity and premature ejaculation are extremely common, and have been tolerated by society, particularly dysfunction in the female, largely because of the taboos which have been placed for many years on free discussion of sexual topics and the lack of realisation of what possibilities there were in terms of therapy. One has only to look at mediaeval literature such as *The Perfumed Garden* or *The Kama Sutra* to realise that such problems have been with the human race since recorded history, and, like baldness, the variety of treatments suggested have reflected the comparative futility of most of them.

In the present social climate, however, such problems are now brought out much more into the open, and as a result the extent of unhappiness within the partnership situation has come to be realised. Many agencies and magazines now offer advice in dealing with such problems, and sufferers may visit marriage guidance counsellors, family planning associations, the home doctor, and a wide variety of other people, to seek help.

Furthermore, a number of clinics are being set up—indeed, some have now been functioning under the Health Service for several years—to give treatment under properly supervised conditions. It is the author's view that such problems should be treated by people with proper medical training rather than by lay helpers who happen to have an interest in the subject. The reason for this is that though many of the problems turn out to be perfectly simple ones which educative counselling can deal with, a proportion of the problems which present are, in fact, caused by some underlying physical organic condition, and, without the recognition and proper treatment, superficial, unhelpful and even dangerous advice can be given.

For example, a common cause of impotence or frigidity in middle age is an underlying depressive illness. Some physical diseases, such as diabetes or high blood pressure, can also cause a fall-off of libido and potency. To attempt to treat such a condition without checking that these underlying possibilities have been eliminated is to be negligent; and without a brief physical examination and one or two simple tests there is no way of being sure that the problem is entirely and exclusively an emotional one.

A survey of cases referred through the clinic for psycho-sexual disorders in York during 1972–73 showed that in about 30 per cent of cases some illness or physical disability had a significant bearing on the problem. Furthermore, the treatment often necessitates procedures which non-qualified people are either unable to use, such as the prescription of medication, or physical examination of the patient, which they would be unwise to embark upon, in terms of the medico-legal implications, without the appropriate cover against charges of assault and so on which a Medical Defence Society would give to a medical practitioner.

Many of the cases referred, nevertheless, do turn out to have a very simple aetiology, and treatment is equally uncomplicated. Deeper psychological problems are not all that commonly found in the type of patients seen, and serious physical illness as a cause is comparatively rare. The analytical type of psychotherapy has not in the past proved particularly successful in the treatment of psycho-sexual disorders in any case, and treatment with hormones or aphrodisiacs of various kinds has in most cases been equally unhelpful.

Treatment Programmes

The work of Masters and Johnson in the United States in the last 15 years has revolutionised the treatment of many partnership problems. Until their clinic established the basic norms of behaviour and patterns of response in sexual arousal, the whole subject had been shrouded in old wives' tales and misconceptions. Their pioneering work into the physiology of sexual response led the way to a formulation of a therapy programme which was suitable for couples, and to the eventual production of a classic textbook on the treatment of psycho-sexual difficulties. It is probably fair to say that most clinics now model their treatment programmes to a large extent on the principles Masters and Johnson laid down, and this has resulted in a great improvement in the effectiveness of such treatment for sufferers.

Masters and Johnson base their approach on treating the couple. They emphasise that these problems are partnership problems, and to treat half a couple is a foolish way of attempting to sort out a problem which exists between two people. The emphasis, therefore, is on round-table discussions with the couple and a male and female therapist. In this way neither partner considers that the therapist is biased towards the other through being of the same or opposite sex.

The exact nature of the problem is carefully delineated, to establish whether the erective or arousal failure is primary or secondary—that is to say, whether it has existed from the word go or whether it is something that has started relatively recently—and also whether the problem is total or partial— in other words, the problem may exist at some times and not at others, or indeed may exist with one partner and not with another partner. This last point, of course, might have to be elucidated in separate discussions with the partners, which is done usually at the initial assessment interview also. It is emphasised that the partner who presents with the complaint is not always the one necessarily with the major problem, and that a problem identifiable between a couple might well not exist in other circumstances, or might differ with differing partners.

At the initial round-table discussion the principles of therapy are outlined after the diagnosis has been established, and a simple educational talk, or sex lesson, as it were, is given. The emphasis is on obtaining communication again between the people. Sometimes this may never have been possible between them, and often it has deteriorated as a result of stresses produced by the problem. It is remarkable how often one finds in the clinic that couples have little idea about each other's needs, likes and dislikes. All these things must be brought out in the opening discussions of the therapeutic process.

The next phase in therapy is an attempt to engage the couple in simple pleasuring when they return home, which Masters and Johnson describe as a **sensate focus** technique. This really means a ban on intercourse for the time being and a return to the non-demand cuddling sort of relationship that the couple probably had in the early stages of their courting. The difficulties in treating impotence and frigidity are the secondary anxiety which will exist concerning performance, and the need to accomplish and achieve orgasm on a particular occasion. The individuals become observers of themselves and are unable to relax, and, as has been explained, the anxiety engendered perpetuates the initial problem and sets up a vicious circle.

The aim of therapy, therefore, is to introduce a non-demand situation where performance is not expected but where the couple can simply lie and enjoy the experience of caressing each other, initially ignoring the genital areas. Once the necessary relaxation has been achieved over a number of homework sessions, the couple move on to the second stage of genital pleasuring, again in a non-demand manner, with one partner acting the part of therapist and the other playing the recipient. The couple can change these roles, but basically it is the one with the problem—be it impotence, frigidity or whatever—who acts the part of the patient, and the other takes the dominant role during the therapy programme. In the meantime, discussions continue to be held with the therapists at the clinic, where any problems that crop up can be ironed out and further counselling can be maintained.

The final stage of this part of the therapy comes when normal arousal has been maintained and communication between the couple has become good. At this stage intercourse can be attempted, using the same principles of non-demand pleasuring as in the initial stages. Also at this stage certain special techniques may be applied—for example, to correct problems of premature ejaculation. The attainment of orgasm for those with orgasmic delay can be initiated, if necessary, through manual stimulation by the couple or by the use of techniques, such as vibrators, to heighten arousal.

In addition to this behavioural therapy other factors may need to be taken into account in the therapeutic process. Besides psychotherapy for the more complex type of problem, we must consider the use of drugs and sexual aids.

Medication

Medication may be needed to treat the underlying condition. In this respect we must consider the anti-depressant drugs for use when there is an underlying depressive illness, anxiolytics where there is marked secondary anxiety and some symptom relief seems indicated, and hormone therapy.

For psycho-sexual disorders, hormone therapy has been tried rather unsuccessfully for some years. This was because, until recently, it was not possible to test hormone levels easily in the body, and treatment was, therefore, guesswork. However, it is now possible to identify cases where a hormone deficiency is present, and treatment in such cases can be initiated.

There are various reasons why the normal hormone level in the body may be deficient. In the menopausal and post-menopausal woman a relative deficiency of oestrogen, which can occur, can produce a loss of libido, and tends to result, in due course, in the atrophic vaginitis. This makes intercourse painful and produces dyspareunia, but can be treated fairly simply as long as the condition is recognised. Replacement hormone therapy, over a period of some years, is of great value in such people. A number of suitable oestrogen preparations are available, and often this treatment is all that is required for middle-aged or late-onset frigidity. It is now possible to estimate the oestrogen levels in the body, and this makes planning of treatment much easier than before, as well as adjustment of the dosage.

With male hormone replacement the problem is a little more difficult. Low testosterone levels are not commonly found, even after the so-called male menopause, and impotence is not usually the result of a lowering of these hormone levels in the body. It may sometimes occur, however, if there has been testicular damage, perhaps from acute viral infection, such as mumps, in a younger person, or after trauma. In these cases testosterone levels can be improved by giving testosterone over a period of some months or on a permanent maintenance basis. Libido may, as a result, be improved. Oral testosterone given over a short period may be helpful in stimulating female sexual arousal in cases of frigidity. The preparation causes enlargement of the clitoris and increases, for the time being sexual awareness. It must not be used, however, over too long a period, or secondary complications may result, particularly in the development of a male kind of hair distribution. Usually, therefore, it is only given for four to six weeks as an aid to the therapeutic process.

Other medication with aphrodisiac properties are drugs which act as alpha adrenergic uptake blockers. The well-known, old-fashioned remedy which has recently undergone a period of rehabilitation is Yohimbine. This alkaloid increases the sensitivity of erectile tissue and increases to some degree sexual desire. It is often helpful in putting a patient into 'overdrive' for a number of weeks as part of a programme of redeveloping sexual awareness within a couple, but can be used longer term in some patients with benefit. A number of synthetic drugs of the same chemical type are presently undergoing trials.

Some creams are available on the market often from manufacturers who also make sexual aids, and these creams are claimed to delay orgasm, to increase sexual arousal and to speed up orgasm depending on the effect that is required. One suspects that some contain a local anaesthetic and others contain a skin stimulant rather like the Vick that can be rubbed on one's chest! They do seem to be sold at rather inflated prices if that is what they contain, and are not available through the National Health Service.

Sexual Aids

Sexual aids are designed for various purposes. Some are used as training aids, and some to assist during the act of intercourse itself. The majority are probably sold to do-it-yourself enthusiasts; lonely, partnerless people; or those who wish to put a bit of kinky variety into their love-making if it has become boring. Some, however, are of value in the treatment of sexual dysfunctions, if used intelligently on the advice of a therapist who is familiar with their function and value.

There are four basic varieties which can be classified as follows: (a) clitoral stimulators, (b) vaginal stimulators, or dildoes, (c) penile supports and, (d) vibrators.

Clitoral stimulators may be of value in assisting females with orgasmic delay to increase the level of arousal that occurs during intercourse. They are usually designed as ring structures, to be worn round the shaft of the penis, and have latex protuberances which produce additional stimulation to the clitoris during the movement of intercourse. A vibratory mechanism may be combined with this.

Vaginal stimulators or **dildoes** are of two types. The basic dildoe is simply a penile-shaped gadget of value principally as a masturbatory aid, though unlikely to be popular as such, since female masturbatory behaviour is usually clitoral-orientated. However, the dildoe often has a vibrator within it to produce a rhythmic stimulatory effect, which may be of some value in women who find that more stimulation is required than is obtained during ordinary foreplay in order to reach orgasm during intercourse.

The second type of vaginal stimulators, usually known as **geisha balls**, are latex tampons which can be inserted much like an internal sanitary protection. They are hollow and contain within them a ball-bearing in a fluid medium which oscillates and produces stimulation to the vaginal wall during movement of the pelvis. The rationale of this device is that the stimulation will cause contraction of the musculature surrounding the vaginal barrel, and that this tightening in response to the stimulus will act as a method of strengthening and improving the tone of the muscles in much the same way as any other exerciser will work in strengthening, say, the arm muscles. It is often found that in women who have had a number of children the vaginal wall becomes lax and the muscles stretched, and, therefore, relatively insensitive. It is argued that by improving the muscle tone the sensitivity of the vaginal musculature will be enhanced, and sexual arousal will become easier to obtain. The tampon is worn as a training aid for some hours during each day over a course of some weeks, but some women complain of an audible click, and others that they fall out!

Male aids are designed on the whole to improve erectile ability in those with partial impotence. They work primarily on the basis that erection is produced as a result of an increased blood supply to the erectile tissue, and the enlargement of the penis follows upon more blood entering the organ than leaves it. The blood supply is controlled by small muscles in the arteries and veins, which are in turn controlled by the autonomic nervous system. The veins that return blood from the penis are situated superficially, whereas the arteries which take blood into the penis happen to be fairly deep within the organ, so that, if a ring structure is put around the base of the shaft of the penis to reduce to some extent the amount of blood flowing out from the organ while still allowing blood to flow in, erection will be enhanced. This, of course, in turn produces a relief of anxiety in those with anxiety-induced impotence, and has a beneficial psychological effect.

Ring structures are worn around the base of the penis during intercourse, but there are also training aids, such as the **Blakoe ring**, which are worn for a number of hours each day and are said to improve the tone of the penile muscles. These structures work in a rather similar manner to the vaginal aids, but the Blakoe ring has small metal galvanic plates which produce, when in contact with normal skin moisture, a very small electrical current that stimulates the tissue directly. This aid, which has been tested in a controlled medical trial, was found to be of value in the treatment of some types of impotence.

In addition to the ring structures there are penile prosthetics and artificial penises, which act in a splint-like-manner and are often incorporated in a sheath device. There are also penile developers, in which the penis is placed in a structure which has a small vacuum effect controlled by a pump. These may be combined with vibrators, and are again more commonly used as masturbatory devices.

Finally, there are **vibrators**. In terms of inducing sexual arousal these are probably the most significant advance in the design of such gadgets in recent years. They are mains or battery-driven, and have a small revolving oscillator inside which produces a highly erotic sensation when applied to the erectile tissue. They are developments of the vibrators that have been used by masseurs for muscular treatment for many years.

The value of vibrators in the treatment of sexual dysfunction lies in their ability to produce a highly erotic stimulation when applied to erectile tissues. They are, therefore, of value in the treatment of orgasmic failure, and to enhance arousal when added stimulation is needed. Often they are combined with other aids, and can be used, therefore, in foreplay or during intercourse itself. This will give stimulation to both partners and the maximum effect will be felt on the clitoris. For cases of primary orgasmic failure, particularly in the female, these may be a valuable way of getting things started. They may also be useful in male ejaculatory incompetence. Some individuals, however, find the idea of stimulation in this mechanical manner off-putting, and individual sensitivities must be considered.

Thus, for the effective treatment of this wide and common range of problems a combination of techniques may be needed, including the specific type of behavioural counselling pioneered by Masters and Johnson, psychotherapeutic skills, a knowledge of the effect of general disease and drugs both in the causation and in the treatment of sexual problems, and appropriate advice on general sexuality, technique, and the possible use of aids where these may seem appropriate.

Sexuality is an area of taboos, and inevitably an area where the charlatan or the unqualified counsellor, well-intentioned or otherwise, can have a field day. The sufferer is well advised to seek out a clinic which has the appropriate medical and psychiatric expertise, and people on the staff who are competent and eligible to do proper physical examinations and to prescribe medication, if and when needed, and set in motion the appropriate tests without which in many cases a proper assessment and diagnosis of the problem cannot be made.

Further Reading

Cole, M., 'Sex Therapy: A Critical Appraisal', *British Journal of Psychiatry*, 147. 337, 1985.

Cooper, F. A., 'Advances in the Assessment of Organic Causes of Impotence', *British Journal of Hospital Medicine*, 36. 186, 1986.

Frank, O. S., 'The Therapy of Sexual Dysfunction', *British Journal of Psychiatry*, 140. 78, 1982.

Haslam, M. T. (ed.), *Psycho-Sexual Disorders, A Conference Report*, Smith, Easing-wold, York, 1975.

Haslam, M. T., *Psycho-Sexual Disorders—A Review*, Charles Thomas, New York, 1979.

Haslam, M. T., *Sexual Disorders*, Pitman Medical, London, 1978.

Haughton, K., 'Sex Therapy Current Perspectives', *British Journal of Hospital Medicine*, 37. 11, 1987.

Kinsey, A., *Sexual Behaviour in the Human Female*, Saunders, London, 1950.

Kinsey, A., *Sexual Behaviour in the Human Male*, Saunders, London, 1948.

Masters, W. H., and Johnson, V. E., *Human Sexual Inadequacy*, Churchill-Livingstone, London, 1971.

Masters, W. H., and Johnson, V. E., *Human Sexual Response*, Little Brown & Co., Boston, 1966.

Questions

1. What is the mechanism at a nervous system level which inhibits arousal and provokes premature ejaculation?

2. What are the pubococcygeus muscles and what part do they play in vaginismus?

3. Is there a local clinic in your area for the treatment of psycho-sexual disorders? Who runs it and how long is their waiting list?

4. What types of sexual aid are relevant to the treatment of psycho-sexual problems? Do you have a local shop where these are available?

19
Psycho-Sexual Disorders: Sexual Behavioural Anomalies

Summary

Definition

Behavioural anomalies are disorders of sexual function from the point of view of a hypothetical heterosexual norm, and the problems that arise therefrom.

Classification

1. Homosexuality.
2. Transvestism and trans-sexualism.
3. Devlancy:
   (a) Fetishism.
   (b) Sado-masochism.
   (c) Voyeurism—exhibitionism.
   (d) Paedophilia.
   (e) Bestiality.

Cause

Theories as to inheritance, pre-natal development, and early environmental conditioning, have been advanced. Fluctuation depends on social circumstances in a community.

Treatment

Psychiatry and medicine would not perceive these classifications as demanding of treatment as such but rather management when the patient, or his or her relationships, becomes a problem. Management comprises counselling, referral to specialist counselling agencies and occasionally specific therapies, such as aversion therapy now rather outdated, and for transsexualism sometimes the sex change operation.

Description

In this second chapter on sexual dysfunctions we shall consider the psychiatric problems arising from sexual behavioural anomalies. A wide variety of unusual patterns of sexual behaviour has been described, but many are of interest only for their rarity and forensic value. There are problems that arise about what to include under the heading of deviancy, since some patterns of behaviour, although deviant by standards of normal heterosexuality, are practised by a sizeable minority of the population and, therefore, it can be argued that they are a normal variant of human behaviour. If we define deviancy as the attainment of sexual climax exclusively by a method other than heterosexual intercourse, then we should have to include masturbation and all homosexual behaviour, and certainly the former in adolescence is statistically commoner and, therefore, more 'normal' than heterosexual intercourse. Perhaps the niceties of what one should and should not include are not so much relevant as a consideration of those groups who may seek or need psychiatric help.

The medical profession, psychiatry in particular, has tended to be criticised in recent years by minority groups, such as those representing or purporting to represent homosexuals, who have become more militant in seeking tolerance and understanding from society. There are now socio-political organisations and counselling services which represent many of those groups whose sexual attitudes differ from the general heterosexual population's, and to whom the phrase deviant or perverse is looked upon, perhaps understandably, as insulting. Psychiatrists have in the past tended to take a literal viewpoint in terms of what is deviant by applying the norm of sexual behaviour—namely, heterosexual intercourse—as that practised by the majority of the population under appropriate circumstances and forming the natural function of potential propagation. Anything which deviates from this as a regular or exclusive alternative is then deviant. Perhaps 'uncommon' would be a better word, but insults are not intended. The factual situation is simply being applied.

Similarly, many groups who represent what by this definition are deviant patterns of sexual behaviour consider that referral to a doctor about such matters is inappropriate, and that the type of counselling which they may receive, having been so referred, is biased towards conversion to what society considers normal rather than coming to terms with their problems within the context of their own behaviour patterns. Let it be clearly stated that, certainly within the Health Service, doctors are quite busy enough without wishing to encourage more referrals than are necessary. Nevertheless, any minority group, whether with sexual problems or any other kind of difficulty, is liable to suffer stresses not felt by the general population, and homosexuals like any other members of society may fall ill.

It is, of course, not the 'happy deviants' who visit the doctor. It is more commonly those who may believe themselves to have deviant tendencies but who would rather not be so who consult the doctor. There is a further group who have fallen foul of society or the law who may seek help, and who may well, under certain circumstances, have been encouraged to seek treatment, to change to 'normal' heterosexual behaviour. Certainly in the case of homosexuality this is by no means always a realistic aim, and it is in this group, where people are seeking treatment because of pressures by society, that groups representing homosexuals argue that counselling should help individuals to adjust to their circumstances, and not to change them. The change should be directed towards society's attitudes.

While the author accepts this viewpoint, there are circumstances where treatment in terms of changing attitudes can be undertaken, and if individuals wish this and request it, then it is not the job of the doctor to put them off. In our society, imperfect though it may be, there is little doubt that the happy heterosexual is more acceptable. One wonders what attitudes would be like were there a simple method of treatment to convert black skins to white, or vice versa, and a member of the appropriate minority group approached the doctor asking for a skin change. We shall, therefore, include homosexuality with other deviations from majority sexual behaviour in this chapter, and discuss the types of case that might present and the possible lines of therapy that may be followed.

Sexual behavioural anomalies fall into various subgroups, which can be conveniently classified as follows:

1. Homosexuality.
2. Transvestism and trans-sexualism.
3. Fetishism.
4. Sado-masochism.
5. Exhibitionism and voyeurism.
6. Paedophilia.
7. Bestiality.

Homosexuality

Homosexuality is not a single entity. If we define homosexual behaviour as being any sexual relationship of whatever degree between two people of the same sex, then it would be fair to say that homosexuality is extremely common. The Kinsey Report has shown that a high proportion of people, both men and women, have indulged in some degree of sexual activity with a member of their own sex at some time in their lives. Minor homosexual behaviour of an immature exploratory kind is frequently found in older children and young adolescents, and is part of the process of experimenting and growing up. Homosexual behaviour is found more commonly in groups that are deprived of heterosexual outlets, as in prisons, boarding schools and so on. Thus, the normal drives are displaced under certain circumstances and can revert to heterosexual again with the return to normal circumstances. Similarly, most adolescents who indulge in minor mutual homosexual activity go on to become perfectly normally adjusted heterosexual adults.

However, we may take a definition of homosexuality which is rather more rigid and define it as the development of an emotional relationship between two people of the same sex where there is both physical and mental attraction, and where, if circumstances are appropriate, sexual activity between the two may be indulged in. We then restrict ourselves to a much smaller group of the population, particularly if we exclude those under the age of consent (which by English law for this purpose is 21) and those by whom both heterosexual and homosexual activity may be practised but the main orientation is towards the opposite sex (i.e. there is a degree of bisexual behaviour). Even with this definition we are talking of something around 5–10 per cent of the population.

The question as to the cause of this differing pattern of sexual response now arises. Is it inherited? Is it the result of distorted hormones in the mother carrying the child? Is it acquired as a type of imprinting behaviour by exposure at a critical age, or is it acquired as a result of emotional develop-

ment being distorted at a younger age? It may well be that all these possibilities play a part, and that in some individuals one may be more significant
than the other.

The majority of homosexuals are indistinguishable from heterosexuals in
every aspect of their life and functioning, apart from the sexual one. A proportion, however, identify with the opposite sex in their mannerisms, speech
and behaviour. Such people may not be consciously aware that they are
deliberately taking on the attitudes of the other sex, and are often the butt
of the music hall joke, where the effeminate man or the butch lesbian is
a source of humour.

Much research has gone into attempting to establish whether there are
abnormalities in homosexual people, or whether identifiable patterns in the
early history will emerge. The evidence is so far inconclusive, though certain
trends have been found to suggest that in some homosexuals there may be
hormone disturbances and in others a pattern has developed as a result of
emotional disturbance during formative years. There is also interesting
research where animal studies have shown that homosexual behaviour can
be induced by altering maternal hormone levels at a critical phase in
pregnancy.

In practice it is not the happy homosexual with a satisfactory emotional
relationship with a member of his or her own sex that attends the psychiatric
clinic. Indeed, many of those seen for homosexual problems are not by our
stricter definition homosexual at all. They seem to fall into three groups.

First, there are those who could be called **heterophobes**. These are people
who for various reasons have developed an aversion to contact with the
opposite sex. They are afraid of heterosexual relationships and unable to
mix with the opposite sex. Nevertheless, their sexual drive is possibly quite
high and is displaced to homosexual behaviour as one possible solution.

Secondly, there are those who have had homosexual experiences and been
distressed by them, perhaps finding them enjoyable although in some ways
repulsive, and fear that homosexuality may be their destiny. This may well
not be the case, and counselling and ressurance are often the appropriate
treatment.

Thirdly, there is a group where the behaviour is not so much homosexual
by our definition but rather immature mutual masturbatory behaviour,
purely genitally orientated, where there is only superficial emotional contact.
They commonly include those who have met in some place such as a public
toilet and have been attracted to genital stimulation at a purely physical,
impersonal level. The **true homosexual** occasionally appears at the clinic,
since depressive reactions are not uncommon in minority groups who are
under stress. It is for this group that counselling through the homosexual
agencies, such as 'Friend', is appropriate.

Homosexuality has by no means always been proscribed by the law.
Indeed, in some countries and cultures it has from time to time been
encouraged. Male homosexual sentiment was common to the structure of
Greek society, for example. Female homosexuality, or lesbianism, has never
been illegal in Great Britain, but male homosexuality first became a matter
for the secular courts in 1533, when a statute was introduced under Henry
VIII making sodomy punishable by death. It remained so until the nineteenth
century, when the punishment was reduced to life imprisonment by the
Offences Against the Person Act of 1861, Section 61. This was in force until

1956! In other words, the insertion of the penis into the anal orifice (even with a consenting female partner) was legally, punishable by life imprisonment! Whilst principally a homosexual activity, this practice was a cheap method of heterosexual contraception, and was also occasionally practised with animals in country areas.

Under the Criminal Law Amendment Act of 1885 all sexual acts between males became offences of gross indecency. Equivalent acts between females were not made illegal.

The new Sexual Offences Act of 1967 removed some of the legal penalties for homosexual acts between consenting adults in private. However, sexual acts between males, even of a non-genital kind, are still against the law, and can carry quite severe penalties if one of the parties is under the age of 21, if more than two males are present, or if they occur in what is technically a public place, such as a public lavatory or a parked car on the highway. Equivalent lesbian acts are not illegal, which is why clubs catering for such live shows employ double acts with females only.

A homosexual act with a youth under 21 still has a maximum penalty of 5 years' imprisonment, even if the youth participates willingly; and for a homosexual act with a youth under 16 the maximum penalty remains life imprisonment. It is an interesting anomaly that a sexual act between a man and a juvenile male carries a severer penalty than intercourse between a male and a female under age, despite the effect on the female's virginity and the risk of pregnancy.

Paedophilia

Paedophilia refers to the desire for sexual activity between an adult and a child. The attraction may be to young girls, or may be homosexual if it relates to young boys. The condition, however, is distinct from adult homosexuality, and adult homosexuals are not more paedophiliac than are adult heterosexuals. There is, therefore, really no reason to consider that a homosexual schoolmaster is more likely to seduce his young male pupils than a heterosexual schoolmaster is likely to seduce his young female pupils. Much prejudice relates to lack of understanding of these points.

Fetishism

In fetishism the individual associates sexual arousal with some particular inanimate object, often a piece of clothing or rubber or leather wear. This is usually a learned pattern of response, and sexual activity becomes fixated on to the object, which becomes essential to the ability of the individual to obtain sexual arousal. This pattern of behaviour, unless it becomes an end in itself from which intercourse is excluded, is a harmless enough pursuit, and there seems little reason for medical intervention. Reassurance of a partner and one or two joint counselling sessions may be helpful if the fetish tends to intrude on the normal relationship.

Transvestism

Wearing the clothes of the opposite sex is a not uncommon occurrence in most societies. In some societies such behaviour is tolerated and acceptable, and in Western society the wearing of men's clothes by women attracts little social disapproval.

Cross-dressing may occur as part of a fetishistic type of arousal, and the wearing of clothes of the opposite sex may also be practised by homosexuals who wish to adopt the opposite role. This, however, is not common, and the heterosexual transvestite is by far the commonest of this group. Transvestism in females is difficult to identify but seems to be relatively less common. Transvestism occurs to some degree in between 0.1 and 1 per cent of males. Often the individual develops an awareness of the desire to adopt some female garments in childhood or early adolescence, and experimenting with sister's or mother's clothing may be the first time the individual becomes aware that a sense of gratification is induced by this behaviour. This kind of experimenting is, of course, very common among children and adolescents in any case, and can, therefore, at this stage not be identified as in any way different.

The transvestite, however, is usually aware by his late teens or early twenties that the wearing of female garments produces a sense of satisfaction, and there is a compulsive need to do so from time to time, usually done in secret and often with some guilt feelings. There may initially be a fetishistic element associated with adolescent masturbatory activity, but usually, if it progresses, cross-dressing becomes an end in itself, the satisfaction being in the adopting of the feminine role for a period of time. If circumstances permit, the individual may extend the practice and add to the wardrobe so that the use of wigs and make-up and complete cross-dressing become the only satisfying procedure. There is often a desire to go public and to take on this feminine role outdoors.

At the same time, the sexual needs of individuals are purely heterosexual in orientation. Many are married or have steady girl friends, and this poses a problem in that the majority of women are likely to prefer their male to be masculine in dress and attitudes; that their partner puts on female garb may well put them off. Thus transvestites may have difficulty in maintaining satisfactory heterosexual relationships, since their ideal would be to be accepted as female in terms of dress but to have a female who still is able to relate to them sexually, despite this anomaly.

A married man of 27 had been aware of the pleasure of cross-dressing since he had experimented with his sister's clothes in secret when a child. He felt in such circumstances that he was able to express the feminine side of his character in a way which he could not do when in the male role. He had never dared tell his fiancée of this quirk for fear that she would reject him and anticipated that when he had married he would in any case be able to give up the habit. This had indeed been the case for a while but the temptation of his wife's clothing and make-up at times could be very strong. He began to dress occasionally in secret again and found that it gave him a feeling of ease and contentment when he was dressed which lasted for some time.

On one occasion he had had a few days' holiday and his wife had gone out for the day with a friend. He took the opportunity to cross-dress but she returned home earlier than expected and the secret was out. The wife felt threatened, not understanding the situation and misinterpreting the actions as implying homosexuality, which it did not, or that he was about to rush off and have a sex change operation. She approached her doctor and the couple were referred to counselling and able to be reassured that the behaviour had no need to imply the break-up of her relationship, and perhaps caused fewer marital breakdowns than did the male addiction to golf playing!

Although cross-dressing in itself is not, strictly speaking, illegal, and, of course, is adopted in drag acts and pantomimes, where it is tolerated with amusement, for the man who masquerades in public as a woman there are certain legal difficulties. He may well find himself on a charge of a breach of the peace or, even worse, may be suspected or importuning or soliciting.

A particular problem arises with the entering of public toilets. If a male dressed as a female enters a ladies' toilet and is 'read', he may well be had up for a breach of the peace. Equally, if he enters a male toilet while dressed as a female (Heaven help him!) he may well again be apprehended, possibly with the additional charge of soliciting or importuning. The moral perhaps is to ensure that one visits the toilet before venturing outdoors.

It is difficult to see why the desire to dress in the clothes of the opposite sex should be so frowned upon by society, and why the transvestite should be legally proscribed. The desire would seem to be singularly harmless, but, of course, social problems will arise if a wife or girl friend previously unaware of the tendency discovers such a practice accidentally when the relationship is already of some standing. Here counselling may well be needed to enable the partner to adjust to this problem, and transvestites may attend the clinic in an attempt to seek treatment. Usually counselling and a referral to appropriate specialist helping agencies is the best line of help. For this purpose the Beaumont Society and a number of other small organisations exist to help the transvestites. They provide opportunities for social activities in safe surroundings while cross-dressed, and also provide a counselling service for cross-dressers, their wives and girl friends who may feel in need of this.

Trans-sexualism

Trans-sexualism is the term given to those who take matters rather further and see themselves as locked in a body of the wrong sex. They wish for sex change operations to live full-time in their chosen role. The sex incidence of this condition is more equal between male and female than transvestism, and the condition may be distinct from it.

A young man of 28, anatomically and hormonally seemingly a normal male, had been aware of an inner conviction of being female in the sense of his personality and inner self from early childhood. He had always felt a misfit in male activities and had found that being in the company of females felt more natural to him. He had tended to dress as a female in his teens when opportunity presented but did not feel any compulsion towards this, rather taking it as the natural thing. For a time he tried to over-compensate by taking up daring types of outdoor pursuits and spent a few years in the forces. He began to realise, however, that his inner conviction would need more opportunity for expression and that he could not be content leading what he saw to be a false existence. He gave up his job and began to live full-time in the female role and approached medical help with regard to gender re-orientation surgery. In due course he persuaded the appropriate services that this was in his best interests and had operative intervention in two-stage procedure, the first being amputation of the penis and removal of the testicles and the second the fashioning of a false vagina using the scrotal skin. Female hormones allowed the development of a reasonable bust and although such an operation can never really convert somebody into a female it enabled the patient to satisfy his desire to live legitimately the rest of his life in the female role.

Some recent research evidence would suggest that trans-sexuals and some transvestites do in fact have a female type of hypothalamic function—that is to say, a gland within the central nervous system is operating in a way appropriate to females, even though the individual is otherwise normal male. Since this differentiation occurs before the birth, the reason for the trans-sexualism cannot be ascribed entirely to early environmental experience.

Female trans-sexuals less commonly appear for medical help and the incidence is probably rather smaller than in the male. The gender reorientation surgery for the female is on the whole less satisfactory, embracing as it does amputation of the breasts and removal of the womb and vagina, fashioning a false scrotum from the stitched up labial skin. Male hormones will enlarge the clitoris out of which can be fashioned a miniature penis but it has not proved possible yet to make the passageway from the bladder pass through it, thus allowing the individual to stand and pass water at a urinal, nor does the clitoris produce an erection sufficient to allow penetration of the female during intercourse.

Exhibitionism and Voyeurism

Exhibitionism is the obtaining of sexual gratification by displaying the genitalia to others as an end in itself. **Voyeurism**, somewhat similarly, is the obtaining of sexual gratification by watching others undressing or in sexually stimulating situations. Both these may be illegal when done without the consent of the other parties concerned. Voyeurism may be prosecuted under the Peeping Tom Act, which has been on the statute book since the seventeenth century.

The earliest reference to exhibitionism is in a communication from the commission against blasphemy, dated 3 January 1550, in which a man in Venice was accused of having repeatedly exposed himself to women in church during mass and was sentenced to six months in gaol and ten years in exile. Again the conditions are found much more commonly in men, but it may well be that society tolerates such behaviour much more readily in women and would be unlikely to report it; furthermore, women who have the need to exhibit themselves do so not only in public but also on the stage and get paid for it.

Usually, individuals who indulge in such behaviour are relatively harmless and are not of the type to indulge in rape. It is commonly the inability of an inadequate individual to form a stable heterosexual relationship which leads him to attempt to satisfy his sexual needs in this non-involved way. Treatment by psychotherapy, behaviour therapy, or the use of drugs is usually helpful. Many of the needs of this group, the fetishists, and the final group of sado-masochists, are satisfied by the prostitutes in the larger cities who advertise in kinky dating journals and cater for such outlets, for those who can afford their prices.

Sado-masochism

Sado-masochism derives its name from two persons: the Marquis de Sade, whose writings described the sexual arousal which such individuals feel by the inflicting of pain; and Masoch, whose name is lent to the desire to be humiliated, put in bondage, or have pain inflicted as a means towards sexual gratification. Often the two go together to some extent, and, again, unless a criminal act is committed in the course of such behaviour, it is unlikely that such individuals will reach the psychiatrist. They are well catered for in kinky dating journals. To a minor degree the condition is not apparently all that uncommon. Some individuals are prepared to pay quite a lot of money to have some other person whip them or subject them to various indignities.

Other less common deviancies may occasionally come the psychiatrist's way. **Bestiality** carries the same sort of legal prohibitions as does the offence of sodomy. For either sex to have sexual relations with an animal is a serious offence and occasionally, therefore, cases are referred from the courts. Usually the individuals concerned are either persons of low I.Q. living in a rural farming community, or the occasional person out for particularly bizarre kicks. The latter group are catered for occasionally by prostitutes and pornographic films.

Prostitution might also be considered deviant behaviour, in that sex is allowed for purely financial gain. Similarly, **pornography**, if used for sexual stimulation as an end in itself rather than to titillate the tired palate of the sexually sophisticated, might also be considered in this category. Rare forms of sexual deviation are sometimes seen in psychotic individuals, such as **necrophilia**, in which intercourse is carried out on a dead person. An unusual perversion, which has been described in classical literature, is that of **pygmalianism**, where the love object is a statue or doll. Some authors include rape, incest and other socially proscribed acts in deviancy, but these are somewhat outside the scope of this chapter.

Treatment

Perhaps a better word to use when discussing sexual behavioural anomalies would be that of management rather than treatment. To what extent should the doctor devote his energies to helping this heterogenous group of people? Those who come to the doctor, and particularly to the psychiatrist, for help fall into certain specific groups. There are those who think themselves homosexual because of an isolated experience or a small degree of bisexuality in their behaviour, and who may be suitably reassured. There are individuals who clearly follow a homosexual life-style but who wish that they were heterosexual. Unfortunately, there is no really effective method of changing a person's sexual orientation, any more than the colour of his skin or eyes. Some treatment procedures, which we shall discuss later in the chapter, have been attempted, but on the whole in this group they have been unsuccessful, and in any case it is doubtful whether ethically there is any more reason to try to alter sexual orientation than to alter the interests of a golf enthusiast or to dye all redheads black or blonde on the basis that they deviate from the black–blonde continuum.

Thirdly, there are the loo-lurker group who have taken part in illegal practices as an extension of mutual masturbatory behaviour, where sexual orientation is not so much the problem as the control of the deviant actions. This group may genuinely seek relief from such practices, if only to avoid getting into trouble. The paedophiliac is in a similar position, as are some who may be referred through the courts because of convictions relating, for example, to fetishistic practices, where perhaps underwear has been stolen from clothes-lines, or the exhibitionist who has been caught exposing in a public place. The motivation for these groups may be a genuine one of seeking treatment, or may be simply a means of trying to get out of trouble, the motive being to avoid a criminal conviction rather than to remove the deviancy.

The younger transvestite may appear with similar worries, thinking himself to be the only one with such a problem. Again, counselling would seem to be most appropriate here, and more particularly for the transvestite with a partner who may find difficulty in coming to terms with her male's rather odd behaviour, as she might see it.

It is often appropriate, particularly with homosexuality and transvestism, to refer such individuals to the counselling agencies which have been set up by these groups themselves, and which have developed a better expertise than psychiatrists. The campaign for homosexual equality (CHE) in Britain has a counselling and befriending organisation known as 'Friend', with experienced, trained counsellors who often man a telephone service, rather like the Samaritans. Similarly, the transvestites in Britain have an organisation known as the Beaumont Society, and this has a counselling service through the Beaumont Trust, a charitable trust set up to help those who experience problems and also to act as a befriending agency for those solitary individuals who feel the need to meet others with similar interests.

Particular methods of treatment, other than counselling and psychotherapy, may sometimes be desirable or necessary for those who wish to reduce their level of sexual drive, which can be done by medication or behavioural methods of treatment, for those who wish to extinguish particular maladaptive behaviour patterns or habits. Some of the phenothiazine drugs, such as thioridazine, tend to reduce sexual drive by their action on the mono-amine dopamine. Haloperidol has been useful in reducing aggressive drive, and, more recently, other butyrophenones, such as benperidol, have been marketed specifically to reduce libido. These can be helpful in the short-term treatment of those with uncontrolled aggressive or deviant drive.

Therapy with female hormones, such as oestrogen, also reduces sexual drive in males but tends to produce feminising side-effects, such as breast development, which can be a nuisance. On the other hand, some trans-sexuals, for example, may request such medication in order to do just that. Cyproterone, a specific anti-androgen, also reduces sexual drive without such marked feminising effects.

Aversion Therapy

Various behaviour modification treatments have been devised to help people who wish to extinguish particular sexual drive patterns. The best known of these, but perhaps least understood, is that of aversion therapy. This has been discussed in Chapter 15. While its use was pioneered in the treatment of alcoholism, its effectiveness in extinguishing particular response patterns as may occur in some types of deviancy is undoubtedly a more effective role for the treatment. Thus it may be used for the fetishist, the loo-lurker and exhibitionist, and has been tried, though with less justification, in transvestism in the past.

Critics will fall back on the argument that a patient is coerced into accepting treatment by a hostile society and prohibitive legislation. To some extent, of course, this is true, insofar as societies do tend to be intolerant of those who do not conform sufficiently to the general viewpoint, and also that society, in order to maintain its structure and, therefore, its strength, will usually legislate to prevent what it sees as antisocial acts. The balance of such a society can, of course, become over-restrictive, so that minorities may be oppressed.

One could, however, take this argument to absurd extremes. For example there are certain social pressures on individuals to maintain a reasonable level of cleanliness, or a reasonable level of dental hygiene, or style their hair into a certain fashion. However, it is surely not the task of the hairdresser to dissuade those who come to him to obtain a haircut similar to that of the majority on the grounds that his customer might have been coerced into such a style by society's pressures! This decision must be left to the individual. Some will prefer to conform to society if they can, and some will prefer to be rebels. It is not the doctors' task to attempt to influence the individual who wishes to be one or the other, but it is his task to offer help to those who seek it.

If an individual has learned a response pattern to provide immediate gratification, but would prefer to be able to control the gratification because of its longer-term implications, help may be given by devising a method of treatment whereby the gratification obtained from the act it outweighed by the unpleasantness of something which can be associated with it. The electrically aversive negative reward perfectly timed to follow response to an erotic stimulus can be utilised in this way. Appropriate pictures, clothing or, if appropriate, a real life situation can be devised to produce the erotic effect, and the aversive stimulus is then administered.

Once the technique is being learned the patients can administer it to themselves in order to continue to reinforce the effect. Attempts must, of course, be made during treatment to help the individual to develop more positive feelings towards heterosexual responses of an appropriate kind, particularly where there are anxieties about heterosexual relationships in the patient. Group therapy may here also be an advantage.

The results of treatment for selected cases are good. It is, however, quite unrealistic to think that one could or should change a reasonably adjusted homosexual into a heterosexual, any more than the reverse.

Sex Change Operations

The trans-sexual tends to see the transvestite as one who indulges in dressing up games. Trans-sexuals see themselves locked in the wrong body, and the use of clothes, therefore, is simply one part of expressing what seems to them the normality of their personality and psyche.

Until the advent of plastic surgery, with sophisticated techniques which enabled gender re-assignment surgery to become a realistic proposition, the matter was somewhat academic. There was no more prospect of changing from one sex to another than from one race to another. If we were in a position that a negro could come into the clinic and ask for treatment to become a white man, or vice versa, we would have to explain that in no way was this possible. Should some treatment suddenly become available, however, which enabled skin colour to be altered permanently, then it might well be that a new class of clients would begin to appear requesting race change treatment.

With the advent in the last 10–15 years of practical ways in which gender re-assignment surgery can be undertaken by plastic surgeons, an increasing number of trans-sexuals are now requesting such therapy, which simply makes the individual rather more like their chosen sex than before. In no way do they actually become functional as a physically normal member of the other sex, however, so that the situation must still be a fantasy.

The male to female operation consists basically of the use of female hormones to encourage breast development and hair softening, the removal of the penis and testicles and the use of the scrotal skin to fashion artificial labia and an artificial opening which may be able to function as a vagina. The male to female operation is requested rather more frequently than the female to male.

The female to male operation is as yet less successful, since a functioning penis cannot be fashioned. The procedure includes the removal of the breasts, removal of the womb, fallopian tubes and ovaries. The labial folds are joined together and, with the aid of two artificial testicles, can be made to seem like a reasonably normal scrotal sac. Male hormones are given to cause clitoral enlargement, and the clitoris is separated from its attachment under the female foreskin and comes to look like a small immature penis. Attempts to make the passageway from the bladder, the urethra, pass out through the clitoris have not, however, been successful so far, and such individuals, therefore, are still unable to stand successfully at a urinal. This is a considerable drawback.

The operation itself is by no means the only or even most important part of 'sex change'. The learning of the attributes and characteristics of the opposite sex, so that behaviour and deportment become appropriate and second nature, combined with all the social factors—changing identity papers, car licences, etc.—are the most important part of the total process. In fact all documents can be changed except the birth certificate; but legally individuals remain their sex of birth at present in terms of pensions and marriage.

Further Reading

Haslam, M. T. (ed.), *Psycho-Sexual Disorders, A Conference Report*, Smith, Easingwold, York, 1975.
Haslam, M. T., *Psycho-Sexual Disorders—A Review*, Charles Thomas, New York, 1979.
Storr, A., *Sexual Deviation*, Penguin, Harmondsworth, 1964.
West, D. J., *Homosexuality*, Duckworth, London; and Penguin, Harmondsworth, 1955.
West, D. J., *Homosexuality Re-examined*, Duckworth, London, 1978.
Wolff, C., *Love Between Women*, Duckworth, London, 1971.

Questions

1. Is homosexuality a minority variant like red hair or a disease?
2. Do you have a local branch of CHE (Campaign for Homosexual Equality), the BS (Beaumont Society) or similar organisations in your town?
3. Analyse your attitudes to deviant minority groups.

20
Child Psychiatry

Summary

A sub-speciality of general psychiatry, child psychiatry draws not only on general psychiatric concepts but touches on paediatrics and assessment of retardation in children. Diagnostic criteria are much less easily defined than in the adult field, and developmental problems of behaviour account for a large part of the child psychiatrists' work.

Causation must take into account genetic factors, the effect of physical disease in the infant, and personal and interpersonal factors, in particular the importance of early life experiences, deprivation phenomena and the quality of bonding which may take place between child and parents. Much of child psychiatry is about family therapy.

Classification

1. Behavioural disturbances.
2. Neurotic traits.
3. Psychotic illness (juvenile schizophrenia and depression).
4. Special syndromes found in childhood and adolescence:
   (a) Anorexia nervosa and bulimia.
   (b) School phobia.
   (c) Tics and the tourette syndrome.
   (d) Autism.
   (e) Hyperkinesis.
   (f) Dyslexia and problems of brain damage.
5. Special problems of adolescence (truancy, delinquency, adolescent crisis).

Treatment

Special types of skills, such as play therapy, must be introduced, both for diagnostic and therapeutic ends. Thus special types of out-patient facility are required.

Description

Rutter's study in the Isle of Wight, which screened the total population of 10-year-olds, showed that the prevalence of psychiatric disorder was 7 per cent of those studied. Intellectual and educational retardation also produced approximately this number, within which 4 per cent had specific retardation reading difficulties. This compared with 5 per cent who showed some chronic physical disorder, and means that about one child in six lives with some form of chronic or recurrent handicap. An equivalent study in the East End of London showed a rate of psychiatric disorder twice as high.

A quarter of all out-patient clinic referrals in the United States are for the adolescent age group. The admission rate of psychiatric hospitals in the UK in the 10–19 age group has increased considerably in the last 20 years to well over 7,000 admissions per annum, representing a bed need of something around 30 beds per million population. There has been an alarming increase in juvenile crime, and the suicide rate in adolescence has increased to 43 per million population per annum. Drug dependence has also increased alarmingly in this age group.

The national child development study of 17,000 children born in one particular week in 1958 had shown that 10 per cent had emotional maladjustment by the age of 7. A third of these showed serious anti-social behaviour.

Thus the size of the problem is considerable, and one would like to think that this is an area in which preventive psychiatry could be at its most effective. The child psychiatrist must be skilled at relating to children, and must develop techniques of history taking and examination quite different from those dealing with the adult. Much work must be done through the parents, whose confidence will need to be obtained; some units have become specialised in handling family therapy, where the whole family, the child along with parents and other siblings, are treated as one unit in a counselling situation.

Child psychiatry is a sub-speciality of its own. In one sense it is perhaps allied more to paediatrics than to adult psychiatry, but in Britain the training for medical staff requires that they take the normal psychiatric qualifications, after passing their medical examinations, and doing a year's pre-registration house jobs. A period of time spent doing general paediatrics and a diploma in child health are often helpful to candidates for consultant posts. The in-patient units are usually run on area lines, since not many beds are needed, most of the work being done through the child guidance services in the community.

A separate unit for adolescents is usually available on an area or regional basis. These units are commonly staffed on a multidisciplinary basis, with psychologists, either clinical or educational, psychiatrists, social workers and nursing staff all engaged. Teaching facilities are usually also needed. The facilities for child and adolescent psychiatry in Britain are rather poor, both in terms of numbers of staff qualified to deal with the problems, and the facilities in terms of beds and units available to them.

The type of cases seen are also rather different from those seen in adult psychiatry. Although children who develop typical depressive illnesses or an early type of schizophrenia are occasionally seen, most of the cases are disturbances of behaviour of personality associated with childhood neurotic traits, bed-wetting, and such problems as refusal to go to school or failure to eat and thrive. Special illnesses which vaguely resemble schizophrenia, such as autism, may be found in children, although they probably have a different aetiology. There is a big overlap with subnormality in terms of assessing the intellectual capacity of children who are slow developers.

The Royal College of Psychiatrists recognises sub-specialities in terms of its examination requirements for the membership examination. These include child psychiatry, subnormality, forensic psychiatry, and psychotherapy.

The child is particularly vulnerable to the difficulties arising out of deprivation experiences, since it is immature and still very dependent for its care on other people. Should the parents fail the child, either through neglect or default, or indeed through no fault of their own, but through force of circumstances, such as accident, illness or death, then the child may at a critical age suffer emotional deprivation which, as we have discussed in Chapter 14, can lead to a variety of problems at a later stage. Thus much of the work of the child psychiatrist is concerned with the attempted resolution of the results of deprivation experiences, and the emotional trauma which this causes to the growing child.

Deprivation and Disrupted Relationships

Since a large proportion of psychiatric problems have their roots or their early development in childhood and adolescence, there is a big field here for preventive medicine, if only the resources and expertise were available. The ability to deal successfully with the crises that may occur could create a great saving in the development of certain types of adult psychiatric problems at a later stage. Often by the time the psychiatrist sees an individual at 16 or 17 with a severe behaviour disturbance, personality disorder, the development of anxiety states or even schizophrenia, it is too late to turn the clock back in terms of deprivation experiences.

Ethologists have shown that **the process of maturation in many species, including man, may be arrested, and later stimulation of the maturing process be ineffective, if severe stresses or deprivation occurred at a critical age in the development of the young**. Köhler states that abnormalities are produced by attacking at just the right time a region in which profound growth activity is under way. Injuries inflicted early will, in general, produce widespread disturbance of growth, both physical and emotional, whereas later injuries will tend to produce more localised defects. If the child suffers such pain through making relationships and having them interrupted that he is reluctant ever again to give his heart to anyone for fear of it being broken, his relationships with people from then on will tend to be under considerable strain. His desire for love, repressed though it is, persists, and often results in behaviour such as promiscuity and theft. A feeling of revenge may also smoulder on and lead to other antisocial acts.

Harlow studied the development of affectional patterns in infant monkeys and showed some highly significant results. Monkeys which had been separated from their mothers at birth, and reared either in the absence of a mother surrogate or with only an inanimate cloth mother surrogate, failed at maturity to show normal sexual patterns of behaviour. Despite this lack of responsiveness, four females in the series were mated, but when their infants were born, they showed a strikingly abnormal absence of maternal behaviour. **This provides an instance of a hidden effect of an early deprivation experience only becoming apparent in later life.**

While one cannot extrapolate these results fully to human behaviour, there is little doubt that there is great relevance to human patterns of response. Bowlby showed that children under the age of 7 seemed to be particularly vulnerable to deprivation, and some of the effects are clearly discernible even within the first few weeks of life. Infants under 6 months of age who have been institutionally reared often present a well-defined picture of listlessness, emaciation and pallor, with relative immobility, quietness and unresponsiveness to stimuli such as a smile. Spitz and Wolfe named this clinical picture, seen in the six- to twelve-month age group, **anaclitic depression**.

Very adverse results can be partially avoided during the first year of life by adequate substitute mothering. However, once imprinting has occurred with one mother figure, a subsequent change to a stranger, however well-meaning and caring, may produce considerable strain and subsequent emotional trauma in the child. This is, of course, sometimes unavoidable, and one can only do one's best to ameliorate the possible effects; but much more care should be given in deciding what is in the best interests of a young child in these matters before irrevocable decisions are made.

Goldfarb has shown that children aged 3 who have been separated from their parents may, for some weeks or months after return, show separation anxiety and not allow their mother out of their sight. They regress to babyish habits; if this is unsympathetically handled, a vicious circle can be set up in the child's relationship to the mother, and in this way an unstable neurotic personality may develop. The period of some 3 months to 5–6 years of age is a vital one in the aetiology of many later problems, and many authors have shown that in a few children, even 6 months or more after the separation has concluded, ill effects are still to be seen. Furthermore, some lasting effects are only manifested later in life under trigger circumstances which may reactivate the pathological processes originally set in train by the early deprivation experience.

Behavioural Disorders

Behavioural disorders in children may occur for a variety of reasons. They may be simply of nuisance value, or compensatory, or reactions of resentment in the family situation. Reactions of excessive dependency or timidity may occur, and acting-out behaviours, such as aggression or delinquency. Anxiety, guilt and regressive behaviour may also be seen. Such symptoms are usually a signal of disturbance within the family, and may be seen as a maladaptive piece of problem-solving behaviour. The child is often brought to the doctor against its will, without knowing the purpose. One needs to know the dynamics within the family if a proper appraisal is to be made. Parents may be hostile or negativistic. One must ask whether the regression fulfils the parents' need rather than the child's, since the symptom can be used by the parents to encourage dependence.

One of the commonest of behavioural problems seen in the child is that of **bed-wetting (enuresis)**. The age at which the child develops the ability to avoid wetting varies considerably, depending on the innate process of maturation, of bladder control, but also such environmental factors as parental efforts at training and emotional problems which the child may encounter. Few children are dry before the age of 2 and 10 per cent are still wetting at 5. Some 5 per cent still wetting at the age of 10, the incidence continuing to fall with age. Often parents' unrealistic expectations of dry beds compound the problem, since their attempts at dealing with it, particularly in the less intelligent of the population, with their reactions of hostility and resentment, cause the helpless child to become terrified of their response to the next wet bed. Often this vicious circle can only be broken by a period of in-patient care. Treatment with buzzers or drug therapy may sometimes be necessary, but usually reassurance of the child, and simple training procedures with family case work are what is most needed.

Physical causes of enuresis are rare, but bladder or kidney infections, unidentified spina bifida, and night epilepsy may need to be excluded.

After the age of 2 **encopresis** (soiling with faeces) becomes rare, and, if persistent, is usually a sign of severe emotional disturbance.

Other common problems seen besides enuresis are **disorders of sleep rhythm**, where night terrors, sleep-walking and other expressions of conflict in the child's emotional state may be seen. Disorders of **food intake** are another common problem, and refusal of food may be used by the child as a weapon in a battle with its parents. Disorders of excretion may occur, with problems over toilet training, and the child may retain faeces because it becomes aware of the anxiety which this may cause to those looking after it. Many parents become concerned that toilet training is not completed as soon as that of their neighbour's child, and, therefore, try to force a situation which the child is emotionally not yet able to cope with. This can lead to further problems, and, of course, in psychoanalytic thinking is a possible cause of the later anal character which shows rigid obsessional personality traits.

Genital manipulation or masturbatory activity in children is often a source of unnecessary concern to parents, who must be reassured that in most cases this is a normal aspect of development.

Disorders of speech are common in children, and minor stammering developing in the third and fourth years of life or at other critical emotional periods, such as starting school, are quite common. Anxiety is usually the underlying feature, since pressure has often been put on the child in an educational sense which is taxing it beyond its immediate capacity. There may be a genetic element, however, in speech disturbance, in that left-handedness is said to be associated with such problems, especially where there has been an attempt to force the child to be right-handed when the natural inclination is to be left-handed. The condition is commoner in boys.

Habit spasms such as **tics** are akin to this and relate to other obsessional compulsive states. They may be anxiety-relieving in origin, along with such symptoms as clearing of the throat, blinking, nail-biting and thumb-sucking. It may be worth pointing out to parents that the adult equivalents of thumb-sucking—namely, cigarette smoking and the chewing of substances such as gum—are also commonly found.

It will be apparent that much of the treatment must be directed at the parents, since behavioural disturbances, while stemming in some cases from an inherant genetic tendency to react to stress in such a way, must, stem to a large degree from insecurities that may exist within the child's environment. Manipulation of the environment, therefore, is likely in most cases to produce the most promising results. Nevertheless, there are occasions where illnesses which are not environmentally determined may occur. It is important to recognise these, which can only be done through proper medical assessment if errors in therapy are to be avoided. It, therefore, seems unwise that clinics attempting to deal with such emotional problems should be set up under non-medical auspices. This is tending to occur in some areas where there is a shortage of child-psychiatry facilities, and where social workers and educational psychologists may be encouraged, because of their own particular skills, to make decisions on problems which may sometimes have a medical aspect, without having acquired the necessary expertise in their training.

Childhood Neuroses

Anxiety in children commonly manifests itself in physical symptoms: for example, muscular tension, headaches and abdominal pain, though fearfulness and phobias of situations are frequent. Ritualistic symptoms comparable to the adult obsessive compulsive state are also frequently seen and commonly are transient phenomena.

Monosymptomatic phobias arising from single frightening experiences are frequently seen. While these often wear off with reassurance and the patient's unknowing application of simple behaviour therapy, their origins may become repressed and sow the seeds of something which in adolescence or adulthood can become a phobic anxiety state with the arrival of some new trigger situation.

The child's fears of illness or death, both in themselves and in those who care for them, may be unexpressed but profound. Bullying and academic pressures at school may be present but not admitted to, and anxieties associated with parental quarrelling can lead to strong insecurities. Depressive reactions can lead to antisocial behaviour, failure to learn at school, and regression to such earlier patterns of behaviour as bedwetting.

A child of 7, previously fit and happy, began to complain of recurrent abdominal pain for which no physical cause could be found. One or two episodes of bedwetting occurred which had not happened for four years. She was noted to be biting her nails and had developed a twitch of the nose which she tended to do repetitively during interview. Anxiety reactions in this age group usually relate either to school or home insecurities, and in this case the problem eventually proved to be some level of ill-treatment by the child's step-father, the mother having remarried after divorcing her first husband when the child had been 5. While family therapy would probably have been appropriate in such a case it did not prove practical, and the therapist's aim was then to allow the child to act out some of its fears through play therapy and what was in effect befriending while trying through the help of the local Social Services Department to bring some improvement to the child's home environment by establishing with the parents why a breakdown in the relationship between the stepfather and the child had occurred.

Treatment of childhood neuroses should not be ignored; drug therapy is rarely needed though help with sleep and mild anxiolytics may sometimes be useful on a short-term basis. Supportive counselling and a consideration of stresses within the family are, however, the keystone to success.

Anorexia Nervosa

Anorexia means simply loss of appetite and can occur for a variety of reasons, both physical and psychological, particularly in depressive states, as seen in the adult. Food refusal as a manipulative measure in the younger child comes in a different category. Anorexia nervosa refers to a condition which, while relatively rare, appears to be specific and most commonly found in teenage girls.

The specific symptoms found in anorexia nervosa are a morbid attitude to weight, which may be associated with a faulty body image, whereby the adolescent believes herself to be fatter than she really is; secondly, there is a marked weight loss of some 25 per cent below the ideal weight; and, thirdly, in the female the cessation of periods or amenorrhoea. The illness commonly occurs in the second decade of life, with a mean age of onset of 17 years. Females are affected some ten times as frequently as males. The condition seems to occur more commonly in the higher social groups, and there is sometimes a family history.

Not infrequently the condition seems to begin with a period of dieting in a sensitive, somewhat over-weight adolescent. Soon, however, food avoidance becomes extreme. In contrast to the patient with a depressive illness, the sufferer from anorexia nervosa usually protests how well she is, and claims erroneously to be full of energy. Thus the mechanism of denial is operating. Often vomiting is induced as a way of getting rid of food and is done in secret.

A girl of 16 who was a little over-plump had tended to be teased by some of her school-mates and initiated a course of dieting. Her appetite and weight, however, began to give cause for concern after some three or four months when it continued to drop below the level of what would have been reasonable for her age and height. Endeavours by her parents to encourage her to eat more sensibly were met with rebuff and the mother discovered that the girl was vomiting up her food in the lavatory after a meal if she had been persuaded to eat more than she felt was appropriate. Her periods, which had previously been normal, stopped and she became increasingly wasted. Throughout this time, however, she gave the impression of cheerful energy and there was no evidence to suggest an underlying depressive state. She had a distorted body image in that she still saw herself in the mirror as overweight, even though to everybody else she was becoming emaciated. Attempts at out-patient treatment proved ineffective and she eventually required admission to hospital in order that a controlled diet and medication could be imposed and more intensive psychotherapy initiated.

The cause of the condition is not clearly known. While occasionally anorexia may occur as part of a pituitary disease or a malabsorption syndrome, tests of patients with anorexia nervosa as a rule fail to establish any physical connection of this type. Some authorities consider that there is a hormonal explanation for the illness, or, in other words, that there is a 'physical' aetiology.

Other workers, particularly in the USA and Sweden, have a socio-cultural explanation, noting that conscious dieting frequently precedes the development of anorexia nervosa, and that its frequency goes to some extent with fashion. Bruch identifies a psychodynamic theory pointing to the disturbance of body image, the sense of ineffectiveness, and the failure to recognise nutritional need as going with certain abnormal interactions within the anorexic's family. Such families fail to transmit an adequate sense of self-value to the child, and the mother tends to superimpose her own wishes.

Crisp sees anorexia nervosa as representing a psychobiological regression to childhood in the face of the conflict of developing womanhood. The illness thus represents a retreat and denial of puberty. The family characteristics of over-protectiveness, often with a less dominant father, seem frequently to be found.

This divergence of opinion as to cause leads to similar divergences in ideas of treatment. The first major hurdle is obtaining the adolescent's cooperation and recognition of the need for some form of intervention. Some means must then be devised for enabling the adolescent to regain a reasonably normal weight, and to prevent relapse.

Some units adopt a behavioural approach, whereby the adolescent is admitted to a prison-like unit where privileges such as visitors or 'phone calls are contingent upon weight gain. Feeding is intensive and carefully supervised, and discharge only allowed when weight has been restored. Unfortunately, in the author's experience, most patients relapse on discharge, and the length of in-patient stay often causes considerable disruption to the adolescent's schooling and prospects for passing examinations.

The more psychotherapeutically minded may utilise family therapy or intensive individual therapy, even hypnotherapy or group methods. Again, this may be time-consuming and prolonged.

In the author's view a more satisfactory method of treatment is along physical lines. In any case, if there is a physical aetiology of hormonal type to the disease, it is unlikely that other methods would be particularly successful. This notwithstanding, supportive psychotherapy is certainly important. Empathy should be gained with the patient, but excessive feeding is not initially attempted. The patient is placed on a combination of a small dose of thioridazine, which has tranquillising and weight-inducing properties, together with small doses of a tricyclic anti-depressant, such as amitriptyline 25 mgms, at night. In the severer cases which require in-patient care this may be extended by boosting the appetite with a modified insulin programme, whereby small doses of insulin, gradually increasing, are administered each morning to stimulate the appetite through developing a sense of hunger, after which a substantial meal is encouraged. In the majority of cases a feeling of well-being develops and weight is gained. In the meantime supportive individual psychotherapy or counselling is employed. Patients are encouraged to eat what they like rather than kept on a balanced diet at this stage. The family is not brought in to treatment but, on the contrary, the adolescent is encouraged to make outside relationships, and problems which may be encountered in this direction, particularly those of eroticism, can be explored in the therapeutic interview. Long-term follow-up is desirable.

With this regime the majority of cases appear to do well. Anorexia nervosa must not be under-estimated, however, as in some cases extremely severe weight loss can occur and death is not unknown.

In bulimia, a similar condition, episodes of binge eating with vomiting can occur.

School Phobia

Another condition occasionally found in children is that of school phobia. The refusal to go to school in this case must be distinguished from ordinary truancy. The child who leaves home in the morning to attend school but prefers to spend his day fishing and returns in the evening pretending to his parents that he has attended school is not suffering from school phobia. Nor is the child who fears to go to school for purely practical reasons of being bullied. Rather, in the school phobic there is a fear of separation from the mother, a neurotic anxiety similar to other phobic anxiety states and often unrelated to school performance as such. The incidence is said to be some one per 1,000 students, and varies in severity. A typical school phobic will avoid school and seek to remain in the confines of home. He or she may develop a variety of psychosomatic complaints, such as stomach-ache or headache, and invent various devices to avoid being sent to school. Stresses are often found in the family situation, the child fearing that some harm may befall the parent while he or she is away or that the parent may die or disappear. Some feel that the smaller nuclear family, with the disappearance of patriarchal authority, may have contributed to an increase in the condition; others feel that the parents are unrealistic in their expectations of the child.

In treatment, therefore, again family therapy may be of most value. Psychotherapy with the child is needed, and this may be analytical or behavioural in its approach. Sometimes a brief admission to an in-patient unit may be desirable to break the secondary gain that may have developed. One must discover how school phobia is being rewarded.

Other workers, however, using drug therapy (small doses of an anti-depressant, such as imipramine, or a phenothiazine derivative, such as sulpiride) have found more rapid improvement and avoided the necessity for in-patient care. One must watch that one is not missing a mild adolescent depressive psychosis. This may explain the success of treatment with anti-depressants in some cases.

Tics and the Gilles de la Tourette Syndrome

Habit spasms with bodily movements of various kinds may be seen in many children who go through a phase of compulsive behaviour of this type. Twitches, coughs, grunts and a variety of types of anxiety-produced or attention-seeking behaviour may occur as transient episodes. Most disappear spontaneously, but may be maintained by secondary gain and sometimes require medical attention. The Tourette syndrome is a rare but intriguing type of tic, sometimes associated with fragmentary ejaculation of words, especially obscenities. There are sometimes signs of minimal cerebral dysfunction, suggesting an organic factor, and sometimes other symptoms related to respiration or appetite, with bulimia, may be found.

Sometimes the syndrome may become severe enough to be quite disruptive to the child's schooling and social life. Fortunately, treatment with halo-peridol or pimozide has been remarkably successful in recent years.

Autism

An important but rare psychotic condition found in children is that of infantile autism. The word autism refers to the symptom of withdrawal into oneself and the aloofness that is found in such a state.

Autism usually starts within the first year or two of life, with an incidence of some 5 per 10,000 children. It seems commoner in boys than in girls, and in parents of higher social class. Children appear normal until the onset except that they often seem to be unresponsive to cuddling or social inter-action as babies. The characteristic features as the illness develops, however, are a profound social withdrawal from gaze, touch and any contact. The child becomes mute, or speech becomes fragmentary and bizarre. Ritual behaviour occurs, with obsessional concentration on sameness, in play with-out the normal use of toys. Any attempt to alter this sameness leads to an acute emotional reaction. There are often odd grimacings and posturings, but, within all this, islets of normality may remain, and the child does not seem to be of low I.Q. or show other features suggestive of subnormality, though formal testing of intelligence is usually impossible.

A mother had a normal delivery of her second child. Initial milestones were reached at the average time and the child began to walk and to learn a small vocabulary.

At around the age of three, however, the parents became aware that the child was not progressing in terms of language and indeed was using words less. His behaviour became increasingly odd and stereotyped. It became less and less concerned with relating to other human beings such as its parents and more withdrawn, spending hours at repetitive games, putting toys and other objects in long lines and making no attempt to use them for their proper purpose—for instance, toy cars. Any attempt to alter this pattern of behaviour or to interrupt the game led to severe temper tantrums and difficult behaviour. The mother noticed that the child never now met her gaze or attempted to be cuddled.

Behaviour remained at this level despite various attempts at therapy over the next few years. As the child grew into early adolescence it became im-possible for the parents to cope with the difficult behaviour and, there being no special unit in the area at that time, it eventually became necessary for the child to be admitted to the local mental handicap hospital. Although the intelligence could be presumed to have been normal and there were some islets of normality which allowed this estimate to be made, any formal testing of intelligence now inevitably produced a score within the subnormal range, largely because of the child's inability to cope with the test situation. Within the children's unit at this hospital the child remained withdrawn and solitary and unable to relate with the other children. Its behaviour was manneristic and often incongruous, and there was a tendency to violent reactions when nurses or therapists attempted to intervene in any activity that might be taking place or to get the child to come to meals.

The cause is at present unknown but does not seem to be related to adult schizophrenia, although many features are similar. There is nothing to suggest abnormality in parents, and previous ideas on this subject related to the secondary effects on the parents of having a child of this type rather than the other way round. It may well be that there is some organically determined subtle receptive dysphasia and lack of comprehension.

Treatment and outcome are not good. Phenothiazines and related drugs may help control behaviour but do not seem to be curative. Behavioural approaches towards the acquiring of social skills and training must be intensive, but the child usually remains handicapped into adolescence and adult life. Special units for treating these children are rare, and many will be admitted to hospitals specialising in the treatment of mental retardation if parents are unable to cope. This placement is, unfortunately, not ideally appropriate, since the type of care they get on the ward geared for 'normal' subnormal children is rather different from their specialised needs. But there are not sufficient cases in any one area to justify the establishment of special units within easy distance of such children's homes.

Hyperkinesis

This is a syndrome which appears in the late toddler through to puberty, and denotes the restless activity, distractibility and aggressive disruption which such children show, producing exhaustion of the family and, as a result, increasing rejection. Education is hampered, and the fact that they are on the go all the time, are often clumsy, and upset other children in classes at school, may lead to their exclusion. Hence secondary handicaps can develop. Certain types of epilepsy are occasionally found in this group, and EEGs may be abnormal. They are probably another example of the results of minimal brain damage at birth or for some other reason, but some cases appear to be emotional in origin and are primarily neurotic. The over-active behaviour is the main problem, for which punishment is, of course, ineffective. Treatment with family therapy and with drugs designed to settle the child, so that he or she can benefit from the social interaction of learning, are the treatments of choice. Again, haloperidol may be effective but, paradoxically, stimulant drugs, such as the amphetamines or methyl phenidate, in this age group may control symptoms most effectively.

Dyslexia

Manneristic behaviour, such as nail-biting, head banging and rocking are often see in the younger child, and disorders of speech development, such as stammering, occur in about 4 per cent of children at some time, much more commonly in boys than girls and possibly related to incomplete cerebral dominance or to some delay in brain development. Dyslexia is a specific disability in reading, which may occur in association with other features of delayed maturation, commonly in left-handed children, and with associated difficulties in speech, suggesting that the disability may be attributable to late development of the parietal lobe in such children.

It is vitally important to the child's schooling that this specific reading and writing difficulty should be recognised for what it is, and appropriate remedial action taken. Such children often reverse letters or do mirror writing, and may show some of the other features of delayed maturation, such as clumsiness. Often the child becomes the butt of ill-informed teasing from his fellows and may be accused by teachers of laziness or not trying. This adds to the child's misfortunes and, until the condition is identified, remedial teaching, better understanding and loving care from those who should be helping the child are unlikely to materialise.

Late maturation of certain parts of the brain, and minimal degrees of brain damage arising from birth trauma or trauma during pregnancy or in the immediate post-natal phase, are commoner than is realised. Virus infections causing a mild encephalitis can produce personality changes without necessarily producing subnormality of intelligence. Specific types of epilepsy, such as the petit-mal attacks and psychomotor or temporal lobe seizures, are not uncommon in this age group, and handicaps associated with partial hearing or partial vision are not always spotted, particularly if child health services are minimal, as indeed they are in many parts of the world. Thus the child's failure to make progress at school may be attributed to lack of effort on his part. As Stafford Clark says, the nature of the child's response to his disability, and equally the response of parents and school, can play a profound part in influencing the course of such disorders. The child with minor degrees of damage may be regarded by his parents and teachers as lazy and difficult; he is then rejected and punished, and reacts with frustration, anger, and anxiety, which may increase the disturbance and the failure of concentration.

Such misfortunes can, undetected, drag on for years, and completely ruin the child and adolescent's future. If in doubt get a check up! A proper physical examination, with a vigilant search for neurological signs, and tests of motor coordination and concentration, are essential. Effective treatment at this age can make all the difference to the child's career.

Psychosis in Children

Juvenile Schizophrenia

This condition, which may occur in the somewhat older child, was described by Kolvin and is, in effect, a schizophrenia of adult type that happens to develop in a young person. In this respect there are similarities to the symptoms found in adult schizophrenia, though modified by the youthfulness and immaturity of the patient. This condition is distinct from autism, and tends to come on more in the school age group, being characterised by a fall-off in work efficiency and a deterioration of behaviour which may first be noticed by teachers, although it may be mistaken for lack of interest or laziness. Such symptoms occur in a child who formerly may have been somewhat schizoid and withdrawn, but has not been a troublemaker nor antisocial in the way that a personality-disordered child might be, but has often been intelligent and a good worker. The significant factor is that the child previously functioned at a more effective level, and there is a noticeable deterioration.

We must remember that hebephrenia not infrequently starts in adolescence, and, indeed, the old term *dementia praecox* was coined for just this reason. In rare cases, however, the juvenile schizophrenia may start as young as the 7 or 8 year old child, and in such cases diagnosis, certainly in the early stage, may be difficult. Treatment will follow the lines employed for treating schizophrenia in the adult.

Acute psychotic reactions may occur following the physical illness, particularly viral infections, which may have produced a toxic confusional state with sub-acute delirium, or a mild encephalitis without gross neurological changes. Furthermore, hysterical conversion reactions are not uncommon in children, and need to be distinguished from psychotic illness. Children may complain of pain or inability to walk or to perform various bodily activities in response to environmental stress situations, with psychosomatic complaints similar to those found in school phobia. Bizarre reactions may produce sympathy and attention from adults, and the psychodynamics of such a situation need careful appraisal.

In the treatment of such cases it is as well to remember that the child, or, indeed, any person who is attention-seeking, is in need of attention. The need for attention may not relate to the degree of hurt which a child feels physically but rather to his sense of rejection. While one should not encourage the perpetuation of such conversion symptoms, therefore, by attention only given at the time that the disturbed behaviour shows up, one should recognise that such children are feeling emotionally starved, and give them adequate attention at all other times, so that they begin to feel the love and care of adults rather than isolation.

Affective Psychoses

Despite the protestations of some workers in child psychiatry, psychotic depression can and does occur sometimes in children. Unfortunately, it is often not recognised at the time and, therefore, is inadequately treated, being misinterpreted as another case of school phobia, anorexia, growing pains, moodiness, adolescent love or what you will. Practitioners working in adult psychiatry, however, are often struck by a history, in patients presenting with a clear-cut adult depressive illness, of an episode in late childhood or early adolescence when a child was off school for many weeks labelled with some neurotic designation but clearly feeling depressed, and in due course recovering and returning to school work.

It is difficult to diagnose depressive illness of psychotic type in children, since it does not present solely with the classical features found in the more fixed personality of the older individual. Nevertheless, therapy with antidepressants can be highly successful, and prevent such a child from wasting time and losing schooling. If, in fact, this is the diagnosis in a particular case, then the use of psychotherapeutic methods of treatment will be useless. Furthermore, the danger of suicide in children and adolescents must not be minimised.

A girl of 11, in whom there was a strong family history of affective disturbance, suffered an attack of 'flu in one of the winter epidemics. A week or two after the illness, despite the fact that physically she seemed to be recovering and had only a residual cough, she became less interested in her food, frequently weepy and irritable for no reason and was not sleeping. She developed attacks of dizziness and complained of headaches. Much of her thought content became depressive in flavour and she felt unable to return to school. She lost weight and began to have episodes of weeping which might start at 10.00 p.m. and were continuing at one o'clock in the morning, the parents being in no way able to get through to her or comfort her.

Reluctance on the part of some of those who were advising her to start anti-depressant therapy led to some delay in anything constructive being initiated. As a result she missed a term's schooling but when she was eventually placed on doxepin, an anti-depressant related to the tricyclic group but with minimal side-effects, she rapidly improved and within the space of three weeks was fully recovered, cheerful and eating well. Medication was continued for a three-month period to be on the safe side and then gradually withdrawn with no recurrence.

The hypomanic reaction is even rarer, but again cases are seen where the over-activity, hyperkinesis, loss of concentration and irritation to others caused by these symptoms may well be put down to a disturbed environment. Often the clue to the diagnosis in such cases lies in a careful appraisal of the family history, since the bipolar affective disorders have a high genetic component, and the presence of such an illness in other members of the family in quite likely. Treatment again is as for manic-depressive illness in the adult.

Adolescence

Finally, we look briefly at the special problems of adolescence. Generally, adolescent units are maintained separately from children's units, since the types of problem and the differing age range make this desirable. Most areas have an adolescent unit, but there is still a considerable shortage of facilities for such cases. Some adolescents have to be admitted to general adult wards in the psychiatric hospital, but this is not always a bad thing, depending on the type of case. Indeed, it is really not possible to cater for all adolescents in one type of in-patient unit, since they will have to contain four basic problems. First, there is the neurotic, anxious child, with such problems as school phobia. Secondly, there are aggressive delinquent, acting-out personality problems in the teenager. Thirdly, there is the occasional child with a typical adult illness, such as schizophrenia, but occurring young. It is also necessary to cater for a fourth special group, those adolescents of low I.Q. whose teaching and training needs will differ from those of the other groups. The type of staffing in such units is important. A high staff -patient ratio is required, and teaching facilities are needed for those who may be in the unit for some weeks.

Adolescence is a critical period in the development of many psychiatric illnesses, and diagnosis is notoriously unreliable. This has been shown by a number of authors and is reviewed in a book by the author entitled *Psychiatric Illness in Adolescence*.

Because diagnosis is difficult, indicators with regard to outcome are also difficult. The personality is not yet fully matured, so that hope of personality modification is, therefore, still reasonable. We have seen in our chapter on personality disorders that the admission rate of young people was some 4,500 in 1970. Twenty-six beds per million population were in use, and there had been an alarming increase in juvenile crime. The suicide rate in this group had nearly doubled. Addiction to drugs was rising rapidly. In January 1964 the Ministry of Health stated that there were only 157 psychiatric beds in the whole country specifically earmarked for adolescents, contained within seven individual units. This was a rate of three beds per million population, and way below that needed to cope adequately with the demand.

A leading article in the *Lancet* in 1967 showed that, in a national child development study of 1,700 children who had been born in one week in 1953, 10 per cent had shown emotional maladjustment by the age of 7, and 6 per cent of those aged 10 to 11 had a definite psychiatric disorder. Suicide has been shown to be the fifth commonest cause of death in adolescence, 12 per cent of suicide attempts come in adolescence, and the fatal to non-fatal ratio is 1 to 50. A very high proportion of the total crimes in Britain are committed by adolescents.

It does seem vital that measures should be attempted to identify and prevent such problems from developing, and there would seem to be a vast field in child and adolescent psychiatry for preventive medicine, given adequate facilities and powers. Unfortunately, very little money is ploughed into this field. The training of child psychiatrists is far below need, and, as a result, proper numbers of doctors are not coming along to take the senior positions, which are often left vacant. Consultant child psychiatrists must cover a very wide area, and can only touch the tip of the iceberg in terms of their role as preventive physicians. As a result, a lot of the work in child and adolescent units is done by totally untrained nursing assistants, who often have very little supervision from trained staff, with the result that the children in such units may not receive the kind of skilled care which should be available to them. Problems may only be sketchily dealt with. It is a sad reflection on society that so little attention is paid to the improvement of facilities for this group, and that a strong drive is not forthcoming to increase the number of training places for doctors and psychologists in this area.

Much of the treatment of the adolescent must depend on the development of relationships between therapist and patient, through which the adolescent can mature, and to develop confidence. It has been shown that a large number of cases admitted in this age range had a dearth of satisfactory human relationships with people they could trust and confide in. The outlook for those with a low score on a scale of 'adequate relationships' was worse than in those who had a number of relationships on whom they could depend. Furthermore, prognosis was found to be improved in cases where an empathetic relationship could be developed with a therapist, particularly in the personality disorder group.

Fortunately, in recent years considerable expansion of facilities has continued in Great Britain. It is too early to say yet how much this will affect adult emotional disturbance later.

Diagnostic labels are not very satisfactory in adolescence, any more than in child psychiatry. Some authors have attempted to delineate special diagnostic categories peculiar to adolescence: for example, the terms 'reactive psychosis', coined by Warren and Cameron, and 'adolescent turmoil', coined by Masterson. Often the syndromes seen in adolescence are ill-defined, and are admixtures of symptoms found in more crystallised form in the adult.

A survey done in 1953 at St Ebba's Hospital showed that a third of those diagnosed in this age group were found subsequently to be incorrectly labelled. Half could not be diagnosed at all at first interview. In general, however, some 7 per cent of those adolescents severely disturbed enough to need in-patient care show psychotic illness, 20 per cent neuroses of one sort of another, and some 48 per cent adolescent personality problems.

The author's series in Newcastle showed that, of in-patients, there were two female to each male, 20 per cent were psychotic, 42 per cent were neuroses of various types, and 38 per cent personality disorders. It is probable that the reason for the higher number of female in-patients relates to the fact that female personality disorders tend to be handled in our society through the medical services, whereas juvenile male personality disorders, with their more aggressive content, tend to be dealt with through the courts and borstals. If these latter were to be added, then the incidence would be much more fifty-fifty.

Further Reading

Barker, P., *Basic Child Psychiatry*, Staples, London, 1971.

Bell, R. W., *Maternal Influences and Early Behaviour*, M.T.P. Press, Lancaster, England, 1980.

Bowlby, J., *Maternal Care and Mental Health*, WHO, Geneva, 1951.

Goldfarb, W., 'Effects of early institutional care in adolescent personality', *Journal of Experimental Education*, 12, 106, 1943.

Harlow, H. F., *Mother-infant Interactions in Monkeys*, Tavistock, London, 1961.

Haslam, M. T., *Psychiatric Illness in Adolescence*, Butterworth, London, 1975.

Howells, J. G., *Principles of Family Psychiatry*, Pitman Medical, London, 1974.

Rutter, M., *Maternal Deprivation Re-assessed*, Penguin, Harmondsworth, 1972.

Rutter, M. and Henson, L., *Child Psychiatry Modern Approaches*, Blackwell, London, 1978.

Shapiro, A. K., *Gilles de la Tourette Syndrome*, Raven, New York, 1978.

Vigersky, R. A., *Anorexia Nervosa*, Raven Press, New York, 1977.

Wing, L., *Autistic Children, a guide for parents*, Constable, London, 1980.

Wing, L., *Early Childhood Autism*, Pergamon, Oxford, 1976.

Questions

1. Is there a child psychiatric facility in your area? Where is it sited? How many in-patient beds are there for the population area served?

2. Is there an adolescent unit? What age range does it serve?

3. What work shows the importance of early deprivation phenomena in the incidence of adolescent breakdown?

4. How important is suicide as a cause of death in minors?

21
Mental Handicap (Impairment)

Summary

Definition

Mental impairment, also known as mental handicap, subnormality, mental retardation, or amentia, is a condition which is present from birth or thereabouts, and implies maldevelopment or damage to the brain, and thus intellectual function, before the brain can mature. This contrasts with dementia, which occurs after a period of normal functioning.

A separate service exists in Great Britain to deal with the needs of this group.

Legal Aspects

The 1983 Mental Health Act recognises two categories of mental impairment, namely severe mental impairment and mental impairment.

Requirements

1. Education.
2. Training.
3. Care.
4. Diagnostic facilities.

Cause

Causes of mental handicap are wide and varied. Consideration must be given to identifying remediable conditions early. Problems may be inherited, infective, toxic, due to trauma, due to maldevelopment, glandular, or environmental.

The majority of milder subnormal problems are the people at the lower end of the normal curve of distribution of intelligence. Particular recognisable syndromes are rarer, tending to fall into the severely subnormal category. Important syndromes considered are the following.

1. Tuberose sclerosis.
2. Phenylketonuria.
3. Wilson's disease.

4. Galactosaemia.
5. Cretinism.
6. Tay Sach's disease.
7. Gargoylism (Hunter Hurler syndrome).
8. Klinefelter's syndrome.
9. Turner's syndrome.
10. Hydrocephalus.
11. Mongolism (Down's syndrome).
12. Rubella (German measles)
13. Toxoplasmosis.
14. Syphilis.

Description

Subnormality, mental retardation or mental deficiency are synonyms for those problems of amentia where intellectual function is below normal range and has been from birth or thereabouts. This distinguishes it from dementia, where intellectual deterioration occurs in someone who has previously had a normal intelligence but whose intelligence declines because of illness or injury.

Subnormality is a speciality of its own, which, like child psychiatry, requires special training. Psychiatrists are expected in training to obtain a diagnostic and therapeutic knowledge of the problems of subnormality, and, if wishing to specialise in the subject, will usually take a post in a subnormality hospital at some period during their training, either before or after the membership examination of the Royal College of Psychiatrists or the Diploma in Psychological Medicine.

Subnormality hospitals are usually separate from psychiatric hospitals, which by and large makes sense, as their needs differ. There is a tendency these days to attempt to group all patients into one large district general hospital catering for every speciality. Unfortunately, different problems require a different design of building, with more or less day space, more or less opportunity for outdoor activities, and more or less length of time spent within the hospital. Thus the needs of acute surgery, midwifery, children, psychiatry and subnormality all require differing nursing techniques and a different building design, in particular with regard to the availability of outside activities and grounds in which longer-stay patients can spend some of their time. Recreational activities, such as football, for example, are rarely catered for in the design of more recent hospital buildings.

A sizeable proportion of patients in subnormality hospitals is at present long-stay, and many are likely to be there for life. The tendency to increase hostel accommodation in the community for such people is laudable, but with the proviso that the facilities created are such as to improve the quality of the patient's life, compared with that of the hospital environment, rather than to detract from it. The idea of discharging people into 'the community' is fine as long as they are not removed from 'a community' to 'no community'.

The hospital provides a community, with companionship, social activities, three good meals a day, television, probably a swimming pool and, most important, friends with whom one can mix and feel at home. A small hostel of twenty or so people situated in a town, possibly with neighbours who reject the idea of such a placement, may well prove a very unfriendly place, and it is economically impossible to provide these small groups with all the facilities available in a larger hospital. Much the same problem applies to elderly people, who the author has seen discharged from hospital care and placed into local authority accommodation, where, instead of having an active day with occupational therapy and social activities, they return, in effect, to the bad old days of sitting around a room staring at each other.

Unfortunately, DHSS policy has been to increase the discharge of patients into the community, and, as a corollary to this, to resist the idea of improving or increasing the hospital facilities available for such patients, without providing the necessary community facilities, which are left to the ratepayer to finance. Thus, those who have to stay in hospital, either because they are just not well enough to cope in the community or because the community has no facilities to take them, are denied in some cases the opportunity of their environment being bettered under the care of people who really understand their problems.

This is not to say that many of the less severely subnormal patients could not be in the community, given proper facilities, such as well-staffed hostels, day centres and sheltered workshops. This is certainly desirable, for keeping some less severely subnormal people in hospital clogs up existing beds to such a degree that the more severely disturbed cases have to remain in the community because there is no room to admit them. This situation is obviously quite illogical and economically unsound.

Training Needs

Until recently, nurses who were working in hospitals for the mentally retarded had a different type of training for a different nursing diploma from those working in general psychiatry. Psychiatric nurses take a diploma known as RMN (Registered Mental Nurse), whereas those in subnormality hospitals took a diploma of their own. The training is now being revised.

Nevertheless, the needs of subnormal patients who are likely to be in hospital much longer will vary quite considerably from those in general psychiatric beds: they will need more of a home. Much more training in everyday living will be required, and education will play a greater part in those who are educable. There will also be more physical nursing, for many mentally handicapped have physical handicaps as well.

While the longer-stay patient may well be adult chronologically, if not emotionally, much of the assessment and, therefore, the problems of the new admission and shorter-stay patient in the subnormality hospital will be work with children, since it is likely that this is the time at which such problems will be diagnosed. Indeed, the children may be in the toddler stage, or even younger. Thus, there is a considerable overlap with paediatrics and child psychiatry, and in the better run hospitals for subnormality, out-patient clinics are often combined with the local facilities in these other specialities.

Legal Aspects of Mental Retardation

The legal aspects of subnormality have also differed from general psychiatry, and have been covered by different Acts of Parliament. The 1927 Mental Deficiency Act, which was based on concepts introduced in the Lunacy Act of 1890 and the Mental Deficiency Act of 1913, defined four categories of subnormality. These were as follows:

1. **Idiocy.** This referred to a group who were unable to protect themselves from common dangers. They were as a rule unable to speak or to guard themselves against burning, fire and such things. Their I.Q. was generally under 25.
2. **Imbecility.** This was a lesser grade of severe subnormality. The patient could not lead an independent existence but might learn to communicate by speech and to avoid common dangers. The I.Q. was between 25 and 50.
3. **Moronic.** This group could benefit from formal education but was educationally subnormal and required special schooling. Their I.Q. was likely to be from 50 to 75.
4. A category of **moral defective** was used for the group of patients now described under the term psychopathy. This category was needed later as a result of the encephalitis lethargica epidemic of 1919.

These definitions have been scrapped since the 1959 Mental Health Act, and two new categories have been defined. The first is that of **severe subnormality**, which is a state of arrested or incomplete development of mind that includes subnormality of intelligence, and is of such nature or degree that the patient is incapable of living an independent life or guarding himself against serious exploitation, or would be so incapable when of an age to do so. The second category is that of **subnormality**, defined as a state of arrested or incomplete development of mind not amounting to severe subnormality but including subnormality of intelligence, and of a nature or degree which requires or is susceptible to medical treatment or other special care or training. The third category, that of psychopathy, is, of course, now included under mental illness, and has been described in earlier chapters.

The 1983 Mental Health Act again revised the definitions. 'Severe mental impairment' now means a state of arrested or incomplete development of mind which includes severe impairment of intelligence and social functioning and is associated with abnormally aggressive or seriously irresponsible conduct on the part of the person concerned, and 'severely mentally impaired' shall be construed accordingly, and 'mental impairment' means a state of arrested or incomplete development of mind not amounting to severe mental impairment which includes significant impairment of intelligence and social functioning and is associated with abnormally aggressive or seriously irresponsible conduct on the part of the person concerned, and 'mentally impaired' shall be construed accordingly. This means, therefore, that in the recent Act so far as the detention of a patient in hospital is concerned under the Mental Health Act, such an individual should not only be of low IQ but should also show aggressive or seriously irresponsible conduct, in which sense this definition is now rather similar to the new definition of psychopathy.

In general terms the mentally impaired group is likely to consist of those people who fall at the lower end of the normal curve of distribution of intelligence. They are the opposite of the genius, and their condition has occurred by chance. However, a number in this category will have had minor degrees of brain damage at birth from a variety of causes, or may have suffered an infection, such as meningitis, in babyhood which has resulted in arrested development of their intellectual ability.

The severely mentally impaired group is likely to comprise those who have a particular cause for their subnormality. It will include such syndromes as mongolism and the severer forms of birth trauma.

The division, therefore, provides a rough guide to the type of problem which will be encountered and the type of treatment best followed. The members of the impaired group are likely to be able to live in a sheltered environment, perhaps at home or in hostels, and will in general probably not need long-term hospital care, though admission may be desirable for a period of assessment and diagnosis and to control abnormal behaviour.

Those in the severely mentally impaired group are likely to need permanent hospital care, and will form the bulk of the long-stay patients in subnormality units of the future. They are likely to have concurrent physical disabilities besides the brain damage. They may well have congenital heart conditions or a variety of locomotor problems, such as spasticity. Their life expectancy will be lower than that of the normal population. They will need full nursing care, and are in many cases likely to be incontinent of urine and faeces. Speech and communication are likely to be minimal in the severest group, i.e. those who would originally have come in the idiocy classification. Many, however, who came in the upper range of the imbecility group, which would include some of the more intelligent mongols, can certainly live an independent existence, given proper training, and many are able to live at home as long as there is a caring family.

Early diagnosis is a most important factor. Treatment in the medical sense is not yet possible in a large number of cases. Preventive measures in the form of genetic counselling and advice to families are all-important, and the early diagnosis of some types of subnormality is vital, since, in a few conditions, treatment is now possible to prevent the further development of brain damage.

The bulk of subnormal children, however, do not fit into a diagnostic category which is easily recognisable, such as mongolism, or into a genetic disturbance which has characteristic features. They are mostly found to have a failure of development of brain substance, which cannot be accounted for by any present known cause, and this is certainly the case in the subnormal as opposed to the severely subnormal group, who are simply at the lowest range of normal distribution.

Investigation of the chromosome or genetic make-up, which can be done easily by taking a smear of cells from the mucosa of the mouth, is an essential feature. Palm prints can be useful, and a full physical examination is essential to establish the possibility of deafness or partial sightedness, and any other internal physical deformity, such as congenital heart disease, that may be present.

Although it is not possible to pinpoint I.Q. accurately in a very small child, an estimate of the likely level of intelligence can be made by simple psychological testing and by observing the stage at which milestones of development have been reached. Certain blood tests may be valuable—for example, to assess thyroid function—as will investigation of the urine for abnormal metabolites, which are found in some subnormality syndromes.

Causation

We shall now consider briefly some of the possible causes of subnormal intelligence apart from those found in the normal variation in the general population.

Inheritance

Here the cause is through the action of a rare single dominant or recessive gene. Such conditions are usually transmitted through families, though occasionally sporadic mutations produce a case 'out of the blue'. Those that are inherited as a **dominant** characteristic will occur in 50 per cent of the children where one parent is affected. The condition will never skip a generation. Only those who have the disease can pass it on to their children.

In the **recessive** type of inheritance, however, individuals may be carriers without themselves showing signs of the disease. If one parent carries the faulty gene and the other is normal in this respect, then 50 per cent of the offspring may be carriers; but if both parents carry the faulty gene, then 25 per cent of the children will be affected by the disease and a further 50 per cent will be carriers. If someone who shows the disease marries a person with normal genes, then all their offspring will be carriers. If someone with the disease marries someone who is a carrier, then 50 per cent of the children will be affected by the disease and 50 per cent will be carriers. In the unlikely event of two people with the disease marrying each other, then all the children will be affected.

Recessive inherited diseases are more likely to occur if closely related people marry, such as cousins, where the genetic make-up of their cells is probably fairly similar, and such problems, therefore, occur more commonly in consanguineous marriages. This is no doubt why some religious groups have developed systems whereby such marriages are not allowed.

Sometimes the inheritance is **sex-linked**—that is to say, it may occur only in the male child and the female child is a carrier. This is because the fault is on the X chromosome and the male XY always shows the condition.

Recessive inherited diseases are rare. The commonest is **phenylketonuria**, and this only occurs in about 1 in 15,000 births. **Tuberose sclerosis** and **acrocephaly** are examples of dominant types of inheritance which produce mental retardation. A condition known as **gargoylism** or Hunter Hurler syndrome is an example of a sex-linked disorder.

The above are examples of subnormality produced by an inherited genetic defect. But the commonest recognisable cause of subnormality, **mongolism**, is a genetic defect of a different type. The chromosome defect in mongolism, or **Down's syndrome**, was only described as recently as 1959 by Lejeune, who showed the condition to be associated with an abnormal extra chromosome which fails to divide properly when the maternal ovum undergoes cell division. The addition of this extra chromosome to the normal set produces the syndrome known as mongolism. This extra chromosome in the gene usually lies free, but occasionally it is found fused to another, and this appears to be due to a defect carried through the mother's cell structure in the egg.

The first and common type of mongolism occurs in some 1 in 700 births,

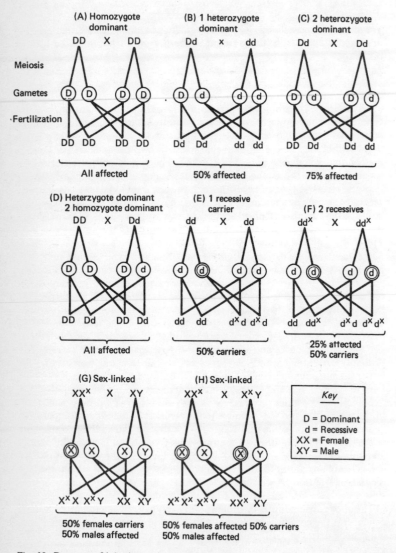

Fig. 10. Patterns of inheritance in mental handicap.

but becomes much more common as the age of the mother at the baby's birth increases. The father's age is of no consequence in this respect. Mothers who have a baby when they are over the age of 45 have a 1 in 40 chance of a mongol child. This type of mongolism is a chance occurrence related to maternal age. The other and rarer type of mongolism (1 in 100) can occur at any age, since the defect is already present in the maternal ovum. It is in this type that there is a possibility of further mongol children being born to the same family. Here, therefore, the doctor has an important role in establishing which type of mongolism is present and in giving counselling to the parents.

Other syndromes which can produce subnormality because of a chromosome defect are the **Cri-du-Chat syndrome, Turner's syndrome** and **Klinefelter's syndrome**. The latter two relate to abnormalities of the sex chromosomes where there are either too many (XXY in Klinefelter's) or too few. Intelligence may, in fact, sometimes be normal in such cases.

Infection

A further possible cause of subnormality is infection of the foetus while still within the mother's womb. The classic example of this is **German measles**, which, if caught by the mother in the first three months of pregnancy, may result in congenital defects in the baby. Apart from brain damage, there may also be deafness, blindness or deformities of the limbs. Other virus infections, however, can also occasionally produce the same result. Some bacterial infections, in particular the venereal diseases such as syphilis, and toxoplasmosis, can produce congenital abnormalities in the foetus.

Toxicity

Foetal damage can occur from poisonous substances taken by the mother, again during the first three months of pregnancy. The classic example of this is lead. Poisoning of the foetus can occur from excessive smoking during the early part of pregnancy. Damage can be done by abnormal breakdown products of blood cells in those babies who have a rhesus incompatibility with the mother—that is to say, the baby's blood group differs from the mother's in such a way that the blood cells in the baby's circulation are broken down and an exchange transfusion is necessary. The breakdown of the blood cells can produce jaundice, and if the bile salts which cause the jaundiced colour reach too high a level, this can have a toxic effect on the brain cells and cause subnormality. Again, this is now a rare problem, since the condition is recognisable during the ante-natal visits by the mother, and something can be done to set it right before the damage occurs.

Trauma

Another common problem causing subnormality arises from the results of birth trauma. With improved obstetric procedures, this should be a decreasing problem, but delay in labour and failure to breathe adequately immediately after delivery, damage caused by an unusual presentation in the birth, and related problems, can occasionally result in minor irreversible brain damage. There is indeed evidence from recent research by Venables that some psychotic illnesses of schizophrenic type can occur more commonly where there has been a history of minor brain damage at delivery.

Maldevelopment

Another possible cause of mental retardation is maldevelopment of the skull structure, the blood vessels, or the central nervous system itself, which may prevent the full development of the cortex of the brain. **Hydrocephalus**, for example, is a condition where the cerebrospinal fluid is unable to flow properly because of malformation of the spaces in which it is normally contained, and this results in a build-up of pressure within the skull. The result is enlargement of the head and also compression of the brain substance, preventing proper development and causing death of cortical cells. If this problem is recognised, early treatment can now be instituted through surgery to correct the congenital defect.

Glandular Disturbance

Subnormality may be caused through endocrine disturbances. The best known of these is the condition of **cretinism**, which is due to absence of thyroid tissue in the infant. This produces a well-identified pattern of retardation because of juvenile myxoedema. The child has a typical facial expression, is dwarfed, slowed in its motor activity, and severely retarded.

Other rarer endocrine disturbances of the glands can also produce subnormality. Here again is an example of a potential cause of mental retardation which can be prevented with early diagnosis and treatment, in this case with replacement of thyroid hormone.

Environment

Finally, in our list of potential causes of subnormality we must discuss environmental deprivation. There is evidence to show that severe emotional deprivation occurring in infancy can reduce the potential intellectual development of the child, probably within the region of 20 or 30 points on the I.Q. scale. Apart from the stunting of emotional development, the sensory deprivation which may occur through isolation and lack of proper maternal care seems to be an important factor, particularly in children who are born deaf or blind or both.

Thus, intellectual retardation may be the result of genetic defects either inherited through the parents or as a result of chromosomal changes, trauma to the foetus before or during birth and infection and toxic processes again either while in the uterus or at an early stage after birth before intellectual development has fully got going.

Diagnosis

We shall now consider briefly the diagnostic procedures which are relevant in establishing these possibilities in a child who is brought to the clinic suspected of subnormality because of its failure perhaps to reach normal milestones.

Diagnostic investigations must be made in two separate fields, the physical and the psychological. Much depends upon an accurate case history, which must include a record of maternal health and the elements of a pedigree investigation in every case. Age, dates of birth, and the mental status of parents and siblings must be considered, miscarriages and stillbirths recorded and a note made of any consanguinity. Details of maternal health during pregnancy should be noted, as must the progress of the suspected defect.

Apart from routine physical examination, chest X-rays, and routine blood tests, certain special tests need to be used. For example, the condition of the cornea in the eye, optic atrophy, or the presence of pigmentation will need to be noted. X-rays may show early abnormalities in the cranial vault, as in microcephaly and hydrocephaly, and an EEG may be required to demonstrate cerebral abnormalities associated with epilepsy. Urine tests will prove the diagnosis of phenylketonuria, and chromatography may show more complex amino-acid disturbances. Palm prints and chromosome analyses have become of vital interest. Psychological testing is designed to assess intelligence. The Stanford Binet, Merrill Palmer, and other scales to measure intelligence may be used.

Treatment

Treatment of impairment falls partly in the realm of prevention, partly in the control of disturbed behaviour and thinking, and partly in educative procedures to develop what potential is present. An important aspect of drug therapy lies in the control of aberrant or overactive behaviour, since, if effective, this allows of a more normal social milieu being maintained. Anticonvulsants are of great value, since epilepsy is a common concomitant of many subnormality syndromes.

The use of barbiturates is generally contra-indicated in retarded children and those with brain damage, for they often cause a paradoxical increase in motor restlessness and, in consequence, disturbed behaviour. Curiously, stimulants, such as amphetamines, may, however, be used in the treatment of the hyperkinetic overactive child. They cause less impairment of learning than the tranquillisers.

Behaviour modification is a term used to describe treatment derived from various learning theories, but, in particular, those of Skinner, which are based upon operant conditioning techniques. The essential feature here is that reinforcement or reward is made contingent upon achieving the behaviour that is being promoted. Reward may take the form of attention, affection or praise, or may be tangible, such as food, or money tokens for those of higher I.Q. Such techniques may be applied to behaviour modification, to toilet training, and to language development.

In April 1971 responsibility for the education of the mentally handicapped child in England passed from the health authority to the education authorities; the 35,000 children who were transferred joined the 60,000 who are regarded as educationally subnormal (ESN). Selection is not on I.Q. alone, but by reference to educational need. In many of the lower grade, 'training' is perhaps a more appropriate word, for the social accept-ability of being allowed to live at home is the main aim, if this is possible.

Families of ESN children come predominantly from lower social groups, whereas the severely subnormal tend to be more evenly distributed. Many suffer from multiple handicaps.

When a child requires admission to a subnormality hospital, it is most important to ensure that the parents maintain contact, visiting regularly and being encouraged to think in terms of discharge. Nevertheless, as things stand, many occupants of subnormality hospitals will remain there, so that a proper therapeutic community must be set up within the hospital to allow the maximum development of these patients' personalities. The environment must be child-centred, with stuctured teaching, proper social activities, and a wide range of stimuli. Much of the doctor's role must be in advice and counselling parents, particularly with regard to those children seen in out-patients, as to whether the more severely subnormal child should be able to stay at home or whether it seems more reasonable, taking everything into account—including the welfare of other children within that family—that the child should board at a hospital. Much will depend on the social circum-stances and the degree of handicap. Units within subnormality hospitals should adopt a 'substitute home' concept, and an individual adult–child relationship within the hospital environment, if possible, will be ideal.

In one experiment two units of twenty-five places each have been set up to provide for all residential care needs of the mentally handicapped children for a total population of 100,000, one in Southampton and one in Ports-mouth. They are situated in the centre of the area served and they are, there-fore, near the children's families. The children are cared for by staff whose main specialities are in child care. The front-line medical care is provided by local general practitioners, with additional help from social workers, educa-tional psychologists, and the local community medical officer. A consultant in subnormality, working from the local hospital, is in control.

Mental handicap or impairment is proceeding along the same lines, or suffering the same fate depending on one's point of view, as is psychiatric illness, in that the closure of the old subnormality hospitals is proceeding a pace. Most of the previous in-mates are being transferred into small community hostels where they may or may not prove to have a better quality of life and few admissions to such hospitals are not being accepted. The problems will be that there are not enough hostels, and there are considerable difficulties in providing a good quality of life for so many small scattered peripheral units. An additional problem will arise as and when such individuals develop periods of acutely disturbed behaviour or psychiatric illness when it is unlikely that there will be in-patient facilities in what are then left of the psychiatric in-patient hospital facilities for them to be properly and temporarily cared for.

Individual Syndromes

In the remainder of this chapter we shall consider in a little more detail some of the commoner syndromes which occur in the subnormality field. We have already stated that the majority of cases show no specific syndrome that can be identified as causative. A sizeable minority, however, do show syndromes for which the cause is understood, and in some cases the early identification of these can allow of treatment.

Genetic Defects

Tuberose Sclerosis (Epiloia)

Of the **autosomal gene defects** with a dominant pattern, **tuberose sclerosis**, or epiloia, is the commonest. Potato-like tumour growths are found within the brain and in other parts of the body. A typical rash, found on the cheeks, is usually easily recognisable. The degree of mental impairment is variable. The incidence is some 1 in 15,000 births. Sterility is generally associated with this condition. In a number of cases there appears to have been a fresh mutation, i.e. no inherited history is found. Epilepsy is commonly present, as it is in many of these syndromes.

A child of 6 was brought to the surgery having had an epileptic fit. The child had been slow to reach normal milestones but was coping at a nursery school. Her vocabulary was small but she seemed reasonably alert. Physical examination revealed a number of nodular lumps scattered over the body surface and the child had a reddened butterfly-shaped area on the cheeks and nose which made epiloia be suspected. A brain scan revealed two similar nodules within the substance of the central nervous system. Supportive treatment with antiepileptic drugs was instituted.

A number of other deformities, such as acrocephaly and some forms of dwarfism, may be associated with a dominant inheritance. **Marfan's syndrome** is occasionally associated with subnormality: in this condition there are long spidery fingers and toes, often with lens abnormalities in the eye and associated congenital heart defects.

Phenylketonuria

Many of the biochemical causes of subnormality are inherited by a recessive pattern. Of these **phenylketonuria** is perhaps the most important, since this is one of the treatable conditions. It was described in 1934 by Fölling. Abnormal metabolites are found in the urine, these being tested for in the urine of babies as a routine soon after birth. The incidence is some 1 in 15,000, and it is found especially in cousin marriages. Typical features of this syndrome include blonde hair and blue eyes, with widely set teeth and a characteristic type of hand movement. Epilepsy may be present.

An adolescent girl was seen in the ward of the local mental handicap hospital. Her behaviour had become more disturbed and she was being aggressive with the other residents. She sat on a chair grinning affably but rather fatuously at those about her. Her hands were continually on the go, making odd little movements. She showed the typical *facies* with widespread teeth and very fair complexion and hair. Her I.Q. had been estimated at around 45. Unfortunately this girl had been born at a time before the cause of phenylketonuria had been identified and no one had known, therefore, to give her a special diet which could have prevented the development of the subnormality of intelligence. The disease was no longer progressive but she was likely to need life-long supportive care in a sheltered environment such as the hospital offered.

The cause of this condition is the absence of an enzyme capable of splitting phenylalanine, which is an amino-acid in the diet. A diet free of phenylalanine will prevent the poisoning of the tissues by the high levels which otherwise would occur.

Maple syrup urine disease, **Hartnup** disease and a number of others have also been identified.

Wilson's Disease (Hepato-lenticular Degeneration)

In **Wilson's disease**, or hepato-lenticular degeneration, described in 1912, there is a progressive development of neurological symptoms, which produce subnormality or, perhaps more strictly, a dementia of childhood. There are difficulty in swallowing, spasticity in the limbs, and characteristic signs in the eyes, due to an enzyme failure which results in an excessive deposition of copper in the brain, liver and other tissues. Again, this is treatable, if the excessive copper can be removed by drugs known as chelating agents.

Galactosaemia

In **galactosaemia**, described in 1908, problems arise from an allergy to milk feeding, which produces symptoms of diarrhoea and vomiting, lethargy and jaundice. If untreated, this can result in mental retardation, but it can be dealt with by a galactose-free diet. Galactose, a sugar, is not properly dealt with by the body's enzymes in this condition. It is possible here to identify carriers, and diagnosis can be made by a blood test from cord blood at birth.

Cretinism

Cretinism is important historically. A number of types occur but one of them is inherited recessively. The lesions result from a deficiency of thyroid hormone, in this case owing to the absence of a particular enzyme, dehalogenase. Characteristic features are mental defects, sluggish behaviour, dwarfism, a coarse dry skin and hair, and large protruding tongue. This condition can be corrected in the early stages by treatment with thyroid hormone.

Tay Sach's Disease (Amaurotic Family Idiocy)

In **Tay Sach's disease**, or **amaurotic family idiocy**, described in 1881, there is a disturbance of fat metabolism which may occur in infancy or in early childhood. There are abnormal movements and difficulty in vision. Part of the retina tends to degenerate, and this can be recognised through an ophthalmoscope. The brain contains an abnormal accumulation of fatty substances, which the body is unable to utilise. The incidence is about 1 in 40,000.

Gargoylism (Hunter Hurler Syndrome)

In **gargoylism**, or **Hunter Hurler syndrome**, there is a disturbance of connective tissue in the body, owing to a disturbance in carbohydrate metabolism, which causes the typical features that give the syndrome its name. The face is coarsened and the skull is mildly misshapen. The stature is dwarfed and generally there is deafness.

Sex-linked Causes

As we have stated, some conditions show as a **sex-linked genetic abnormality** not always associated with subnormality.

In **Turner's syndrome** there is an absence of the male sex chromosome. The individual is female, but there is an absence of ovarian tissue and usually dwarfism, a typical webbed neck and sometimes other abnormalities. Complications may occur with other chromosome abnormalities when, for instance, there are three X chromosomes, or female chromosomes, in the cell, or in **Klinefelter's syndrome**, where there are two Xs and an additional male Y chromosome in the cell. Here the patient is male and often develops normally until puberty, but there is absence of testicular tissue, causing infertility and partial impotence. The condition is often associated with psychopathic behaviour and sometimes subnormality.

Finally, in this group, **hydrocephalus** is rarely found as a sex-linked inherited feature. Blockage of the flow of cerebrospinal fluid causes enlargement of the head due to pressure inside the skull, and results in degeneration of brain tissue if not treated. These days, however, operative treatment is possible to by-pass the blockage.

Foetal Abnormalities of Developmental Origin

Our fourth group are those **foetal abnormalities** which are of **developmental** origin. Abnormalities such as **anencephaly** and **spina bifida** fall into this category, and there are often gross malformations not compatible with long survival.

Naevoid Amentia (Sturge-Weber Dimitri Syndrome)

Here one sees a characteristic birthmark on the face and neck, affecting one side. It may affect the brain underneath, and calcification can be seen by X-ray. If the brain is affected, subnormality is often present, sometimes with a paralysis of one side and epilepsy.

Mongolism (Langdon Down's Syndrome)

The most important condition and commonest of the syndromes we have been describing is that of **mongolism** or **Down's syndrome**, described by Langdon Down in 1886.

It is increasingly probable that soon we shall be able to carry out screening tests on all foetuses, particularly in the age group where the mother is at risk, in order to establish whether the condition is present in the foetus at a stage when termination of pregnancy is still reasonable. In this way, assuming this to be an acceptable reason for termination of the pregnancy, the incidence of mongolism in the community could be considerably reduced.

Many mongol children are sterile when they have grown to adulthood. Some women who suffer from mongolism have become pregnant, however, and, in these cases, it is usually found that 50 per cent of the children who are born will be mongols themselves.

The features characteristic of mongolism are most obviously the shapes of the face and eyes, which give the name to the syndrome because of the Asiatic look of the slanting eyes. There is usually a degree of dwarfism and the I.Q. is usually less than 50. There is a small head and what is known as an 'epicanthic fold' in the eyes, which gives a slanted effect. The tongue is often large and fissured, and tends to protrude. The ears have a pixie sort of shape. There are abnormalities in the palm prints and palm creases, and also in the toes, where the fissure between the first and second toes shows a deeper cleft than normal. There are often associated congenital abnormalities of the internal organs of the body, such as congenital heart disease. The life expectancy in mongols is lower than in the normal population.

A child seen at a clinic in an overseas country in a less developed part of Africa had been slow to walk and was not talking. Although now 6 he had not learned to control bowel habit properly but was an amiable cheerful little character who was quite popular in spite of all his problems with his fellow children. Despite the negroid complexion, the slanting eyes and large tongue typical of the mongol child were plainly present. A general physical examination revealed other typical features of the condition. It was noted in this case that the mother was relatively young but this was her third child. Genetic investigation was able to confirm that this was a coincidental finding and not likely to recur in another child. The child's I.Q. was assessed at around 50 and it was probable that within the village community the child would be able to live a reasonable existence supported by caring relatives.

The temperament of mongol children is usually placid and happy, unlike the overactivity often found in some subnormal children. For this reason, and the fact that the I.Q. is not all that low, some education may be possible. The children are often musically appreciative, and the outlook, although not bright in terms of a subsequent independent existence, is certainly such that parents can be reassured of being able to develop a good relationship, with the knowledge that a family life will be beneficial to the child and rewarding to the parents.

The effect of such a child on the family unit as a whole, and on the other children must, of course, be considered, and the possibility of boarding in a subnormality unit so that special educational needs can be provided may be the best course. The facilities in the area and the standards available in the local unit must be weighed against the home problems. A full discussion with the local consultant psychiatrist specialising in subnormality should, therefore, be arranged on an out-patient basis once the diagnosis has been established.

As has been mentioned earlier, the cause of mongolism is a faulty development of the genetic structure of the cell, and this can come about in a number of ways but produces the same end result. In the common type, an extra chromosome 21 is found (there are 23 chromosome pairs in a human cell). This is usually the result of failure of separation of the chromosome during cell division, and it is this type that increases with the age of the mother. Sometimes a break takes place near the centre of the chromosome as it divides and the wrong pair of ends rejoin. This may occur at chromosome 13 or 15. A mongol of this type has all 46 chromosomes, and the mother is found to have 45 chromosomes with the same translocation. She is in this sense a carrier, although normal herself. In another type of mongolism there is a translocation of chromosomes 21 and 22, which can be paternal or maternal. Occasionally the fault is found in some cells and not in others, which is known as **mosaicism**. In these rarer types maternal age is of no relevance.

Environmentally Determined Causes

Finally, in our more detailed review of causes of subnormality, we must mention environmentally determined disabilities due, for example, to **prenatal injury** from a variety of causes. Temporary failure of the oxygen supply to the baby's brain during birth is perhaps the commonest, or used to be when obstetric facilities were not so well developed. This is commonly accompanied by traumatic injuries, with physical damage to the skull.

Radiation has been found to affect the infant, and for this reason X-rays of a mother carrying a child are now kept to a minimum. **Chemical agents** and some **drugs** have been found to be toxic to the foetus, as are the effects of **nicotine** in heavy smokers. A number of **poisons** can cross the placental barrier and get into the foetal circulation from the mother.

Certain **vitamin deficiencies** can result pre-natally in subsequent subnormality, and vitamin A deficiency is particularly relevant here. Toxic effects from rhesus incompatability, producing **kernicterus** with jaundice, due to the deposit of bile pigment in the brain cells, can occur if exchange transfusion is unsuccessful. Foetal infections can be caught from the mother. In particular, German measles or **rubella** in the first three months of pregnancy can be hazardous, and is now recognised as a valid reason for termination. **Toxoplasmosis**, which can be caught from animals, such as dogs, and may affect the mother and be transferred to the foetus, is another fairly rare cause of subnormality. This infection is produced by organisms known as protozoa, and epilepsy is common in survivors.

Finally, **congenital syphilis** may be caught from mothers with the infection. In all those who attend ante-natal clinics this will have been eliminated by appropriate tests, which are carried out as a routine, but the condition does still occasionally turn up. It is of considerable historical interest. Typical physical abnormalities which help diagnosis are found. There are keratitis; abnormalities of the pupils, which do not react to light as does the normal pupil by contracting; a particular type of deformity of the teeth; a bossing of the skull; and scarring of the nose and palatal tissue. Effective treatment of the mother in pregnancy will prevent this condition developing.

Subnormality has tended to be a neglected field in medicine. Far too little money has been spent on subnormality hospitals, with the result that some have been overcrowded and acquired a bad reputation, and medical and nursing staff have been difficult to find. This has led to politically induced moves to convince people that all patients in subnormality hospitals would be better in the community. We have discussed this argument earlier in the chapter, and drawn attention to some of the hazards that this kind of thinking can produce if applied too extensively. It has always seemed strange to the author that a hospital catering for the acutely sick who may only be in the ward for some ten days should have considerable facilities provided in the shape of bedside telephones, radio sets and colour television, when patients who may be in hospital for years are expected to live in substandard surroundings. Somewhere society, or the Department of Health, has got its priorities wrong. Much more attention should be paid to community services developed from the hospital, with properly run out-patient departments in association with other psychiatric and general hospital clinics. Surprisingly, this facility is still not available in many areas. Far too few doctors are given the opportunity or the encouragement to train in subnormality, and it has thus tended to be a Cinderella of the profession. One can only hope that somebody will have the vision and foresight to steer a better course.

Further Reading

Better Services for the Mentally Handicapped, Cmnd. 4683, HMSO, London, 1971.
O'Gorman, C. O., *Modern Trends in Mental Health and Subnormality*, Butterworth, London, 1978.
Penrose, L. S., *The Biology of Mental Defect*, Sidgwick and Jackson, London, 1977.
Simon, B. G., *Modern Management of Mental Handicap*, M.T.P. Press, Lancaster, England, 1980.
Tredgold, R. F., and Soddy, K., *Mental Retardation*, Aberdeen University Press, 1970.

Questions

1. Where is your local subnormality unit? How many beds has it? Do they have out-patient facilities at your local hospital?
2. Do the Social Services provide hostel care and sheltered workshop facilities in your nearest large town?
3. What are the basic reasons for the development of mental retardation?

22
Forensic Psychiatry

Summary

Definition

Forensic psychiatry is the study of those areas where psychiatry and the law overlap: the psychiatric aspects of criminal behaviour, aggression and responsibility in law

Special Hospitals

Rampton, Broadmoor, Moss Side, Park Lane, and Carstairs are set aside for the mentally ill criminal.

Important Legislation

The 1983 Mental Health Act.
Homicide Act 1957.
Criminal Lunatics Act 1800.
Criminal Procedure (Insanity) Act 1964.
Offences Against the Person Act 1861.
Criminal Justice Acts 1948 and 1967.
Magistrates' Court Act 1952.
Suicide—1961 Suicide Act.
Infanticide—1938 Infanticide Act.
Termination of pregnancy—1967 Abortion Act.
Legislation on drugs—Misuse of Drugs Act 1971.
Sexual offences—Criminal Law Amendment Act 1885, Sexual Offences Acts 1956 and 1967.

Other Relevant Problems

The 'battered baby' and 'battered wife' syndromes, shoplifting, and epilepsy must be taken into consideration.

Description

Our final subject, forensic psychiatry, is the last of the sub-specialities which are examined separately in the examination for the membership of the Royal College of Psychiatrists. Consultants and trainees are appointed to posts within the Health Service in Forensic Psychiatry, and sometimes joint appointments are held with the Home Office or within the prison service. In addition, there is a Diploma in Medical Jurisprudence, much of which is concerned with the forensic aspects of psychiatry, and this diploma can be taken separately by suitable candidates with the necessary experience, through the Society of Apothecaries in London.

Forensic psychiatry is concerned with the study of those areas where psychiatry and the law overlap. It is thus concerned with the psychiatric aspects of criminal behaviour, the study of aggression, and questions of responsibility. A knowledge of the relevant legal Acts is required, and this includes a wide range of subjects, such as suicide, legal definitions of insanity, termination of pregnancy, the law with relation to epilepsy and driving, and all topics to do with mentally disordered offenders. Psychopathy and delinquency and the laws relating to drug offences and sexual offences must also be studied, and such offences as baby battering and shoplifting, and such crimes as murder, often have a psychiatric component.

Some of these areas have already been covered in the appropriate chapters but here we shall try to coordinate the various items and look at the sub-speciality in a little more detail.

Health Service psychiatric units in Britain are now almost universally open ones—there are no locked wards, and by and large provision is not made for dealing with any criminal problems. From time to time admissions to the hospital may include patients who, because of the nature of their illness, are unpredictable or even violent, but this is normally a temporary problem, soon resolved by appropriate medication. It is, therefore, neither appropriate nor desirable that district psychiatric units should be expected in any sense to act as gaols.

At the same time, there may be people who have committed criminal offences, such as murder, who are obviously mentally sick and for whom prison sentences would be inappropriate without proper medical care being provided. This care cannot be carried out in the normal prison environment, and special hospitals administered under the Home Office have been set up in Britain to cater for this kind of problem. The vast majority of patients in these hospitals, which are strict security hospitals with locked wards, are psychiatrically ill but have committed offences of a nature that requires their detention under secure conditions. Some of these patients may be of subnormal intelligence, and some psychopathic. Some are suffering from psychotic illnesses, such as schizophrenia or manic-depressive psychosis. In England these hospitals are at Park Lane, Rampton, Broadmoor and Moss Side. The State Hospital at Carstairs caters for similar patients in Scotland.

There may, however, be patients who require temporary secure conditions but have not committed any offence which would allow the courts to make such an order. It would hardly be reasonable to wait until a possible offence had become reality before making such an order, but, at the same time, to deprive someone of their liberty on the basis of a hunch is hardly fair. To deal with these cases, principally the severer personality disorders, who may be very disruptive in an open-ward environment, some regions have set up special units where there is a degree of security and where patients can be temporarily transferred for special care until such time as the ordinary psychiatric unit can more appropriately contain them. This programme is at present under way, but is often held up by lack of finance, so that the courts are often put in the position of making a recommendation that patients receive such care without having somewhere appropriate to send them. This continuing social problem will only be resolved with the injection of further money into this branch of the Health Service. It is particularly true of the delinquent disturbed adolescent group. It is impossible for the psychiatrist asked to provide advice to the court on such a case to give a recommendation for the kind of care which he knows full well, however desirable it may be, is in practice unobtainable.

The state hospitals have their own medical and nursing staff, where those doctors specialising in forensic psychiatry are likely to be working. The kind of case they see will, as has been explained, be rather different from the general run of psychiatry, and requires its own expertise.

Psychiatrists have often been criticised by the courts and the press that such dangerous patients have been allowed loose, or that people who should be criminally responsible for their actions are given excuses by psychiatrists who blame it all on to deprivation of upbringing. As will be made clear in this chapter, **the question of criminal responsibility is a legal one and not a medical one**, and what constitutes responsibility or absence of responsibility has been laid down by judges in the past. A psychiatrist is, therefore, merely asked for advice, and the court can choose to take cognisance or disregard it as it sees fit. It is not unreasonable to assume that early environmental deprivation is quite likely to have an effect on the causation of much criminal behaviour, and, indeed, there is ample evidence to show that this is so. Whether this should be considered as diminishing responsibility for a person's actions is a matter for society and for the courts, and decisions made by them should not subsequently be blamed on the medical profession.

A similar situation arises in regard to the discharge of patients from special hospitals. If an individual suffering from schizophrenia or mania has, as a result of that illness, committed an offence which may perhaps have led to the death of another person, he may well not have been considered responsible for his actions, and may have been admitted to the state hospital on a court order through the Mental Health Act. If such an illness subsequently responds satisfactorily to treatment, and the patient is, therefore, in this sense cured, the question of what to do next will arise: whether he should be allowed to leave the state hospital in view of the gravity of the previous offence, or should be transferred to an open unit, or should be forced to remain, even though the reason for his offence is no longer pertinent.

At this point, when the case comes up for review, the doctor in charge of the patient will be asked for his report on the patient's mental state. He will do this on the basis of his medical judgement as to the effectiveness of cure and the likelihood or otherwise of relapse. This report is passed to the Home Office for consideration by a panel of advisers and ultimately by the Home Secretary. The release of any patient is, therefore, a decision not made basically by the medical staff but does, of course, take into account their advice.

When on very rare occasions a patient so released does commit a further offence, this, of course, hits the headlines and the vast majority who lead perfectly satisfactory lives following discharge tend to be forgotten. This is not to say, of course, that the strictest precautions should not be taken to protect the public if there should be any degree of doubt at all. Such decisions carry considerable responsibility, and it is, therefore, important that hospitals should be encouraged to have the highest quality of staff. The only way to do this is by providing adequate conditions and salaries to attract the best people, and unfortunately, this is not always the case.

An additional problem is faced by the open hospital at district or area level attempting to run a service for the psychiatrically ill of its local population. Local communities and community health councils, and, more particularly, patients and their relatives, are by no means keen to have a discharged special hospital patient in the bed next door or the unit just down the road. While the special hospital may assure us that there is no longer risk, such patients would probably in the past have been dangerously aggressive and may well have killed somebody. The community feels threatened, and its members 'do not want our sick loved ones to be nursed in the same place as them'. The formation of special interim units, therefore, is essential if such patients are to be properly cared for and the overcrowding at special hospitals to be reduced.

One must, however, keep the matter in proportion. There are some 200,000 admissions to psychiatric hospitals in Great Britain per year, whereas the admissions to all the special hospitals amount only to some 200. Admissions to Broadmoor Hospital, about which there has recently been some ill-founded criticism, amount to some 80 patients per annum, and the hospital contains only some 600 male and 120 female patients at any given time. This total is, however, some 200 more patients than the hospital was originally meant to provide for, and adverse publicity has a bad effect on recruitment of staffing. Thus there is said to be a shortage of nursing staff. It is also said that some 200 patients no longer need the level of security which such a hospital provides, and could perfectly well be in less secure regional units within the community. This situation is currently receiving considered attention.

Legal Responsibility

Let us now take up some points of forensic interest in more detail. We have mentioned the question of criminal responsibility. This has a long legal history.

In 1723 an English court declared that for an accused to escape punishment he **'must not know what he was doing, no more than a wild beast'**. In other words, total want of reason was required as a defence if the individual were to be found not guilty by reason of insanity. This state of affairs, in fact, very rarely exists, and is of little practical consequence in the majority of cases that come before the courts. However, an attempt on the life of George III by a psychotic individual led to the passing of the **Criminal Lunatics Act 1800**, and in 1843 Daniel McNaughton was tried for the wilful murder of Edward Drummond, private secretary to Sir Robert

Peel. McNaughton was a paranoid schizophrenic, and, arising from this case, the House of Lords proposed five questions to the fifteen judges of England regarding the law of insanity. This proposal has been quoted in the form of two rules known as the **McNaughton rules**.

To establish a defence on the grounds of insanity it must be clearly proved that at the time of committing the act the party accused was labouring under **such a defect of reason from disease of the mind as not to know the nature and quality of his act or if he did know it that he did not know that what he was doing was wrong**.

These rules have for the last 100 years had a wide influence on trials of individuals with psychiatric illnesses who have committed criminal offences of a serious nature, but again the severity of the illness demanded for such a strict legal ruling of insanity (really a legal concept rather than a medical one) made many murder trials appear farcical to the medical profession. The legal arguments became hair-splitting, and considerable importance had to be attached to such points, particularly in the days when capital punishment was still in force.

It was not, however, until the **Homicide Act 1957** that a plea of **diminished responsibility** was allowed. Under this Act, if the offence was committed when the subject's mental stability was impaired by a mental disorder, the charge could be reduced from murder to manslaughter. This defence has largely replaced the plea of insanity, and the sentence, which is left to the discretion of the court, can be probation, imprisonment or detention in hospital under one of the appropriate Mental Health Act sections.

This plea seems much more logical than the previous plea of insanity, and in line with current medical thinking; it has been used in cases where the individual has suffered from a psychopathic personality disorder. Its use has, however, led to some abuse of psychiatrists by lay people who have felt that the criminal has in a sense been let off on what might appear rather flimsy grounds. Detention in Broadmoor for an unlimited period of time, however, is hardly what most people would consider being let off, and may well imply longer detention than would the life sentence they might otherwise be given.

The **Criminal Procedure (Insanity) Act 1964** changed the verdict of 'guilty but insane', which had been brought in under the 1883 Trial of Lunatics Act, to 'not guilty by reason of insanity'—in other words, a form of acquittal. This also allows for an appeal, and such a patient can be committed to a special hospital under Section 97 of the Act.

Murder and Manslaughter

It is interesting to note the definition of murder: 'Where a person of sound memory and discretion unlawfully kills any reasonable creature in being and under the Queen's peace with malice aforethought, expressed or implied, death following within a year and a day'. This is common law. The essential element of murder is 'malice aforethought'. One must examine what the accused intended. He must either intend to kill or cause grievous bodily harm, but the accused's act need not be the only factor. And the intent to kill is usually required.

The definition of manslaughter comes under Section 7 of **Offences Against the Person Act 1861**. It is defined in common law as the unlawful killing of a person in circumstances which are not so heinous as to make it murder and not amounting to infanticide or child destruction. There are two types, voluntary and involuntary. The **Infanticide Act 1938**, which refers to the killing of a child under one year of age by its mother if she is suffering from a mental illness, allows such cases to be dealt with as manslaughter instead of murder.

Under the **Criminal Justice Act 1967**, a majority verdict on the part of the jury became sufficient. Also note that in Section 8 the court must judge what was in the patient's mind subjectively and not objectively (i.e. malice aforethought), and in Section 39 allowance is made for suspended sentences. These again are all of significance in terms of psychiatrists' recommendations and the possible disposal of a patient who is in this unfortunate situation.

Suicide

Let us now turn our attention from the serious charge of homicide to a consideration of the questions surrounding suicide.

To commit or attempt suicide until 1961 was, in Britain, a criminal offence. Different countries and different societies vary widely in their attitude to this subject, custom depending largely on religious attitudes and the ecclesiastical law which exists. The Christian church, in particular Roman Catholics, has considered that to take one's own life is a mortal sin.

It had, however, been recognised for many years before 1961 that a large proportion of suicides and attempted suicides occurred, not surprisingly, in the context of psychiatric illness. This is particularly so with psychotic depressive illness, where the mental state of patients might be such that their responsibility for their actions in civil law would certainly have been questioned, and to charge someone in court with attempted suicide would have been ridiculous. For this reason, before 1961, the majority of cases were referred to hospital, and those that came to court were similarly dealt with.

Legal and religious considerations have made it extremely difficult to obtain reliable statistical information on the incidence and prevalence of suicide and attempted suicide, since, in some countries, the figures will be artificially low through the desire on the part of the courts and relatives not to bring in such a verdict, if there are social and moral prohibitions operating, whenever there is the slightest doubt. Comparsions, therefore, of the incidence of suicide and attempted suicide between different countries are by and large rather meaningless.

Under the **1961 Suicide Act**, suicide and attempted suicide ceased to be criminal offence. It is, however, still a criminal offence to enter into a suicide pact, and the survivor of such a pact between two or more individuals can still be charged. It is also an offence to aid or abet a suicide, and this could certainly apply to a relative, a doctor or a nurse who, for example, gave a lethal dose of tablets to an individual knowing that they were suicidally inclined and were intending to take them. This or even the more serious charge of murder could certainly be applied to any participation in such an act as euthanasia.

Termination of Pregnancy, Child Destruction and Infanticide

Child destruction differs from abortion and infanticide. The offence occurs before the child is completely born, i.e. before it has had a separate existence, no instrument or drug being used. The child must be capable of being born alive, which is in effect an assumption of a 28-week pregnancy. Any wilful act which causes the child to die before an independent existence has started may be prosecuted in Britain under this offence.

It has been recognised since the **Infanticide Act 1938** that women who have a puerperal psychosis—a psychotic illness that comes on in the puerperium or the first few weeks following childbirth—may behave in a manner which is abnormal and which diminishes their responsibility. This is particularly the case in acute depressive illnesses and in schizophrenia coming on after childbirth. Under these circumstances, if the mother kills her baby within a year from the time of delivery, and is recognised as suffering from a puerperal psychosis, then the case will be treated as manslaughter instead of murder. It will not be so treated after this period of time, nor does the Act apply to a murder committed on any other person or any other child of that woman other than the newly born one. Under these circumstances the woman would be tried for murder, but, of course, the fact that she had a psychotic illness would be considered, as outlined earlier.

Termination of pregnancy had always been illegal under the Offences Against the Person Act 1861, and under common law, until the **Abortion Act of 1967**. Case law had, in fact, set certain precedents before this, by which doctors had been acquitted of charges where the pregnancy had been terminated for strong medical reasons. The case of *Bourne v Rex* in 1939 no longer applies, but this was important historically, since it was a case in which a gynaecologist challenged the law publically by aborting a girl who had become pregnant under the age of consent, as a result of rape. In this case the gynaecologist was acquitted, which is interesting, because there were strictly no medical grounds for termination, such as are required now under the 1967 Act.

The 1967 Act is permissive only. It came into force in April 1968 and applies to England, Scotland and Wales. Abortion as such remains a criminal offence under Sections 58 and 59 of the Offences Against the Person Act 1861. The Abortion Act merely makes certain exceptions to these Sections.

Under the 1967 Act two medical practitioners must in good faith give an opinion that termination of pregnancy is necessary in accordance with the regulations under Section 2 of the Act, and that one or more of the following four categories apply:

1. That the continuance of the pregnancy would involve risk to the life of the pregnant woman greater than if the pregnancy were terminated.

2. That it would involve risk of injury to the physical or mental health of the pregnant woman greater than if the pregnancy were terminated.

3. That it would involve risk of injury to the physical or mental health of any existing children of the pregnant woman's family greater than if the pregnancy were terminated.

4. That there is a substantial risk that if the child were born it would suffer from such physical or mental abnormalities as to be seriously handicapped.

The wording of the Act leaves a lot open to personal opinion. The third clause above has been rather controversial, and the so-called social reasons for termination of pregnancy have in many doctors' view been unethical.

Apart from social reasons for wishing termination—such as the woman being unmarried or already having a large family, or being unable to afford further children—what are the medical reasons for termination? Severe heart disease, or severe lung disease, such as open tuberculosis, would probably be considered a medical indication, but in practice the general medical indications for termination of pregnancy are rare. The grounds on which termination is usually sought are psychiatric, or more commonly pseudo-psychiatric grounds where the social reasons outlined above are often the real issue. Are there any strictly psychiatric grounds for termination?

Some authors, such as Myre Sim, would suggest there are virtually none, while others would give a wide range of reasons. Often a depressive state is given as a reason for termination. In practice, however, the woman who threatens suicide if someone does not give her an abortion is usually being manipulative. In any case, depression is these days relatively easily treated, and most cases will recover completely, so that, strictly speaking, according to the wording of the Act, depression is not a very good reason. Nevertheless, it is an acceptable reason and has never been challenged; the woman who is having difficulty only need swallow a small number of tranquillisers to prove her point, and termination is usually arranged.

A better reason is a diagnosis of schizophrenia, where it is recognised that continuation of pregnancy in some cases may induce a relapse of the schizophrenic illness. Since this may result in long-term personality change, it could be argued that a history of schizophrenia is adequate reason for termination if the patient so wishes.

The more difficult, but in the author's view more reasonable, case for termination is found in the severer personality disorders, where it may be apparent that the woman is incapable of properly looking after or bringing up a child; and, of course, this may apply to the severer, ongoing psychotic illnesses as well. It could be argued, however, that this is more a reason for compulsory adoption than for termination of pregnancy, although it may be unlikely that the children of such parents would be adoptable.

The psychiatrist who specialises in subnormality may also have to consider termination issues, in particular where there is a risk of the child being born subnormal—for example, through mongolism—or where the pregnant woman is herself subnormal and considered to be unable to rear a child. Within subnormality, in order to prevent such births or the need for termination of pregnancy, some doctors have argued that sterilisation should be undertaken, and this issue recently caused considerable discussion and ethical heart-searching when it was proposed that such an operation should be carried out on a girl under age. There have also been those who wanted to change the present law, some wishing to tighten it up to prevent so many terminations and others wishing to loosen it to allow more. No doubt these attitudes depend on the intrinsic morality structure of those who are arguing. To the author the issue seems a fairly simple one. Either terminating a pregnancy is murder, and if you believe that, you should not do it at all; or it is not murder, in which case it seems reasonable that the issue should be decided by the woman herself, which, in effect, means abortion on demand.

If the latter attitude is taken, then it is no more unreasonable or improper to run an abortion clinic and to invite fee-paying patients to have such an operation if they wish it than it is to run a similar clinic for straightening noses, enlarging bosoms, or, indeed, more life-saving measures, such as heart operations on the wealthy. There is a lot of talk about ethics by people who have personal opinions to voice. It seems unfortunate that the psychiatrist has to be caught up in giving psychiatric justification for an operation which is quite clearly demanded by the public for reasons which are usually not remotely psychiatric.

Mentally Disordered Offenders

Let us now take a look at the law as it relates to mentally disordered offenders, apart from those serious charges such as murder, which have already been discussed.

Under Section 4 of the **Criminal Justice Act 1948**, treatment in a psychiatric hospital for a period of not more than 12 months by or under the direction of a named doctor may be made a condition of probation. This must have been recommended in written or oral evidence by a doctor approved under Section 28, and the court must be satisfied that proper arrangements have been made. Such a provision is useful in cases where medical supervision seems desirable for the individual's long-term welfare, but, through the nature of the condition, is unlikely to be carried out regularly on a voluntary basis. It also means that if this condition of probation is broken, the court is empowered to take a further look at the case and, if necessary, make alternative recommendations.

Equally, magistrates can, under Sections 14 and 105 of the **Magistrates' Court Act 1952**, remand the patient in hospital as an alternative to custody or bail, for the purposes of a medical report before a further hearing of the case.

Certain sections of the **1983 Mental Health Act** apply to the courts. These are contained under Part Three of the Act 'patients concerned in criminal proceedings or under sentence'. Under Section 37, magistrates' or higher courts can make a hospital or guardianship order if the offence is punishable by imprisonment, and if there is evidence from two doctors, one of whom must be recognised as having special experience in the diagnosis and treatment of mental disorder, as long as there is a hospital willing to take him and this seems the most suitable method of disposal. The provisions are much as in Section 3, which has been discussed previously, except that the nearest relative cannot under these circumstances order the patient's discharge.

Under Section 41, the crown court can make a hospital order, with a restriction on discharge, for a specific period or without limit of time. Again, the medical safeguards and evidence must be given, but under these circumstances discharge, transfer or leave of absence from the hospital can only be given with the consent of the Home Secretary, and application to a Mental Health Review Tribunal cannot be made. This Section is rather a nuisance in terms of an open psychiatric hospital, since the restrictions on discharge and on leave make use of a therapeutic community almost impossible. For this reason most hospitals prefer to avoid taking cases on such conditions, preferring that they should go to a special state hospital. It may be, however, that the offence is not considered so grave as to merit this, and in these cases the absence of secure units in many regions is a considerable drawback to these people's proper care.

Section 47 of the Mental Health Act allows a sentenced prisoner to be transferred to a mental hospital for compulsory detention until the end of his sentence, and Section 36 provides for immediate transfer to hospital of a prisoner awaiting trial if this seems urgently necessary for the appropriate treatment of such a person. Section 22 of the Prison Act 1952 allows the Home Secretary to release a prisoner temporarily for mental treatment.

Under Section 136 of the Mental Health Act, a police constable is allowed to convey a person found mentally disordered while in a public place to a place of safety, which may be interpreted as a psychiatric hospital, where he may be detained for 72 hours for observation and for proper medical assessment. The hospital is empowered to discharge such an individual before 72 hours if this is considered appropriate.

Despite criticism from some quarters, it should be recognised that these laws have been formulated both for the protection of society and for the protection of the sick individual, who may, because of his sickness, have committed some kind of criminal offence. It should not, therefore, be looked upon as part of a sentence but rather a means of ensuring that such a disordered individual obtains the benefit of a proper appraisal and treatment where appropriate.

Legislation on Drugs

Consideration of the problems of drug addiction has already been given in Chapter 15. Legislation on drugs has been considerably brought up to date in the last ten years. The **1971 Misuse of Drugs Act** replaced the Drugs (Prevention of Misuse) Act 1964 and the Dangerous Drugs Acts 1965 and 1967. The 1964 Act dealt with amphetamines and hallucinogens, and the 1965 Act with hard drugs. The 1967 Act was the controversial 'Stop and Search' Act, which gave the police wider powers and gave the Secretary of State authority to make regulations for the safe custody of drugs. Some of the sections in these Acts were rather inconsistent and inflexible, but under the 1971 Act an advisory council was established to keep the drug situation under review.

Controlled drugs are divided into three categories. In category A come the so-called hard drugs, such as opium derivatives, pethidine, morphine and cocaine, together with LSD and other hallucinogens. Category B includes amphetamines, cannabis and codeine derivatives. Category C includes methaqualone, phentermine and a few others. Curiously, barbiturates were not included, even though most doctors would recognise that they are much more addictive than some of the preparations listed.

The penalties in the Act are different for possession of, for intent to supply, and for production of, a controlled drug, and vary with the category in which the drug comes. The forensic psychiatrist is likely to come across the psychiatric problems associated with drug offenders frequently, both because of some of the effects produced by the drugs and also because of the personality disturbance often found in drug offenders—which, of course, is the principal reason for taking to drugs in the first place.

Sexual Offences

The medico-legal aspects of sexual offences have also been discussed in some detail, in Chapter 19. The forensic psychiatrist is likely to meet a rather different group of people with psycho-sexual problems, since he will see the sexual offenders. Thus, he will be dealing principally with the psychiatric aspects of rape, incest, offences associated with prostitution, and with the more bizarre of the deviancies. It must be remembered, however, that most of the minor sexual offences occur as breaches of the peace or relate to voyeurism under the Peeping Tom Act or to indecent exposure.

As we have said, the law regarding many sexual offences and, in particular, some of those considered more serious, have penalties which seem by present-day standards to be quite unrelated to anything which requires any kind of control at all. Certainly many are often treated more seriously than offences of an aggressive nature against the person, or cases of vandalism, which on the whole would seem a graver social problem than the occasional kinky pursuits, usually of lonely individuals who are hurting nobody, not even themselves! It must be realised, however, that we live in a peculiar society, where to depict one person killing another on a television screen is considered acceptable but to demonstrate two people making love to each other produces cries of abhorrence in some sections of the population. One would have thought it would be the lesser of two evils for children to watch people loving each other than hurting each other, but such seems not the case.

The 'Battered Baby' Syndrome

The psychiatrist may come into contact with 'battered baby' cases through requests for reports on treatment for the parents. Sometimes parents claim that bruises, etc. were acquired naturally, and deny the charge. It may be possible to uncover such histories if the patient is willing, by the use of thiopentone or so-called 'truth drug' methods. Evidence so obtained would, of course, put the doctor in a difficult position, since ethically he would not be able to reveal what had been told him by a patient without his or her consent. Equally, the courts do not accept evidence which has been obtained through the use of drugs.

The 'Battered Wife' Syndrome

More topically, the **'battered wife' syndrome** has recently been in the headlines. This syndrome is usually the result of a woman's marriage to an immature male whose aggressive instincts are poorly controlled, and may be worsened by alcohol. The problems some women face in this situation, particularly if they are also caring for their children, are considerable.

Child Abuse

In 1988 and 1989 problems relating to child abuse and particularly child sexual abuse received considerable publicity from the media, largely because of the probable excessive diagnosis of such cases, in particular parts of the United Kingdom by particular groups of doctors and social workers. This whole issue became known as the Cleveland Experience and led to an enquiry and subsequently the Butler-Sloss report.

Child abuse and particularly sexual abuse is an emotive subject. In any abuse situation there is always the dilemma on the one hand of the child continuing with its parents and on the other the danger of separation and the destruction of bonding, however imperfect this bonding may be which may on occasions cause more damage than the abuse itself.

A further dilemma arises whereby the damage to the child of the court appearance or the awareness that his or her confessions have perhaps caused a father or close relative of whom the child may be fond to go to prison may create a level of guilt and disturbance which is far worse in its long-term effects than was the sexual abuse in the first place. Where, therefore, should one draw the line?

The removal of a child from its parents must always be considered as a serious matter, and the League of Nations report as far back as 1938 laid down a principle that: 'it may be regarded as axiomatic in child care that no child should be removed from the care of otherwise competent parents when the provision of material aid should make such a removal unnecessary.'

Since the Cleveland Child Abuse enquiry the ability of professional care organisers to respond and treat sexual abuse has been questioned, and received continuing publicity by the media. The possible reasons for sexual abuse have been considered. The interviewing of a sexually-abused child and parental problems have all been covered in books published in recent months. The definition of abuse remains a difficult one. A child is considered to be abused if he or she is treated by an adult in a way that is unacceptable in a given culture at a given time. These last two clauses are important because not only are children treated differently in different countries but within a country or even within a city there are sub-cultures of behaviour and variations of opinion about what constitutes abuse of children. Moreover, standards change over the years and the significance or otherwise of sexual taboos changes with them.

We might remind ourselves of the words of Lord Shaftsbury who in 1880 when talking of the problem of child abuse in the home said, 'The evils are enormous and indisputable but they are so private, internal and domestic a creator as to be beyond the reach of legislation, and the subject would not I think be entertained in either Houses of Parliament.' In Britain the first charter for children appeared in 1887 some 67 years after the introduction of legislation to protect animals!

The clinical literature suggests that sexual abuse during childhood can play a role in the development of serious problems ranging from anorexia nervosa to prostitution. However, researched confirmation of these effects has often been lacking. The phenomenon of child sexual abuse has been defined in different ways be different investigators. Some have included coerced sexual experiences within a peer group, and others look only at sexual abuse perpetrated by adults and family members. Indeed in some societies within historical times sexual activity between adults and juveniles has been considered desirable as a means of training the young in sexual expertise. Some cultures have also accepted incest as being normal within certain sub-groups.

One may argue that it is not the sexual abuse as such but societies' attitudes that may cause a subsequent trauma to the young person. A survey of adult women showed a variety of traumatic effects relating to the type of abuse and the length of time during which it continued. Some have suggested that less serious forms of sexual contact are associated with less trauma. Many suggest that penetration is much more traumatic than other types of experience and that force and aggression are strong factors in causing traumatic consequences.

Shoplifting

Gibbens has written a monograph on this subject. There is an association with personality disorder, but also, interestingly, shoplifting is sometimes found in middle-aged women with depression who have previously had a completely blameless record. If a psychiatric report on such a patient establishes evidence of psychiatric illness and, in particular, menopausal depression, the courts may take cognisance of this in considering their verdict.

Research work has also shown that there is an association between shoplifting offences and the pre-menstrual phase in the cycle of women. This may relate to an increase in shoplifting crimes at this time, or may, of course, relate to an increase in the probability of getting caught.

Epilepsy

This condition has some important medico-legal implications. These relate to the road traffic laws, to the question of automatism and offences alleged to have been committed while in such a fugue state, and the legality of marriages contracted by couples when one partner had failed to reveal that he or she suffered from epilepsy before the marriage.

Slightly more epileptics are in prison than are found in the general population. Epileptic automatism, however, is rarely a satisfactory defence for a crime committed, since automatisms when truly epileptic are usually stereotypes and not sophisticated patterns of behaviour. Aggressive acts, however, may take place in the post-fit phase in some individuals. The establishment of a diagnosis of epilepsy would usually be within the province of the neurologist rather than the psychiatrist, but the problem of assessing disturbed behaviour, of course, may well come the way of the psychiatrist working for the courts. Epilepsy of temporal lobe type may be associated with episodic meaningless aggressive outbursts, without a seizure being present at all, and can sometimes be identified by abnormal EEG findings and treated with anti-TLE drugs.

Further Reading

Butler Report (Report of the Committee on Mentally Abnormal Offenders), Cmnd. 6233, HMSO, London, 1975.

Gay Search, *The Last Taboo Sexual Abuse of Children*, Penguin, 1986.

Great Ormond Street Sexual Abuse Team, *Child Sexual Abuse Within the Family, Assessment of Treatment*, Norman Wright, 1988.

Gibbens, T. C. N., *Mental Health Aspects of Shoplifting*, British Medical Journal monograph, 1971.

Glaister, J., and Renton, E., *Medical Jurisprudence and Toxicology*, Livingstone, London, 1966.

The Mental Health Act 1983 Memorandum on Parts 1–6, 8 and 10, Department of Health and Social Security 1983, HM Stationery Office, HM (W) 1912.

Prins, H., *Criminal Behaviour*, Pitman, London, 1973.

The Report of the Enquiry into Child Abuse in Cleveland 1987, HMSO, CM 413, June 1988.

Rollin, H. R., *The Mentally Abnormal Offender and the Law*, Pergamon, Oxford, 1963.

Sales, B. D., *The Law and Human Behaviour*, Plenum Press, London, 1980.

Speller, S. R., *The Mental Health Act, 1959*, Institute of Hospital Administrators, London, 1964.

Walker, N., and McCabe, S., *Crime and Insanity in England*, Edinburgh University Press, 1973.

Whitlock, F. A., *Criminal Responsibility and Mental Illness*, Butterworth, London, 1963.

Questions

1. What developments have led to the concept of diminished responsibility?

2. How may a convicted criminal be legally detained in a psychiatric unit?

3. Where is your local prison? Is there a forensic psychiatrist employed in your area? Do you possess a 'Secure Unit' for special care and treatment of the abnormal offender? Where is it sited?

4. What are the McNaughton Rules?

5. What is 'child destruction'?

6. What are the grounds under which termination of pregnancy may legally be carried out?

23
Future Trends

We have attempted so far in this book to portray the current scene in psychiatry within the National Health Service in Britain. In the appropriate chapters we have tried to show in brief historical perspective the key factors which have led up to our current position. We have tried to be factual and to show the deficiencies as well as the virtues of this system.

It is to be hoped we have avoided the pitfall of being over-erudite in a book designed to give the public an insight into a complex but fascinating area of human concern. We have particularly avoided giving an idealised picture, based on practice in the centres of excellence or in, as some might describe them, the ivory towers of research-orientated units attached to university departments. Such units may well be better staffed than most, or indeed over-staffed, and will see a selected group of patients rather different from the norm, just as surgical units in an equivalent facility might see a host of rare disorders but never a simple case of appendicitis. To portray such a unit, therefore, would be to distort the general picture, since those working in such units have a distorted case load.

In this final chapter, however, we must look at the way in which psychiatry appears to be developing, taking into account the innovations coming out from such centres of excellence. We must try to see what may happen over the next 10–20 years and predict where developments are most likely to occur.

It is relatively recently that psychiatry has progressed from the era of locked wards, and airing courts, where patients hidden away from the day-to-day stream of life might take some exercise or enjoy the sunshine while still kept captive. Advances in treatment have removed the necessity for such constraints. Indeed, we have heard from some idealists that the mental hospitals should be abolished altogether and that community care, based on sociological premises, can cope with the psychiatrically disordered individual in all but a few cases.

Much of this argument was based on projections of a decreasing need for hospital beds, derived from a time when advances in the medical treatment of psychotic illness, in particular, were making their greatest impact. The community was seen as a caring place, in contrast to the stark grimness which was the outsider's concept of what had once been called an asylum. Unfortunately, the promoters of such ideas have been guilty of some naivety and as often happens the results of advice which had not been thought through has been acted upon, to the detriment of the service available.

Sadly, the community, by which is meant the town or city from which the sufferer comes, is not a particularly caring place. Nor is it practical to finance dozens of small homes, each needing staff and facilities, when it is much more economical to run a larger establishment, where facilities are on the spot and can be shared by greater numbers. All too often one has seen the patient discharged from hospital finding that the community support is a myth. Opposition to the setting up of group homes or hostels for the discharged mentally ill or mentally retarded comes from residents' groups hastily formed to protect the area from what is seen as an undesirable addition. By all means build such establishments anywhere you like except in our street! For the chronically mentally ill or retarded this rejection follows them around. Not many neighbours really want to befriend an eccentric. Employment is difficult for such individuals to come by and references hard to obtain. Sheltered workshops are noteworthy for their absence in many parts of the country, and facilities for daily activities, whether in the homes themselves or at day centres, are often poor in the quality of life they provide.

Thus the patient who, when in hospital, has received three square meals a day, colour television, a comfortable bed and a good social life, with a patients' social club and many organised evening and weekend activities, suddenly finds himself plunged into a non-supportive, big wide world with little money and a very boring, lonely existence. This may seem to be painting the black side of the picture, but it is all too often true, and it seems very doubtful whether we have improved the quality of existence for such an individual by discharging them from hospital.

Unfortunately, the results of such ideas have been to make it very difficult to expand the facilities and open new wards in the hospitals that do care for these people, particularly in the Cinderella of the service, the sub-normality or retardation hospital. Despite government promises of increased funds, the money still tends to go on the glamour services. It is the patient in hospital for two weeks with appendicitis who gets the bedside telephone and individual radio earphones.

In contrast to this gloomy picture, the better-run psychiatric hospital was and is able to provide a community within itself, where friends can be made among the longer-stay patients and a wide range of recreational activities are provided. It is precisely this type of sheltered environment which many people need. When put out and into 'the community', they may stick out like a sore thumb. The old meaning of the word asylum was a place of refuge and caring, and the current emphasis placed on avoiding admission and keeping people in the community, while laudable in many respects, has sometimes meant that patients who genuinely need to be cared for and to be out of circulation for a while, so that they can rest and restore themselves away from the community pressures and their friends and relations, are now denied the opportunity.

One process which has taken place in between the locked door and the open door has been the phase of the revolving door. Thus many patients restored to health in hospital, when discharged, soon relapsed again because follow-up community care was inadequate and the patients themselves discontinued medication. We can only hope that better education of the public and of the public services, with community provision of psychiatrically trained nurses and similar projects, will reduce this trend.

It is sobering, however, to consider the results of a research project carried out in Middlesbrough in recent years as to what had befallen those longer-stay patients who had been discharged from the hospital community in the 10 years during which such a policy had been in practice. Few had been readmitted, not because of a lack of need but because many beds had been dismantled in order to resolve overcrowding, so that their availability was much reduced. Many former patients had finished up in Salvation Army hostels or equivalent doss-house dwelling places. Some were sleeping rough, and a not inconsiderable minority had been imprisoned for recidivist petty offences, the courts having no other options at their disposal and the individuals not being in a position to pay fines.

Only a small number had been totally integrated into the community, and were happy, working and contented within a family unit, or married. The rest formed the bulk of the cheap bed-sitter brigade, where they eked out a living on national insurance money and spent much of their time in the good weather sitting in the park, and in the bad weather sitting in the public library. They could not afford entertainment and often did not feel up to playing a part in local community care projects, even if these existed. Thus in many ways they were more institutionalised within their homes than they had been in the busy day-to-day activity that had existed for them in the specialised community of the hospital. It is well, therefore, to remember this background when looking at the advances which are undoubtedly being made in treatment and care and when trying to point towards trends in the future.

Another argument has raged over the question as to where psychiatric facilities should best be placed. Should they be within the district general hospital or in the specialised psychiatric hospital? There are advantages and disadvantages to both points of view. At the district general hospital all facilities for pathology, radiology, physiotherapy and the expertise of other specialities are on the spot. Medical and nursing staff are within the main stream of medicine and do not feel themselves to be isolated. The district general unit is conveniently situated in the population centre of the district it serves. A new hospital does not have the stigma which may still be attached to the older mental hospitals.

To balance these points, however, one needs to recognise that particular specialities require particular types of facility for the best treatment and caring of their patients. Thus, the type of facility needed for a children's unit or an obstetric department would be quite different from that required for the longer-term care of orthopaedic patients or the treatment of cases with spinal injuries. A main difference between the psychiatric ward and the general ward is that the vast majority of patients in psychiatry are up and about during the day, and need to be occupied in some sort of rehabilitative activity. They are not in general physically ill. Thus what they need is space, particularly day space and pleasant grounds surrounding the hospital, where, in suitable weather, they can enjoy outdoor activities. While this is less important for the patient who will only be in for two or three weeks with a new condition, such as depression, it is very important for the rehabilitation of the longer-stay patients, who still form quite a large proportion of the hospital clientele. The amount of space at night in the sense of room between beds is much less relevant, since they will only be there to sleep. In contrast, in the general hospital the bed and its surroundings form the only private space the patient has while there.

Thus, to apply standards appropriate for the general hospital to a psychiatric unit makes little sense. Unfortunately, the new general hospitals tend to be built on valuable land within towns and tend to build upwards. The opportunity for day space is more limited, and there are unlikely to be grounds outside the hospital where patients may engage in outdoor activities. While one can treat the acute short-stay patient in such surroundings, it is of little use for those two-thirds of the psychiatric patient community who require longer-term attention.

This is even more true when one considers the siting of facilities for the mentally retarded and for specialised units dealing with children, alcoholics, drug addiction and the like. The same argument applies to the chronically physically sick, and it is now being recognised by many who wished to see the district general hospital as the sole base for all facilities that in many ways it is inappropriate to try and combine such different disciplines under one roof. It is to be anticipated, therefore, that the current trend of putting district general hospital psychiatric units in each large town will be tempered by the realisation that there is still a need for a specialist unit with more space. These will probably be at area level, thus allowing the present specialist psychiatric hospitals to continue to function where they are situated within easy reach of appropriate centres of population. Perhaps we shall eventually be able to discard some of the older, more isolated, county mental hospitals.

Paralleling this, one can anticipate an expansion of day care services, in the shape of day hospitals, where treatment can be carried out with qualified medical and nursing staff over the full range of therapies it is practical for an out-patient to embark upon. These day-hospital facilities would be provided at the district general hospital, where there are back-up in-patient facilities, or at the specialist psychiatric hospital, if this is conveniently situated.

To support this facility there will be an expansion of day-centre care, where discharged patients can be given occupational facilities and daily activities as part of their continuing rehabilitation within the community. This care would be organised by social services departments, with access for general practitioners and community nurses, and the specialist as required.

There is likely to be a further expansion of the community psychiatric nursing service to complement these other activities, in order that patients, particularly the long-stay type that have returned to the community, may be able to receive continuing care and supervision, particularly with regard to such matters as receiving monthly injections of the long-acting medication they may need to take. Additional facilities in the shape of social clubs, sheltered workshops, and industrial rehabilitation schemes, all require to be expanded, though financial constraints are likely to delay the full implementation of such schemes in many areas.

It seems probable that the beds required for psychiatric problems have now dropped to a dangerously low level, which is beginning to deprive the people who have real need of a period in hospital of the opportunity. This will apply particularly to the elderly, and it seems probable that the present trend to reduce beds further, largely for economic reasons, will have to be reversed.

Experiments in the improvement of community care have given rise to certain new concepts, which have been put into practice on a trial basis in this country. One of these is the walk-in clinic, which has been tried successfully in the United States. Under this scheme a psychiatric team is in attendance at specified clinic centres at certain times, and patients can seek advice for a wide range of psychiatric problems without requiring a specific appointment or advance notice through a doctor's letter. Whether such a scheme will prove to have real value or will simply be abused by those inadequate personalities with time on their hands, who tend anyway to monopolise the time of any helping agency, be it telephone Samaritans, social services departments, etc., remains to be seen. One obvious snag is that such a scheme would by-pass the general practitioner, who in Britain, with his primary care team, should be the initial referring agency for any patient on his list.

Another development has been the introduction in some areas of the crisis intervention team, which functions rather like its equivalent in the casualty branch of surgical practice—the medical flying squad. The crisis intervention team can go to a house or anywhere in its catchment area and visit a patient at any time, members of this team being on permanent stand-by during the day they are on call for such a purpose. Time can then be spent in trying to resolve the situation as it has occurred, and avoiding the need, in some cases, for hospital admission.

Again it remains to be seen whether such a scheme will prove worthwhile and really do what people hope it will. The concept of a team which may include a social worker, nurse and doctor, all being tied up for this purpose may be somewhat wasteful of trained professional time. Furthermore, the presence of three professionals from different disciplines may give a wider range of expertise to the situation at this crisis time but cannot be other than inhibiting to the patient, who, in the author's experience, usually wants to talk through his difficulties in a one-to-one relationship with a therapist in whom he has confidence rather than to be exposed to a group of people in front of whom he may feel able to say very little.

In revising this book for the second edition it is interesting to reread the five preceding pages on future trends. The first edition of this book was published in 1982 and in the seven years between the first and second editions there have been been many developments in this area. There has been yet another reorganisation of the Health Service providing a managerial structure for the hospitals. Many of the big old psychiatric hospitals have proceeded towards closure at varying speeds and some of them have indeed closed down completely.

The development of small peripheral, so-called community units has also developed apace. In some areas this has met with more success than in others. In areas where there have been more than one psychiatric hospital it has been possible to close the first while transferring the residual, difficult to place patients to the second. In other areas the central hospital has been progressively run down with all the consequences of low morale and lack of funds being provided for the facilities that still remain.

There appear to be two central issues, the first being whether it is possible to provide peripheries of excellence in contrast to centres of excellence and indeed where staff will now gain their training. The job description of many professionals including Consultant Psychiatrists is needing to be rewritten.

The second problem is whether it is in fact practical to peripheralise a service and still maintain the features of daily living care which could be provided within the institution. The institution for all its faults was a community and provided all the essential features of communal or community living. Kathleen Jones (Professor of Social Studies at York University at the time) has drawn attention to what she calls 'word magic' whereby changes in definition hardly produce changes in care. To suppose that a small unit of 20 individuals living in a private house in some inner suburb of a town are more integrated into the community than they were in the larger institutional unit of a psychiatric hospital is largely a myth. It is very easy to become institutionalised in a small, inwardly-looking environment and it is not always easy to make it outward looking. Such practical matters as staff cover, the delivery of facilities, daily activities, such as occupational therapy and sheltered workshops, just do not materialise. The cost is often too great.

As a result, there has been a considerable increase in homelessness in Great Britain in the last few years, particularly apparent in the big cities. The problem was already there in New York five or ten years before that, but learning by experience has never been easy for humanity. There is now a vast increase in vagrancy and we are back to the sort of problems that were dealt with in the 1774 Vagrancy Act by the development of the forerunners of hospital services.

The problem is not simply with the first discharge which is often carefully organised to an appropriate hostel. It is the problem of dealing with problems that crop up (e.g. relapse) once the patient is out in this so-called community. The patient may make a second move and is no longer in a situation where anyone can successfully monitor this, and it is in this second or subsequent move that the residual schizophrenic with all the disabilities that that illness implies finds himself eventually on the streets.

The Multidisciplinary Team

The point made in our last paragraph underlines one of the major areas of conflict in the current development of the psychiatric health service. Before the development of the health service and the 1959 Mental Health Act, all hospitals were run on traditional and conservative lines, by a medical superintendent, perhaps a small number of deputy medical officers, and a matron in charge of nursing staff. The only other professionals concerned with the running of the mental health service were the mental welfare officers, who derived in turn from the duly authorised officers, whose main tasks were to organise the conveyance of patients to hospital and make arrangements for the magistrates' orders, or latterly the compulsory powers under the appropriate legal acts, to be carried out.

Within the last 20 years, however, with the development of the psychiatric hospital as a more open establishment, active out-patient and day-patient departments, and increased turnover of admissions, roles have been found for a number of other professional groups. The medical psychiatric team has been considerably expanded, and, following representation from medical groups at the time of the development of the 1959 Mental Health Act, additional consultants have been appointed to psychiatric hospitals, with full clinical responsibility over their patients (as had already occurred in the general hospital). Junior medical staff were appointed as trainees, and a considerable expansion of staffing came about in this way, spelling the end of the autocratic side of the medical superintendent's role. In fact, this grade in recent years has been phased out as these consultants have retired. With the loss of the medical assistant grade, however, the consultants have acquired on their medical team rather more junior staff than they had before. These junior doctors, while fully trained in general medicine and surgery, are trainees so far as psychiatry is concerned and relatively inexperienced. Much of the day-to-day therapy carried out by the medical teams in the sixties and early seventies in many peripheral non-teaching hospitals inevitably decreased, through lack of experienced people to carry out such programmes as group therapy or individual psychotherapy.

An expansion of nursing staff has also taken place, with an increased emphasis towards community nursing; but, with the better conditions of work and reduced hours, this has not made an appreciable increase in the number of nursing staff available on the wards at any given time. Moreover, the increase in elderly confused patients has resulted in more time needing to be spent on practical physical nursing, and less time available for the development of a psychiatric nurse's particular therapeutic skills in handling the psychiatrically ill.

A new discipline has developed from the generic social worker who, following the Seebohm report, replaced, so far as psychiatry was concerned, the mental welfare officer. The development of career grades within social services, however, meant that many of the psychiatrically more experienced workers went into administration, and new, younger social workers, often experienced in totally different fields, such as child care, were put into the position of having to organise admissions of mentally disturbed individuals and take on a new and sometimes threatening role. The hospital-based social worker and almoner were replaced by social workers whose allegiance was to their employer, the social services department, and who therefore ceased to come under the hospitals' direction. Nevertheless, an expansion of the social work input into psychiatry has been considerable.

Another new professional group, of clinical psychologists, has also appeared on the scene in recent years. Such professionals, derived from individuals who had taken a psychology degree at university and wished to make a career within the abnormal psychology field, were originally concerned with establishing mental norms and assessing intellectual performance, intelligence and personality function. Their particular interest in behavioural therapy resulted in the development of methods of treatment, particularly within the neuroses, concerning which a special expertise was developed. A major part could also be played by psychologists in designing treatment programmes for mentally retarded individuals and rehabilitation programmes in the longer-stay schizophrenic wards. Some of the original enthusiasm for such treatment methods has been tempered through experience, but the treatment role of the clinical psychologists has expanded considerably and they have come to feel that they should be able to have more personal control and a bigger say in what has traditionally been a medical field.

Other professional groups have also developed within the hospital service. There are now occupational therapists, art therapists and rehabilitation officers within the resettlement areas of the hospitals.

This development can have two consequences. It may result in an increased cooperation, to the general benefit of the patients, or it can result in professional jealousies, with the established groups feeling threatened and the newer groups wishing to build their own empires. One rather woolly concept, which has been given much play, is that of the multidisciplinary team. By this is implied that if all the professional groups—social workers, clinical psychologists, psychiatrists, nurses, and occupational therapists—can get together and plan programmes of treatment and rehabilitation, five heads are better than one. While this is true at the planning stage and in organising general programmes, it has been taken by some to imply the same principles should operate in the treatment of the individual patient; in consequence, the patient may be swamped by a lot of professionals all sitting in clinical conferences, each with their differing views, rather than getting on with treating the patient within their own skills.

While the group concept of therapy may be appropriate for some patients, it is not for all, and a ship with five captains, or steered by a management by consensus type of democracy, is likely to go round in circles. We hope, therefore, that the best of the new ideas, having been tried, will be retained, and those that are seen to have been naive and ill thought out will rapidly be discarded.

As a finale to this book, therefore, let us look at what progress can be expected within individual psychiatric syndromes in the next 10–20 years.

Psychoses

It would seem highly probable that, in the schizophrenic syndromes, advances in biochemical research will produce a breakthrough, giving us greater understanding of the underlying biochemical disturbances in these conditions. Greater understanding of the mechanisms of mono-amine neuro-transmitters within the brain will produce results, we hope.

Venables' work in York in establishing the physiological means whereby cases may prove to be identifiable by a confirmatory physical test, and whereby possibly those at risk, carriers or those who will be schizophrenia-susceptible, may be identifiable, is extremely important. Should this type of research produce results which give a clinical application available to hospital medical staff, however, then some particularly difficult ethical problems will arise. The present drugs which relieve the symptoms of schizophrenia are somewhat toxic, and can produce long-term unwanted side-effects. If it becomes possible to identify the schizophrenic at the pre-clinical stage, as is possible now with some other diseases, such as diabetes, then how should we proceed in terms of prevention or prophylaxis? There is as yet no evidence to show that giving such drugs would necessarily prevent the condition developing, even though it might control the outward manifestations of the psychosis. Furthermore, if such a risk of developing the disease can be identified in childhood should we attempt to modify the environment in some way to try to reduce the possibility of the disease developing in this at-risk group? As yet we are not sure what factors are important in triggering off the disease, but recent research shows that stressful personal interactions are certainly highly relevant in determining the relapse rate of recovered and treated schizophrenics.

In the more immediate future this type of research is likely to give us a better insight as to the type of follow-up necessary, and recommendations for the patient's life-style after recovery from such an illness in order to prevent further difficulties. We are likely to see an extension of hostel and supervised lodging accommodation, and a more effective use of day-hospital and day-centre care. Thus the number of patients requiring to reside in hospital for longer than six to eight weeks with a diagnosis of schizophrenia should continue to reduce.

At the same time, disturbing research, such as that quoted earlier from Middlesbrough, may imply that the schizophrenic process can and will still break through in later years, despite the continued usage of current drug therapy and continuity of care in the follow-up period outside hospital. Thus it is possible to visualise a situation where many of those who are discharged from hospital within the last ten years into the community as a result of these more effective methods of treatment may in later life still become ill again to the extent that readmission is necessary. We may then have to see again an expansion of in-patient facilities to cope with the new long stay. If an average district catchment area of 250,000 people were to add to its chronic hospital population by only five patients per year, should the average length of stay prove to be ten years, as was the case 40 years ago, then at least two wards will be needed simply to cope with that long-stay demand.

Turning to the affective psychoses, of depression and the rarer form of mania, the evidence for a genetically determined biochemical disorder affecting mono-amine systems and producing alterations in electrolyte levels in the nerve cells is even stronger. One must anticipate that within the next decade this will be clarified further, leading to a more specific antidote, which would in turn see a marked reduction in the need for electroplexy. At the same time, sociological research has been concentrating on the nature of the triggers which set off an attack in such a depression-prone individual, and we may therefore look for a better understanding of the relationship between the environment and these internal factors, leading to more effective prophylactic measures.

Psychoneuroses

Perhaps the most important factor limiting advances in the treatment of this very widespread group of conditions is a lack of finance, leading to a lack of availability of professional time. A wide range of therapists, however, see neuroses as being within their therapeutic skills. Thus anxiety and psychosomatic conditions are treated by psychiatrists, psychologists of varying disciplines, and schools from analytical and behavioural to the frankly fringe. Social workers see themselves as therapists in this area, as do many other groups ancillary to medicine, and, indeed, the general practitioner perhaps most of all sees a very wide selection of such problems within his surgery caseload. Psychoanalysts, hypnotherapists, lay counsellors within various organisations, such as the Samaritans and marriage guidance, all treat the neuroses. Perhaps the widest benefit from superficial supportive counselling comes from barmaids, hairdressers, masseurs in sauna parlours, and even prostitutes. With all this range of expertise, why is it that neuroses remain so common? Like baldness, there are many hair restorers on the market and still more bald people. Perhaps it is that none of these groups and none of their therapies can do more than alleviate problems. Would a great input of professional time and money make much difference to the 25 per cent of the population who might seek help?

The answer probably lies in the fact that, whether behavioural or analytical in their theoretical orientation, most workers would agree that early experiences have much to do with the later development of neurotic behaviour and personality disorders. By the time most professionals see such people the damage has long since been done. A baby apple marked by the feeding of an insect grows to full maturity, but the scar can be traced through the tissue from its skin to its core.

Prevention under such circumstances could only be realistic if relationships were tackled from infancy onwards, and if parents could be persuaded all to become perfect child rearers. Unfortunately, such idealistic aims are unrealistic. Improving social circumstances and relieving poverty can help, but inadequate parents cannot easily be made adequate, and the interference by social agencies may or may not be tolerated by such parents. Removal of the child from an imperfect environment creates an even greater problem of further emotional deprivation to a child already handicapped.

In different parts of the world experiments have been made with different social systems, where communal welfare, as in the Chinese commune, have been tried on a massive scale. It remains to be seen whether neuroses can be reduced in such a system, or whether they will simply be replaced by neurotic behaviour relating to a different set of stress factors, which are unwittingly produced. Indeed, some would say that some degree of neurotic expression is necessary for progress, and to act as a stimulator for people in the population to strive towards bettering their own lot and that of others.

Where, therefore, can we look for improvement in the next decade? At the level of first aid for acute neurosis drug therapy probably remains the most practically effective method of helping the sufferer. The benzodiazepine drugs, however, are on the decline and other drugs such as Buspirone and others are being introduced. It is likely, however, that no effective drug can be completely free from hazard in dealing with anxiety, since freeing the individual from anxiety is, like alcohol and nicotine, something that may make dependence almost inevitable. We have certainly seen problems arising from the release of inhibition with drugs such as benzodiazepines which allow patients to act in a way which their anxiety may previously have prevented, and this may on occasions be anti-social. At the same time the vast majority of people do obtain relief from anxiolytics and as long as they are not continued overlong they can be a useful first aid remedy.

At the same time, this does not get at the root problems of the neurotic personality; we must recognise, however, that analytical types of therapy are time-consuming and impractical for the majority. We must look, therefore, for improvements in short-term psychotherapy or behavioural therapy, and a clearer cut idea as to who can benefit.

It is to be anticipated that hypnosis, apparently undergoing a revival of interest, may be more widely practised as just this kind of shortcut. Physical methods of treating anxiety, such as the Somlec mentioned in Chapter 12, again may be improved and used more widely.

It is doubtful whether any major breakthroughs can be expected in the traditional psychotherapies, though the increased use of group techniques may allow a greater number of individuals to be reached. Behaviour therapy has not, unfortunately, lived up to the promise and enthusiasm of those who hoped that therein would lie the answer to all neurotic ills.

Inevitably, therefore, for the vast majority of patients with minor neuroses who will see their general practitioner, the use of more effective anxiety-relieving medicaments is likely to be the main first line of attack, with a more widespread awareness of the uses and limitations of hypnosis and short-term counselling leading to a more effective use of these treatment models.

The Elderly (Psycho-geriatrics)

The psychiatric crisis problem of our time is the increasing number of elderly people suffering from senile and other dementias. The increased longevity of the population, and their improved physical health, has not been matched by an ability to contain these disturbances of the central nervous system. Current research, however, is pointing towards the establishment of the metabolic cause of senile dementia. Should this come to pass in the next few years, with the ability, therefore, to provide a rational preventive treatment to stop this deterioration of brain function, this would be of immense value to the whole community, comparable to the breakthrough achieved with the discovery of the syphilitic cause of *dementia paralytica* and its treatment; or, in more recent times, the discovery of electroplexy as an effective method of relieving depression; or the discovery of the phenothiazines as a method of controlling psychotic thought processes. This breakthrough, which may not be too far off, would dramatically change the situation with regard to current psychiatric in-patient needs. Indeed, such a breakthrough is vital if the service is not to be swamped by an ever-increasing number of elderly, severely mentally infirm. At the same time better facilities for treating the elderly both in local community hospitals and in day centres, with maximum community support, must also be developed as an urgent priority in the next few years.

The Personality Disorders

Much of what we have said about the prevention of neuroses and the control of the child's environment applies as much, or even more so, to this group. Much debate at present is centred on whether the psychopathic personality or, indeed, the less severely affected, socially inadequate individual, is the proper brief for the psychiatrist or medical services at all. This is perhaps the area where social counselling through social services departments and prevention through better child care could be best directed. Unfortunately, these departments are already under considerable pressure from their various duties, and the implications in terms of staffing could be considerable.

Undoubtedly, however, individuals suffering from personality disorders of various types get into scrapes more often than the rest of the population, are more prone to depressive mood swings, and may suffer from additional problems, such as minor degrees of epilepsy, emotional deprivation, and various social disorders, more than do the general population. Their problems will bring them into contact with casualty departments, with psychiatrists, because of self-poisoning episodes, and with the police, because of minor delinquent behaviour, more frequently than the general population. The more serious forms of personality disorder in the shape of the psychopathic personality form a prominent part of the population of such special hospitals as Broadmoor and Rampton.

The continued advance of the psychiatric hospital towards a district-based open unit has meant that such individuals, requiring some degree of security, are no longer conveniently housed on the same wards as the general group of patients. Their presence is disruptive, yet their numbers do not justify a special unit in every district. At the same time, the fact that the special hospitals are mostly overcrowded leads to considerable problems, for there is no alternative accommodation available to transfer such individuals out of the special hospitals when they cease to be a gross danger to the community. To this end the Department of Health and Social Security set aside a considerable sum of money for the provision of the necessary secure units, and as a temporary measure the provision of area interim secure units to provide for the type of patient who needed some degree of security, a better nurse-staffing ratio, and a more intensive rehabilitation programme than was necessary or could be provided on routine admission wards. Some of these units are now open, and some of them remain to be completed. In due course, however, each region will have a specialist secure unit, just as each region has a specialist unit for the treatment of alcoholism or drug addiction, psychosexual disorders, or epilepsy and so on. This should relieve the special hospitals to a considerable degree by allowing individuals who do not need the long-term strict secure care of Broadmoor or Rampton to be contained near their own home and relatives. An easier transition can be made between the special hospital and the open unit by having such a halfway-house type of facility.

A number of additional secure units have also now been made available on a regional basis for offenders or for potentially dangerous individuals who have not committed a criminal offence.

It is possible that improvements may be made in the early environment to prevent the development of personality disorders to the extent that they now occur, though, as we indicated, there are limits to the practicality of this ideal. Advances in the medical management of aggressive behaviour through influencing mono-amine or other metabolic systems in the central nervous system can be expected, as can the better recognition of some of the underlying factors, such as psychomotor epilepsy, which may occasionally complicate such cases.

A New Range of Problems ('Liaison Psychiatry')

While psychiatry has been able to contract in terms of total bed numbers, and the control of such diseases as schizophrenia has made a considerable advance, it has, at the same time, expanded into new fields as the result of the opening up of community and out-patient services. With the return of the psychiatric unit to the district general hospital, colleagues from other medical and surgical disciplines increasingly call upon psychiatrists to advise in the management of a variety of conditions, principally of the psychosomatic type, which previously came their way less frequently. One hopes to see an expansion of the availability of psychiatrists also in the management of such cases as asthma, duodenal ulcer, and some of the skin diseases, to mention but a few of the conditions in the general wards which have a psychiatric or psychological component.

With the development of psycho-sexual clinics, a further link has been forged between psychiatry and such specialities as gynaecology, on the one hand, and the expertise of the marriage guidance counsellor, on the other. A wide range of new skills are called upon in dealing with this group of patients, who, until recently, had no area of expertise that they could tap. This is but one example of a series of new fields which are opening up to the psychiatrist, so that there would seem little prospect of a total reduction in workload, despite the promise of an illness-free utopia, envisaged by Bevan, when the Health Service was first conceived.

Advances can only be made by properly conducted research, by constant striving for the better distribution of funds, and an increased public awareness of the needs and deficiencies of the service. Within recent years the National Association of Mental Health (MIND) has devoted considerable energy to the raising of funds and to bringing to the attention of the public and the appropriate government departments the needs of the mentally ill and the maintenance of mental health within society. MIND has drawn attention to existing deficiencies, and has promoted many projects in the area of mental health.

Within psychiatry itself, the Society of Clinical Psychiatrists in Britain, and a similar group in the United States of America, known as the Group for Advancement of Psychiatry, have acted as ginger groups in the development of psychiatric services and the introduction of modern methods within the psychiatric hospital. The SCP has also been instrumental in the promotion of a Royal College of Psychiatrists, which has set up standards for trainees in psychiatry, and accreditation committees, which visit the psychiatric units in the country, ensuring the maintenance of proper standards of training for psychiatric staff, and administer an examination of membership of the College, required before obtaining a senior post.

The Society of Clinical Psychiatrists maintains study groups on matters of current importance within psychiatry, and produces publications on such areas as psychiatry and the social worker or public relations. It has also established a research fund to assist psychiatrists who need financial help in carrying out research into psychiatric problems.

The last two decades have been a time of exciting change and advance in psychiatry. The inclusion of psychiatry within the Health Service, and the advances made possible by new treatment methods and by the legal improvements consequent upon the 1959 Mental Health Act, have made Britain a leader in the development of a psychiatric service. One can look forward in the next two decades to even greater advances, and perhaps even to the final conquering of schizophrenia and the dementias.

Further Reading

Howells, J. E., *Contemporary Issues in Psychiatry*, Butterworth, London, 1974. Available from Society of Clinical Psychiatrists.

Plog, S. C., *The Year 2,000 and Mental Retardation*, Plenum, London, 1980.

Silverstone T., *Contemporary Psychiatry*, Royal College of Psychiatrists, London, 1976.

Spitzer, R. L., and Klein, D. F., *Critical Issues in Psychiatric Diagnosis*, Raven, New York, 1978.

Glossary

Abreaction. The re-experiencing and acting out of repressed emotional material.

Acetyl-choline. One of the mono-amine chemical transmitters in the central nervous system which is important in nerve conduction, particularly in peripheral nerves and the parasympathetic branch of the autonomic nervous supply.

Aetiology. The cause of a disease.

Affect. A continuing emotional state.

Affective disorder. A psychiatric illness whose main feature is a change in emotional state, particularly depression or elation.

Amentia. Subnormality of intelligence, mental retardation or mental deficiency.

Anaclitic depression. The morbid unresponsiveness seen in emotionally deprived young children.

Angiography. A method of X-ray investigation whereby blood vessels are injected with a radiopaque substance which will show up on an X-ray screen as it flows through the vessel.

Anxiolytic. A drug used to relieve states of anxiety.

Autism. An emotional withdrawal into oneself seen in some psychotic states, as in infantile autism.

Autochthonous idea. A primary delusion, suddenly occurring, chiefly in schizophrenia, which arises *de novo* and has an intense conviction of truth.

Autonomic. That part of the nervous system which is concerned with and controls internal bodily function and emotional state.

Benzodiazepines. A group of drugs effective in controlling anxiety states.

Bioenergetics. A group therapy technique.

Bipolar affective disorder. A psychotic illness where both depressive and manic swings of mood occur in the same individual at different times.

Blood brain barrier. The concept which describes the inability of certain substances to pass out of the blood stream into the cerebrospinal fluid.

Bulimia. Compulsive eating.

Butyrophenones. A group of drugs effective in controlling manic behaviour and some aspects of schizophrenia.

Cachexia. A state of severe malnutrition.

Cataplexy. A disorder of the brain whereby a state of emotion tends to induce sudden falling asleep.

Catatonia. A type of schizophrenia, characterised by a disturbance of motor activity, bizarre rituals and behaviour patterns.

Cerebellum. A part of the brain particularly concerned with the balance and coordination, especially well developed in birds.

Cerebrospinal fluid (CSF). The fluid which bathes the brain within the skull, and the spinal chord.

Chorea. A disturbance of the basal ganglia within the brain coordinating centres, concerned among other things with fine movement, which, when damaged, produce choreiform or abnormal jerky movements of the limbs. This is seen in some types of dementia.

Chromosome. The paired genes found in the nucleus of every cell, which are concerned with inheritance.

Clang association. A word associated with another because of its similar sound.

Compulsion. A symptom in some neurotic illnesses whereby the individual feels compelled to act out some ritual piece of behaviour.

Confabulation. A tendency found in some dementias to make up for a deficiency in memory by giving a false, imaginary answer to questions posed.

Conversion reaction. A phenomenon seen in hysteria, where a sudden alteration in belief or behaviour patterns may occur.

Cortex. The outer part of the brain substance, as in cerebral cortex. The white matter.

Cyclothymic. The type of personality characterised by swings of mood between happiness and sadness, for internal rather than environmental reasons.

Delirium. An acute disorder of memory and orientation, often found in high fevers, toxic states, or physical illness of sudden origin.

Delirium tremens. The type of delirium which results from sudden withdrawal of sedative drugs, particularly alcohol.

Delusion. A false belief, contrary to the individual's background and intellect, and not amenable to reasoned argument.

Dementia. An illness resulting from degeneration of brain cells within the cortex from a wide variety of sources, and causing primarily disturbances of memory, orientation and social awareness.

Dementia praecox. The old term for schizophrenia.

Depersonalisation. A condition of altered awareness found in some psychiatric illnesses, where the individual's body seems changed in some way.

Derealisation. A similar condition to depersonalisation except it is the external environment which seems changed or different.

Disinhibition. The loss of normal inhibitions and loosening of social awareness, which is seen in dementias.

Dissociation. A state of altered consciousness seen in hysterical neuroses and anxiety states, as in fugues and hysterical amnesia.

Diurnal. Varying during the day, as in diurnal mood swing; typical of the depressive phase of an affective psychosis, where the mood is more depressed in the mornings than in the evenings.

Drug. Any substance not a food taken into the body which will have an effect on the body's responses or on organisms that have invaded the body.

Electra complex. The female equivalent of the Oedipal complex, a Freudian concept used in the understanding of neuroses.

Electrocoagulation. A technique used in surgery to destroy the unwanted tissue but reduce unnecessary tissue damage or bleeding. The procedure is particularly useful in surgery and in leucotomy operations.

Electroencephalogram (EEG). A technique used for recording electrical activity in the brain, rather similar to the electrocardiogram used to measure heart waves.

Electrolytes. Molecules which break down into electrically charged ions when in solution—such as sodium, potassium or chlorine.

Electroplexy. The technique whereby an electrical current is used to induce a generalised seizure discharge in the brain substance, particularly used in the treatment of affective psychoses.

Electrosleep. A procedure developed for the relief of anxiety and tension states, whereby a small electric current is utilised to induce sleep. It produces an hypnotic effect by synchronising the electrical brain rhythms as seen on the electroencephalogram.

Embryology. The study of the developing foetus or baby before birth.

Empathy. A relationship of mutual sympathy and understanding between two people.

Encephalitis. An infection of the central nervous system or brain by a virus.

Endocrine gland. A hormone-secreting gland, such as the thyroid, pituitary or adrenal.

Endogenous. A condition which arises from a disturbance within the body's own metabolism and not from the external environment. Thus an endogenous depression is a depression arising from within for chemical reasons and not due to outside environmental cause.

Epilepsy. A condition where the nerve cells in the brain become hypersensitive and fire off in an uncontrolled discharge, inducing a seizure or fit.

Exhibitionism. A term usually applied to persons who exhibit themselves sexually for their own gratification.

Forensic psychiatry. A study of the medico-legal and criminal aspects of psychiatric illness.

Fugue. A state of altered consciousness found in epilepsy and in hysterical neuroses, whereby the individual shows automatic behaviour without recall or subsequent memory of the episode.

Functional. A term applied to the schizophrenic and affective psychoses to distinguish them from organic states, where physical illness may be causing psychotic symptoms.

Ganglia. A grouping of nerve cells, often with complicated interconnections and serving particular functions within the central nervous system.

General paralysis of the insane (GPI). An old term for the type of dementia seen as the result of the late effects of syphilis.

Gestalt therapy. A psychotherapeutic technique by Peris.

Goitre. The swelling in the neck associated with enlargement of the thyroid gland.

Hallucination. A false perception, e.g. a voice perceived without there being any external stimulus to cause it.

Hebephrenia. A type of schizophrenia characterised by delusional thinking and hallucinatory experiences.

Hormones. Substances produced in the body by endocrine glands and carried by the blood stream to affect the body metabolism in various ways.

Hyperprolactinaemia. An excessively high level of the hormone prolactin in the body, sometimes associated with growths in the pituitary gland, and with impotence.

Hyperthermia. An excessively high body temperature. This can be created deliberately in the treatment of certain chronic brain infections, such as late syphilis.

Hypoglycaemia. An abnormally low level of sugar in the body, usually resulting either from insulin being given to an individual to induce such a state, by diabetics accidentally giving themselves too much insulin, or from an insulin-secreting growth or tumour in the pancreatic gland.

Hypomania. A condition of abnormally elated mood or euphoria. A milder degree of mania.

Hysteria. A neurotic state where a disordered bodily function exists without appropriate physical cause.

Illusion. A distorted perception due to false recognition of some external stimulus.

Imprinting. A process whereby a young animal learns certain patterns of behaviour at critical stages in its development.

Intravenous. Injection into a vein.

Ionise. The property of some chemicals when in solution to become electrically charged.

Keratitis. A horny hardening of the outer layers of the skin.

Kernicteras. The deposition of bile salts in the brain substance, usually seen in new-born babies when there has been a rhesus blood incompatibility between mother and child.

Lability of mood. A condition found principally in dementias, showing sudden swings from sadness to happiness, or vice versa, which are excessive in the circumstances appertaining at the time.

Leucotomy. A brain operation used to treat severe levels of tension, depression, and obsessional states, whereby certain nerve tracts leading from the limbic lobe to the frontal cortex are divided.

Limbic lobe. That part of the central nervous system, principally in the mid-brain, composed of the amygdaloid nucleus, hippocampus, fornix and other connections, and concerned with the control of emotional levels and responses in the individual.

Mania. A psychiatric illness associated with euphoria and abnormally elated mood, and often seen as part of a bipolar affective psychosis.

Manic-depressive psychosis. The old term for a bipolar affective disorder.

Meiosis. Part of the process of division of the reproductive cell before fertilisation.

Metabolites. The products of chemical processes acting on proteins, carbohydrates, and fats within the body. Often the breakdown products of enzyme proteins.

Milieu therapy. The term to describe the psychotherapeutic process in a therapeutic community.

Mitosis. The process in cell division where the chromosome pairs separate and the cell splits into two new cells.

Mono-amines. A group of chemical transmitter substances in the brain.

Mutation. A change. The process in inheritance where a new factor which was not present in the previous generation occurs.

Narcolepsy. An abnormal or pathological tendency to fall asleep.

Neuropathy. An inflammation or degeneration of nerve cells.

Neurosis (psychoneurosis). A psychiatric disorder, usually of milder type, where anxiety is the predominant feature and insight is retained.

Obsession. The mental preoccupation with something, which in obsessional neurosis usually has ritualistic features.

Oedipus complex. A concept formulated by Freud and given its name from the Greek legend of King Oedipus, to explain the development of some neuroses due to the failure of the male child to be able to resolve its conflicts of love for the opposite-sexed parent, and a jealousy of the same sexed parent.

Oestrogen. The principal female hormone formed in the ovaries.

Organic vulnerability. The situation in an early dementing state when the brain is just functioning effectively in maximal conditions, but where symptoms of confusion begin to occur if other illness should supervene and the metabolic efficiency of the brain be disturbed.

Paediatrics. The study of disease in children.

Paedophilia. Unnatural sexual desire aroused in someone through association with children.

Paranoid. Morbidly suspicious thinking, often of delusional character, with ideas of persecution, as seen in the condition of paranoia and in paranoid schizophrenia.

Paraphrenia. A psychotic paranoid illness resembling schizophrenia, in old age.

Parasympathetic. That branch of the autonomic nervous system concerned with internal glandular secretions and states of sexual arousal or erection.

Parkinsonism. A state of tremor, particularly the pill-rolling tremor of the hands, muscle stiffness, shuffling gait and excessive salivation seen in Parkinson's Disease and in some diseases of the basal ganglia due to hardening of the arteries. Parkinsonism may also be drug-induced as a side-effect of some neuroleptic drugs.

Phenothiazines and butyrophenones may particularly induce this state, but it is reversible and can be cleared up by reducing the dosage or adding an anti-Parkinsonian drug, such as benzhexol.

Pathology. The study of morbid change in the body or body tissues.

Peripheral neuropathy. Damage to the nerve endings supplying the peripheral parts of the body, particularly, therefore, the hands and feet. This can occur from a variety of causes, such as toxic processes, poisons, vitamin deficiencies, or neurological disease, such as multiple sclerosis.

Phenothiazines. A group of chemicals with a basic tricyclic benzyl ring structure which are valuable in the treatment of schizophrenia and other psychotic illness. In small doses they may also be used to control anxiety.

Pilo-erection. The hair standing on end, as it does in some mammals when in a state of anxiety or arousal.

Placebo. An inert substance which is not a drug, given instead of medication for its psychological benefit only. A placebo may be used to compare the effectiveness of a new active drug in treatment, as in a clinical trial.

Prognosis. The outlook or outcome of a disease.

Prophylaxis. Attempting to prevent the onset of a disease, e.g. immunisation.

Psychiatrist. A doctor who specialises in conditions which cause disturbances of mood, thinking or behaviour.

Psychoanalyst. A person not necessarily medically qualified who has undergone a personal training analysis based on Freudian theory.

Psychodrama. A psychotherapeutic technique using play acting.

Psycho-geriatric disorders. Psychiatric problems appertaining to old age.

Psychologist. One who specialises in the study of mental mechanisms and may work in the educational, health service or research fields. He is not medically qualified but may work in association with psychiatrists in hospital on the testing of mental processes in patients or take part in behaviourally orientated treatment programmes.

Psychology. The study of normal mental mechanisms.

Psychopathology. The study of the psychological processes which may be helping to cause disease.

Psychopathy. A condition where the individual shows persistently irresponsible or aggressive behaviour.

Psychosis. A serious psychiatric illness, such as schizophrenia, in which insight is frequently lost.

Psychosomatic. Disease where demonstrable physical change can be found in the body but where there is an association with psychological factors in its cause.

Pubococcygeus muscles. The perineal muscles, which stretch from the pubic bone across the base of the abdominal cavity to the spine, and which surround and form sphincter muscles to control the passage of material through the urethra or rectum. These muscles also surround the vagina and are relevant in the condition of vaginismus.

Pyknic. That type of body configuration characterised by fatty deposits and a square-shaped frame, usually associated with the cyclothymic personality and a tendency to bipolar affective psychotic illness.

Reticular formation. That part of the mid and hind brain associated with levels of arousal, and with intimate connections to the limbic lobe.

Schizophrenia. A psychotic illness or group of illnesses characterised principally by disorders of thinking.

Scoline. A drug used to induce paralysis of the muscles during anaesthesia, and useful in preventing the muscular contractions associated with electroplexy.

Sex-linked. The type of inheritance of a disease factor which is linked to the female or X chromosome. Thus a recessive factor will be manifested in males who have only one X chromosome, but females will be carriers.

Sodium. An atom of importance in its ionised form, along with potassium, in nerve-cell conduction. It is a component of sodium chloride or common salt. Its level is raised in the cell of patients suffering from affective psychosis. The giving of an inert salt, lithium chloride, since lithium does not ionise in solution, causes a reduction in intra-cellular sodium in patients, since the molecules are replaced on a one-for-one basis.

Somatic. Belonging to the body—physical symptoms, such as palpitations, or pain, such as headache.

Somlec. Electrosleep, a treatment used in states of anxiety and tension.

Standard deviation. A statistical concept to describe the degree to which the item to be measured deviates or diverges from the average.

Stereotypy. Stereotyped repetitive behaviour of a meaningless character which may be seen in dementias or in the pseudo-dementia of more serious schizophrenic breakdown.

Subdural haematoma. A collection of blood in the subdural space below the skull, which may collect as a result of a blow or injury to the skull and which, by enlarging, can cause pressure on the brain.

Sympathetic nervous system. That part of the autonomic nervous system which is concerned with preparing the organism for fighting or flight. It mediates fear responses and functions by means of the mono-amine noradrenalin.

Synapse. The nerve-cell junction where the electrical impulse from one cell is transmitted to the next by means of chemical transmitter agents.

Syphilis. A venereal disease, usually contracted by sexual intercourse, which can, if untreated, after many years affect the central nervous system, if the brain substance is invaded by the infecting organism, a spirochaete. If the spinal column is mainly affected, the condition is known as tabes, and if the central nervous system is affected, as general paralysis of the insane or GPI.

Tardive dyskinesia. Abnormal movements of the muscles, particularly of the mouth and tongue, due to degeneration in the basal ganglia as a result in some cases of long-term use of high dosage phenothiazines, particularly the type with an aliphatic side-chain, such as chlorpromazine.

Temporal lobe epilepsy (TLE). A seizure discharge occurring in the temporal lobe of the cerebral cortex in the brain, without generalising to the whole brain substance. Major fits are not, therefore, caused, but bizarre disturbances of motor function or sensation and episodes of disturbed memory may occur.

Testosterone. The principal male sex hormone, produced within the testes.

Thalamus. A collection of ganglia within the central part of the brain which is of considerable importance as a coordinater of responses from various sources, and, in particular, the limbic lobe, which subserves emotional state.

Thiopentone. A rapid-acting barbiturate anaesthetic used in anaesthesia for electroplexy and as an intravenous abreactive technique.

Thioxanthines. A group of drugs similar to phenothiazines and used in the treatment of schizophrenia.

Transference. The development by a patient of an emotional relationship with the therapist during psychotherapy, particularly that of analytical type.

Transvestism. The need or compulsion to cross-dress in clothes normally appropriate to the opposite sex.

Trans-sexualism. Condition of individuals who desire to be of the other sex, and feel that their personality is trapped in the wrong-sexed body. Such individuals may wish to undergo a sex-change operation.

Trauma. Damage to the body or psychological processes of an individual.

Tribadism. Another name for lesbianism or female homosexuality.

Unipolar affective disorder. A psychotic depressive state, endogenous depression, or unipolar depression, where no phases of mania or hypomania occur.

Vaginitis. A painful inflammatory condition of the vagina, often due to bacterial or fungal infection.

Venexperential psychotherapy. A concept in family therapy by Howells.

Visual analogue scale. A method of assessing experience or mood, such as anxiety, by requesting patients to rate themselves on a straight line, with maximum at one end and minimum at the other.

Voyeurism. The obtaining of sexual gratification by watching others undress or perform sexual acts.

Wasserman Reaction (WR). A test used to diagnose syphilis, especially in its later stages, from a blood test.

Index